International Standard Library of Chinese Medicine

Diagnostics
in Chinese Medicine

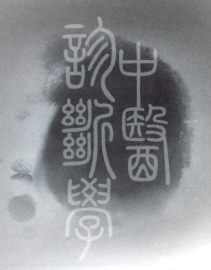

Project Editors: Zhou Ling, Lara Deasy & Liu Shui
Copy Editor: Zhang Meng
Book Designer: Guo Miao & Zhao Jing-jin
Cover Designer: Guo Miao & Zhao Jing-jin
Typesetter: Wei Hong-bo

International Standard Library of Chinese Medicine

Diagnostics
in Chinese Medicine

Chen Jia-xu, Ph.D. TCM
Professor and Chief Physician, Doctoral Supervisor,
Beijing University of Chinese Medicine,
Beijing, China

Jane Frances Wilson, MSc, CAc, FHEA
Senior Lecturer, School of Life Sciences,
University of Westminster,
London, UK

PMPH PEOPLE'S MEDICAL PUBLISHING HOUSE

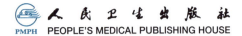
PEOPLE'S MEDICAL PUBLISHING HOUSE

Website: http://www.pmph.com/en

Book Title: Diagnostics in Chinese Medicine
(International Standard Library of Chinese Medicine) (DVD Included)
中医诊断学（国际标准化英文版中医教材）（含光盘）

Copyright © 2011 by People's Medical Publishing House. All rights reserved. No part of this publication may be reproduced, stored in a database or retrieval system, or transmitted in any form or by any electronic, mechanical, photocopy, or other recording means, without the prior written permission of the publisher.

Contact address: No. 19, Pan Jia Yuan Nan Li, Chaoyang District, Beijing 100021, P.R. China, phone/fax: 8610 5978 7338, E-mail: pmph@pmph.com

For text and trade sales, as well as review copy enquiries, please contact PMPH at pmphsales@gmail.com

---

Disclaimer

This book is for educational and reference purposes only. In view of the possibility of human error or changes in medical science, the author, editor, publisher and any other party involved in the publication of this work do not guarantee that the information contained herein is in any respect accurate or complete. The medicinal therapies and treatment techniques presented in this book are provided for the purpose of reference only. If readers wish to attempt any of the techniques or utilize any of the medicinal therapies contained in this book, the publisher assumes no responsibility for any such actions. It is the responsibility of the readers to understand and adhere to local laws and regulations concerning the practice of these techniques and methods. The authors, editors and publishers disclaim all responsibility for any liability, loss, injury, or damage incurred as a consequence, directly or indirectly, of the use and application of any of the contents of this book.

First published: 2011
ISBN: 978-7-117-14650-0/R · 14651

Cataloguing in Publication Data:
A catalogue record for this book is available from the CIP-Database China.

Printed in The People's Republic of China

Contributors (Listed alphabetically by name)

Chen Jia-xu（陈家旭）**, Ph.D. TCM**
Professor and Chief Physician, Doctoral Supervisor, Head of National Key Discipline of Diagnostics of TCM, Beijing University of Chinese Medicine, Beijing, China

Ding Jie（丁杰）**, Ph.D. TCM**
Assistant Professor, Shanghai University of Chinese Medicine, Shanghai, China

Kou Mei-jing（寇美静）**, M.S. TCM**
Assistant Professor, Hubei University of Chinese Medicine, Wuhan, China

Tang Yi-ting（唐已婷）**, M.S.**
Assistant Professor, The Open University of China, Beijing, China

Wang Li-min（王利敏）**, Ph.D. TCM**
Assistant Professor, Beijing University of Chinese Medicine, Beijing, China

Wang Shao-xian（王少贤）**, Ph.D. TCM**
Assistant Professor, College of Integrative Chinese and Western Medicine, Hebei Medical University, Shijiazhuang, China

Zhao Xin（赵歆）**, Ph.D. TCM**
Associate Professor, Beijing University of Chinese Medicine, Beijing, China

Zou Xiao-juan（邹小娟）**, B.S. TCM**
Associate Professor, Head of the Teaching & Research Section of TCM Diagnosis, Hubei University of Chinese Medicine, Wuhan, China

Translators (Listed alphabetically by name)

Chen Jia-xu（陈家旭）**, Ph.D. TCM**
Professor and Chief Physician, Doctoral Supervisor, Head of National Key Discipline of Diagnostics of TCM, Beijing University of Chinese Medicine, Beijing, China

Ding Jie（丁杰）**, Ph.D. TCM**
Assistant Professor, Shanghai University of Chinese Medicine, Shanghai, China

Guo Xiao-ling（郭晓玲）**, M.S. TCM**
Beijing University of Chinese Medicine, Beijing, China.

Jiang You-ming（姜幼明）**, M.S. TCM**
Beijing University of Chinese Medicine, Beijing, China.

Li Jing-jing（李晶晶）**, Ph.D. TCM**
Assistant Professor, Guangxi University of Chinese Medicine, Nanning, China

Liu Yue-yun（刘玥芸）**, M.S. TCM**
Beijing University of Chinese Medicine, Beijing, China.

Yue Li-feng（岳利峰）**, Ph.D. TCM**
Associate Professor, Beijing University of Chinese Medicine, Beijing, China

English Editors

Jane Frances Wilson, MSc, CAc, FHEA
Senior Lecturer of School of Life Sciences, University of Westminster, London, UK

Lara Deasy, Bsc (Hons) TCM,
B.M. (Beijing) TCM, MRCHM, OMBAcC.

About the Authors

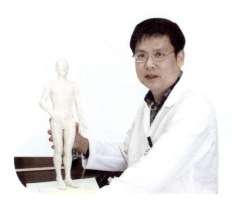

Chen Jia-xu (陈家旭)

Prof. Chen Jia-xu, born in 1966, is native of Hubei, China. He is a professor, state approved doctoral supervisor, and director of the state-level subject of Chinese Medicine Diagnostics in Beijing University of Chinese Medicine (BUCM). He is one of the well-known and highly respected practitioners and teachers with many years of professional experience. Dr. Chen has spent virtually his entire career at this prestigious university, where he has been teaching, conducting research, and practicing at the hospital since 1988.

Dr. Chen is a specialist in Chinese medicine, and a scholar in the diagnostics of Chinese medicine. In recent years, he has been concentrating his efforts on publishing books, academic papers and essays on the diagnostics of Chinese medicine. Dr. Chen brings over twenty years of experience to this book, his most recent work being the *Diagnostics of Chinese Medicine*. This book is a complete, easily available and highly illustrated guide to Chinese medicine diagnostics. Professor Chen has also received many awards in recent years.

In 2004 his *Diagnostics in Chinese Medicine* was awarded as the National Elaborate Course from the Ministry of Education of China, and then was supported by the China National Funds for Distinguished Young Scientists in 2008.

Jane Frances Wilson has been a senior lecturer at Westminster University since 1998 in The School of Life Sciences; Department of Chinese Medicine: Acupuncture. She trained as a physiotherapist at The Royal London Hospital, and has been a member of the Chartered Society of Physiotherapy and the Health Professionals' Council since qualification, as well as an Advanced Member of the Acupuncture Association of Physiotherapy for many years.

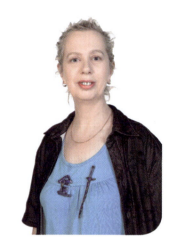

Jane Frances Wilson

Jane worked in the National Health Service from 1977-1987, qualified as a teacher in 1984 and was awarded a Diploma in Teaching Physiotherapy from The Middlesex Hospital in central London, later moving to teach biomedical subjects at the London School of Acupuncture and Traditional Chinese Medicine. Jane completed courses in Shiatsu and spent one year training at Nanjing University of Chinese Medicine: Acupuncture under Prof. Xiao, Prof. Zhou and many others. In 1995 she became a member of the British Acupuncture Council (BAcC) and completed a Master's degree in research methods from Kings College University of London.

In 1994 she started up her own practice, The Treatment Room, which since 1998 is situated in a creative media hub in Shoreditch, near the City of London, where she continues to have a vibrant private practice.

Editorial Board for *International Standard Library of Chinese Medicine*

Executive Directors

Li Zhen-ji（李振吉）
Vice Chairman and Secretary-general, World Federation of Chinese Medical Societies, Beijing, China

Hu Guo-chen（胡国臣）
President and Editor-in-Chief, People's Medical Publishing House, Beijing, China

Directors

You Zhao-ling（尤昭玲）
Former President and Professor of Chinese Medical Gynecology, Hunan University of TCM, Changsha, China

Xie Jian-qun（谢建群）
President and Professor of Chinese Internal Medicine, Shanghai University of TCM, Shanghai, China

General Coordinator

Liu Shui（刘水）
Director of International TCM Publications, People's Medical Publishing House, Beijing, China

Members (Listed alphabetically by last name)

Chang Zhang-fu（常章富）
Professor of Chinese Materia Medica, Beijing University of CM, Beijing, China

Chen Hong-feng（陈红风）**, Ph.D. TCM**
Professor of Chinese External Medicine, Shanghai University of TCM, Shanghai, China

Chen Jia-xu（陈家旭）**, Ph.D. TCM**
Professor of TCM Diagnostics, Beijing University of CM, Beijing, China

Chen Ming（陈明）
Professor of *Shāng Hán Lùn*, Beijing University of CM, Beijing, China

Cui Hai（崔海）**, Ph.D. TCM**
Associate Professor of TCM, Capital Medical University, Beijing, China

Deng Zhong-jia（邓中甲）
Professor of Chinese Medicinal Formulae, Chengdu University of TCM, Chengdu, China

Ding Xiao-hong（丁晓红）
Associate Professor of Tui Na, International Education College, Nanjing University of CM, Nanjing, China

Doug Eisenstark, L.Ac
Professor of Chinese Medicine, Emperors College, Los Angeles, USA

Stephen X. Guo（郭鑫太）**, M.A. International Affairs**
Director of Jande International, New York, USA

Han Chou-ping（韩丑平）
Associate Professor, International Education College, Shanghai University of TCM, Shanghai, China

Hu Jun（胡俊）**, B.A. Medical English**
Currently pursuing Master's of Science in Social History of Medicine, Peking University, Beijing, China

Hu Ke-xin（胡克信）**, Ph.D. TCM**
Professor of Otorhinolaryngology, Keelung City Municipal Hospital, Taiwan, China

Hu Zhen（胡臻）
Professor and Head of Department of Traditional Chinese Medicine, Wenzhou Medical College, Wenzhou, China

Huang Fei-li（黄菲莉）
Professor of Cosmetology, Hong Kong Baptist University, Hong Kong, China

Russell William James, M.S. TCM
IELTS Examiner & Marker, Beijing, China

Jia De-xian（贾德贤）**, Ph.D. TCM**
Professor of Chinese Materia Medica, Beijing University of CM, Beijing, China

Jin Hong-zhu（金宏柱）
Professor of Acupuncture & Tui Na, Nanjing University of CM, Nanjing, China

Lao Li-xing（劳力行）**, Ph.D.**
Professor of Acupuncture and Moxibustion, University of Maryland School of Medicine, Baltimore, USA
Past Co-President of the Society for Acupuncture Research

Hon K. Lee（李汉光）**, Dipl. OM, L.Ac.**
Director of the Jow Ga Shaolin Institute, Herndon, Virginia, USA

Li Dao-fang（李道坊）**, Ph.D. TCM**
President of Florida Acupuncture Association; Executive Board Director, National Federation of Chinese TCM Organizations, Kissimmee, USA

Mei Li（李梅）**, M.S. TOM, L.Ac.**
Translator and Editor, People's Medical Publishing House, Beijing, China

Li Ming-dong（李名栋）**, Ph.D. OMD, L.Ac.**
Professor of Chinese Internal Medicine, Yo San University of Traditional Chinese Medicine, Los Angeles, USA

Li Yun-ning（李云宁）
Qi Gong and TCM Translator, Beijing, China

Liang Li-na（梁丽娜）**, Ph.D. TCM**
Associate Professor of Ophthalmology, Eye Hospital of China Academy of Chinese Medical Sciences, Beijing, China

Liu Zhan-wen（刘占文）
Professor of Chinese Medicine, Beijing University of CM, Beijing, China

Lü Ming（吕明）
Professor of Tui Na, Changchun University of CM, Changchun, China

Mark L. Mondot, B.A. Chinese Language, L.Ac.
Translator and Editor, People's Medical Publishing House, Beijing, China

Jane Lyttleton, Hons, M Phil, Dip TCM, Cert Ac.
Lecturer, University of Western Sydney, Sydney, Australia

Julie Mulin Qiao-Wong（乔木林）
Professor of Chinese Medicine, Victoria University, Melbourne, Australia

Andy Rosenfarb, M.S. TOM, L.Ac.
Acupuncture Health Associates, New Jersey, USA

Paul F. Ryan, M.S. TCM, L.Ac.
Taihu Institute, Jiangsu, China

Martin Schweizer, Ph.D. Molecular Biology, L.Ac.
Emeritus Professor of Medicinal Chemistry, University of Utah, USA

Secondo Scarsella, MD, DDS
Visiting Professor of Tui Na, Nanjing University of CM, China Department of Maxillofacial Surgery, San Salvatore Hospital, L'Aquila, Italy

Tsai Chun-hui, Ph.D.
Associate Professor of Pediatrics, School of Medicine, University of Colorado, Denver, USA

Wang Shou-chuan（汪受传）
Professor of TCM Pediatrics, Nanjing University of CM, Nanjing, China

Douglas Wile, Ph.D.
Former professor of History & Philosophy of Chinese Medicine and of Chinese Language at Pacific College of Oriental Medicine, New York; Professor of Chinese language at Alverno College, Milwaukee, USA

Xiao Ping（肖平）
Associate Professor, Hunan University of TCM, Changsha, China

Yan Dao-nan（严道南）
Professor of Otorhinolaryngology, Nanjing University of CM, Nanjing, China

Zhang Ji（张吉）
Professor of Acupuncture and Moxibustion, Beijing University of CM, Beijing, China

Helen Q. Zhang（张齐）, Ph.D. TCM, L.Ac.
Director of Qi TCM Clinic, New York, USA

Zhao Bai-xiao（赵百孝）, Ph.D. TCM
Professor of Acupuncture and Moxibustion, Dean, School of Acupuncture and Moxibustion, Beijing University of CM, Beijing, China

Zhou Gang（周刚）, Ph.D. TCM
Lecturer of *Shāng Hán Lùn*, Beijing University of CM, Beijing, China

Sun Guang-ren（孙广仁）
Professor of TCM Fundamentals, Shandong University of TCM, Jinan, China

Tu Ya（图娅）
Professor of Acupuncture and Moxibustion, Beijing University of CM, Beijing, China

Wei Qi-ping（韦企平）
Professor of Ophthalmology, Beijing University of CM, Beijing, China

Jane Frances Wilson, M.S., L.Ac.
Senior Lecturer of School of Life Sciences, University of Westminster, London, UK

Xu Shi-zu（徐士祖）, M.A. Chinese Martial Arts
Chinese Traditional Sports and Health Cultivation Instructor, School of Physical Education in Wenzhou Medical College, Wenzhou, China

Ye Qiao-bo（叶俏波）, Ph.D. TCM
Lecturer of Chinese Medicinal Formulae, Chengdu University of TCM, Chengdu, China

Zhang Ji（张季）, Ph.D. TCM
Professor of Chinese Materia Medica, Emperor's College of Oriental Medicine, Alhambra University, Dongguk University, Los Angeles, USA

Zhang Qing-rong（张庆荣）
Professor of TCM Fundamentals, Liaoning University of TCM, Shenyang, China

Zhao Xia（赵霞）, Ph.D. TCM
Professor of TCM Pediatrics, Nanjing University of CM, Nanjing, China

Gregory Donald Zimmerman, M.S., L.Ac.
Lecturer, Southern California University of Health Sciences (formerly LACC), California, USA

Sponsored by
World Federation of Chinese Medical Societies

Preface

Acting as a bridge connecting basic knowledge with clinical practice, the subject of Diagnostics in Chinese Medicine is a requisite course set for students from all majors of Chinese medicine. However, it is known for being difficult to completely understand and fully grasp. Since the diagnostic methods involve both fundamental theory and clinical knowledge and experience of various departments, it is difficult for students to grasp their depth by having just captured the fundamental theories. Its vast knowledge is also difficult to grasp since it covers all fields of medical expertise, which are rarely connected to each other in biomedicine. Therefore, this book is arranged in a highly comprehensive way and includes numerous complete figures and tables. In general, the tables list diagnostic methods and principles and relate them to concrete signs and symptoms as well as different disease's syndrome differentiation. Their connection to the diagnostic system is also significantly emphasised. The content of this complex information was put into simple and straightforward vocabulary to increase the understanding and comprehension of the readers.

Designed for overseas students, the main contents of this book include: the four diagnostic methods in Chinese medicine, pattern differentiation according to the eight principles, pattern differentiation according to pathogenic factors, pattern differentiation according to qi, blood and body fluids, pattern differentiation according to *zang-fu* organs, and other types of pattern differentiation. In addition, the comprehensive application of the four diagnostic methods with pattern differentiation, case record writing, a training course for the four diagnostic methods, as well as a case study are involved, too. This book is written based on the national textbooks of Chinese medicine in China, and combined with the National Elaborate Course given by Professor Chen Jia-xu at Beijing University of Chinese Medicine, to clearly explain the diagnostic principles in order to stimulate faster learning and deepen the understanding of the complicated concepts and principles. In order to facilitate teaching and studying, a DVD is attached which vividly presents various images of the inspection examination.

To continually increase the quality of this manual, I always welcome and greatly appreciate the opinions of and corrections from the readers and experts of the field. I also would like to express my sincere gratitude to all who provided assistance and guidance in the compilation of this edition.

Prof. Chen Jia-xu Ph.D. TCM
Beijing University of CM
2011

TABLE OF CONTENTS

Chapter 1　Introduction 1

Chapter 2　Inspection Examination 6

Section 1　Inspection of the Circumstances of the Entire Body 6
　Inspection of the *Shen* (Spirit) 7
　Inspection of Colour 9
　Inspection of the Form of the Body 14
　Inspection of Posture and Movement 16
Section 2　Inspection of the Circumstances of Various Parts of the Body 19
　Inspection of the Head and Face 19
　Inspection of the Five Sense Organs 22
　Inspection of the Body 29
　Inspection of the Four Limbs 32
　Inspection of the Anterior and Posterior Yin (Genitals and Anus) 33
　Inspection of the Skin 34
Section 3　Inspection of Excreta 38
Section 4　Inspection of the Superficial Vein of the Index Finger 41

Chapter 3　Tongue Examination 43

Section 1　Overview of the Tongue Examination 44

Principles of the Tongue Examination ·· 44
Method of the Tongue Examination ··· 45
Summary of the Important Parts of the Tongue Examination ············ 46

Section 2 Normal Tongue Manifestation and Physiological Differences ··· 47
Normal Tongue Manifestation ·· 47
Physiological Differences of the Tongue Manifestation ······················ 47

Section 3 Contents of the Tongue Examination ··· 48
Inspection of the Tongue Body ··· 48
Inspection of the Tongue Coating ··· 53

Section 4 Main Points for Analysing the Tongue Manifestations ··· 58
Section 5 Clinical Significance of the Tongue Examination ··· 60

Chapter 4 Listening and Smelling Examination — 61

Section 1 Listening to Sounds ··· 61
Normal Sounds ··· 62
Pathological Sounds ·· 62

Section 2 Smelling Odours ··· 70
Body Odours ··· 70
Sickroom Odours ·· 71

Chapter 5 Inquiry Examination — 72

Section 1 Significance and Method of the Inquiry Examination ··· 73
Significance of the Inquiry Examination ··· 73
Method of the Inquiry Examination ·· 73

Section 2 Contents of the Inquiry Examination ··· 74
Section 3 Present Illness History ··· 75
Inquiring into Cold and Heat ·· 76
Inquiring into Sweating ··· 79
Inquiring into Pain ·· 81
Inquiring into the Head, Body, Chest and Abdomen ··························· 85
Inquiring into the Ears and Eyes ··· 88

Inquiring into Sleep ··· 89
Inquiring into Diet and Partiality ··· 90
Inquiring into the Urine and Stool ··· 94
Inquiring into Menstruation and Vaginal Discharge ··· 97
Inquiring of Children ··· 99

Chapter 6 Pulse Examination — 101

Section 1 Overview of the Pulse Examination ··· 102
Principles of the Pulse Examination ··· 102
The Positions of Pulse Examination ··· 102
Methods of Pulse-Taking ··· 105
Elements of the Pulse Image ··· 106

Section 2 A Healthy Pulse Image ··· 107
Characteristics of the Normal Pulse Image ··· 107
Physiological Variation of the Pulse Image ··· 107

Section 3 Abnormal Pulse Images ··· 108
Common Abnormal Pulses ··· 108
Differentiation of the Pulse Images ··· 112

Section 4 Examination of the Pulses of Women and Children ··· 117
The Pulse in Women ··· 117
The Pulse in Children ··· 117

Section 5 Clinical Application and Significance of the Pulse Examination ··· 118
Clinical Application of the Pulse Examination ··· 118
Significance of the Pulse Examination ··· 119

Chapter 7 Palpatory Examination — 120

Section 1 Contents of the Palpatory Examination Including Methods and Significance ··· 120
Section 2 Areas for Palpatory Examination ··· 122

Chapter 8 Pattern Differentiation According to the Eight Principles — 128

Section 1 Concept of Pattern Differentiation According to the Eight Principles — 128
Section 2 The Basic Patterns of the Eight Principles — 128
  Exterior and Interior — 128
  Cold and Heat — 132
  Excess and Deficiency — 135
  Yin and Yang — 138
Section 3 The Relationship Among the Eight Principles Patterns — 146
  Combined Patterns — 146
  Transformation of Patterns — 147
  True and False Pattern — 151

Chapter 9 Differentiation of Patterns According to Pathogenic Factors — 155

Section 1 Pattern Identification of the Six Exogenous Pathogenic Factors — 155
  Wind Pattern — 156
  Cold Pattern — 157
  Summer-Heat Pattern — 157
  Dampness Pattern — 158
  Dryness Pattern — 159
  Fire Pattern — 159
Section 2 Pattern Identification of the Seven Emotions — 160
Section 3 Pattern Differentiation of Diseases due to Improper Diet, Overstrain or Lack of Exercise — 161
Section 4 External Injury or Trauma — 162

Chapter 10 Pattern Differentiation According to Qi, Blood and Body Fluids — 163

Section 1 Patterns of Qi — 163
- Qi Deficiency Pattern — 165
- Qi Sinking Pattern — 166
- Qi Collapse Pattern — 166
- Qi Stagnation Pattern — 167
- Qi Counterflow (Perversion) Pattern — 168
- Qi Blocking Pattern — 169

Section 2 Patterns of Blood — 170
- Blood Deficiency Pattern — 170
- Blood Stasis Pattern — 170
- Blood Heat Pattern — 173
- Blood Cold Pattern — 174

Section 3 Simultaneous Qi and Blood Disease Pattern Identification — 174
- Qi Stagnation and Blood Stasis — 175
- Qi Deficiency and Blood Stasis — 176
- Deficiency of Both Qi and Blood — 176
- Loss of Blood due to Deficiency of Qi (Qi Failing to Control Blood) — 176
- Collapse of Qi Resulting from Haemorrhage — 178

Section 4 Patterns of Body Fluids — 179
- Insufficiency of Body Fluids Pattern — 179
- Retention of Body Fluids Pattern — 180

Chapter 11 Differentiation of Patterns According to the *Zang-Fu* Organs — 189

Section 1 Heart and Small Intestine Pattern Differentiation — 191
- Heart Qi Deficiency Pattern — 193
- Heart Yang Deficiency Pattern — 194
- Sudden Collapse of the Heart Yang Pattern — 194

Heart Blood Deficiency Pattern ··· 197
　　Heart Yin Deficiency Pattern ··· 197
　　Heart Fire Hyperactivity Pattern ·· 198
　　Obstruction of the Heart Vessel Pattern ·· 199
　　Phlegm Misting the Heart Orifices Pattern ··· 201
　　Phlegm Fire Harassing the Heart Pattern ·· 203
　　Blood Stasis Obstructing the Brain Collaterals Pattern ····························· 204
　　Excess Heat in the Small Intestine Pattern ··· 204
Section 2　Lung and Large Intestine Pattern Differentiation ···················· 205
　　Wind-Cold Invading the Lung Pattern ··· 207
　　Wind-Heat Invading the Lung Pattern ··· 208
　　Lung Dryness Pattern (Invasion of the Lung by Dryness Pattern) ·················· 209
　　Cold Pathogen Congesting the Lung Pattern ······································· 210
　　Phlegm-Damp Obstructing the Lung Pattern ······································· 211
　　Heat Pathogen Congesting the Lung Pattern ······································· 211
　　Phlegm-Heat Obstructing the Lung Pattern ·· 214
　　Lung Qi Deficiency Pattern ··· 215
　　Lung Yin Deficiency Pattern ·· 216
　　Large Intestine Damp-Heat Pattern ·· 217
　　Heat Obstructing the Large Intestine Pattern ······································· 218
　　Large Intestine Dryness Pattern ··· 219
　　Large Intestine Deficient-Cold Pattern ··· 221
Section 3　Spleen and Stomach Pattern Differentiation ························· 221
　　Spleen Qi Deficiency Pattern ··· 223
　　Sinking of Spleen Qi Pattern ··· 223
　　Spleen Yang Deficiency Pattern ··· 226
　　Spleen Failing to Control Blood Pattern ·· 227
　　Cold-Damp Encumbering the Spleen Pattern ······································ 228
　　Retention of Damp-Heat in the Spleen Pattern ····································· 229
　　Stomach Cold Pattern ·· 231
　　Stomach Heat Pattern ·· 232
　　Stomach Yin Deficiency Pattern ·· 233
　　Retention of Food in the Stomach Pattern ··· 234
　　Blood Stasis in the Stomach Pattern ··· 235
Section 4　Liver and Gallbladder Pattern Differentiation ······················· 237

XIX

- Liver Blood Deficiency Pattern · 239
- Liver Yin Deficiency Pattern · 240
- Liver Constraint (Depression/Depressed/Stagnated) Pattern · 241
- Liver Fire Blazing Upward Pattern · 243
- Hyperactivity of Liver Yang Pattern · 244
- Liver Wind Stirring Internally Pattern · 246
- Damp-Heat in the Liver and Gallbladder Pattern · 249
- Cold Stagnation in the Liver Channel Pattern · 252
- Depressed Gallbladder with Phlegm Harassing Pattern · 252

Section 5 Kidney and Bladder Pattern Differentiation · 254
- Kidney Yang Deficiency Pattern · 254
- Kidney Yin Deficiency Pattern · 256
- Kidney Essence Deficiency Pattern · 257
- Kidney Qi Deficiency Pattern · 259
- Kidney Failing to Receive Qi Pattern · 260
- Damp Heat in the Bladder Pattern · 261

Section 6 Combined Patterns of *Zang-fu* Organs · 263
- Disharmony between the Heart and Kidney Pattern · 263
- Heart and Kidney Yang Deficiency Pattern · 263
- Heart and Lung Qi Deficiency Pattern · 265
- Deficiency of Both Heart and Spleen Pattern · 266
- Heart and Liver Blood Deficiency Pattern · 267
- Spleen and Lung Qi Deficiency Pattern · 267
- Kidney and Lung Yin Deficiency Pattern · 268
- Liver Fire Insulting the Lung Pattern · 268
- Disharmony between the Liver and Stomach Pattern · 269
- Liver Invading the Spleen Pattern · 270
- Liver and Kidney Yin Deficiency Pattern · 272
- Kidney and Spleen Yang Deficiency Pattern · 274

Chapter 12 Additional Patterns Differentiation · 275

Section 1 Pattern Differentiation According to the Six Channels/Stages · 275

General Introduction ······ 275
Taiyang Pattern ······ 275
Yangming Pattern ······ 280
Shaoyang Pattern ······ 282
Taiyin Pattern ······ 284
Shaoyin Pattern ······ 285
Jueyin Pattern ······ 286
Transmission of the Six Channel Pattern ······ 286

Section 2　Pattern Differentiation According to the *Wei*, Qi, *Ying*, and Blood ······ 288
Wei System Patterns ······ 289
Qi System Patterns ······ 291
Ying System Patterns ······ 291
Blood System Patterns ······ 291
Transmission of the Four Systems Patterns-Warm Heat Patterns ······ 292

Section 3　Pattern Differentiation According to the *Sanjiao* Theory ······ 294
Upper *Jiao* Patterns ······ 295
Middle *Jiao* Patterns ······ 295
Lower *Jiao* Patterns ······ 296
Transmission of *Sanjiao* Patterns ······ 298

Section 4　Pattern Differentiation According to the Twelve Channels ······ 299

Chapter 13　The Case Record　302

Chapter 14　Examples of Traditional Chinese Medical Records　312

Chapter 15　Diagnosis Methods Training and Case Analysis　314

Section 1　Diagnosis Methods Training ······ 314

The Methods of the Inspection Examination ··················314
Method and Guidelines of the Tongue Examination ··················315
The Guidelines for Inquiry and History of the Present Disease ··················317
The Method and Guidelines of the Pulse Examination ··················320
Section 2   Analysis of Cases ··················322

Index   335

CHAPTER I
Introduction

Under the instruction of the basic theory of Chinese Medicine (CM), diagnosis in CM is a subject, which focuses on the basic theories, diagnostic methods, and identification of patterns. As a bridge between the basic theory of CM and all clinical practice, diagnosis in CM can be regarded as the central conceptual process in CM.

In order to provide evidence for prevention and treatment of illness and disease, the contents of diagnosis in CM include: examination; examining the pathological conditions of the disease; analysis by means of proper methods; determining the characteristics of clinical manifestations in various diseases and patterns; and the rules that relate to various stages of an illness.

During the long history of clinical practice, through the accumulation of copious clinical experiences in diagnosis by CM practitioners in various historical times, a characteristic, integrated diagnosis system was well formed in China. This diagnostic system includes the Four Diagnostic Methods – sì zhěn 四诊 (inspection, listening and smelling, inquiry, pulse reading and palpation), and the Identification of Patterns and Diseases. The specific diagnostic methods and the recognition of diagnosis in CM have not only created significant effects in clinical practice but also through their development have lead to certain influences on biomedicine.

1. The main contents of chinese medical diagnosis

The four diagnostic methods, diagnosis of the disease, differentiation of the patterns, and case records can be classified as the main four parts of diagnosis in CM.

(1) Four diagnostic methods

These include inspection, listening (auscultation) and smelling (olfaction), inquiry (interrogation), pulse reading and palpation, which are the four procedures used in examining and collecting data about patients' health conditions (Fig. 1-1).

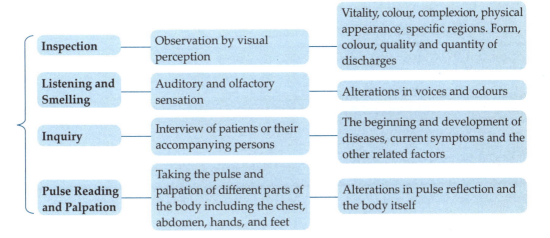

Fig. 1-1　Brief comparison between the four diagnostic methods in CM

2 Diagnostics in Chinese Medicine

(2) Diagnosis of diseases

Aiming at determining the entity of the diseases, diagnosis of a disease can also be called differentiation of a disease. Since the name of the illness is the generalisation of the characteristics and patterns of a certain disease, diagnosis of a disease is the main content in the concepts of clinical medicine such as internal medicine, surgery, gynaecology, paediatrics, etc.

(3) Pattern differentiation

Pattern differentiation is the foundation of Chinese medicine. Firstly, distinguishing between several terms such as symptoms, patterns, and diseases is essential for the better understanding of the deeper meaning of pattern identification and differentiation (Fig. 1-2).

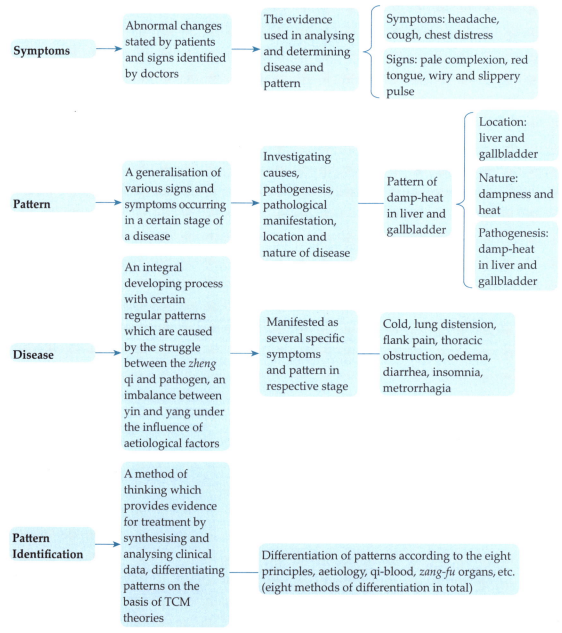

Fig. 1-2 Concepts of symptoms, patterns, disease, and pattern identification in CM

Many methods of pattern differentiation were developed during the long history of clinical practice, such as the eight-principle pattern differentiation, pattern differentiation according to aetiology, qi-blood-body fluid pattern differentiation, *zang-fu* organ pattern differentiation, pattern differentiation according to the theory of six channels, *wei* (defense) - qi - *ying* (nutrient) - blood pattern differentiation, *sanjiao* (triple burner) pattern differentiation, channel and collaterals pattern differentiation. These methods can be utilised individually or in syncretism.

(4) The medical record (TMR)

Written records about diagnosis and treatment in clinical practice, called the "case record" in antiquity, should contain important data for clinical care, scientific research and teaching. Writing the case record is one of the basic skills required for all clinical practitioners. The practitioners should write down fully the details about the patients' conditions, history, diagnosis and treatment.

2. The basic principles in Diagnosis of CM

There are three basic principles in the diagnosis of CM:
① Examination of the human body as an organic whole;
② Use of four diagnostic methods;
③ Combination of disease differentiation and pattern identification.

(1) Examination of entirety (to observe both the internal and external aspects of the body)

Since the human body is an organic whole and constantly communicates with the external environment, the diagnosis of local pathological changes should include the analysis of the overall condition of the body and the influence of the external environment.

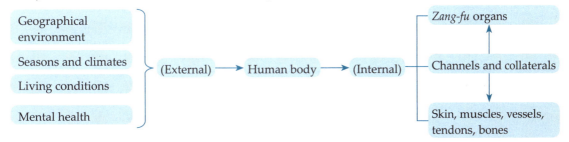

Fig. 1-3　Examination of entirety

(2) Application of the four diagnostic methods

Although inspection, listening and smelling, inquiring, pulse reading and palpation have their characteristic role in the diagnosis of diseases, they still have some limitations and cannot replace each other. So, the comprehensive application of the four diagnostic methods is essential to collect all the necessary data used in pattern identification.

(3) Combination of disease differentiation and pattern identification

This is essential to clarify the nature of diseases by identifying both disease and respective patterns and combining the disease differentiation and pattern identification in diagnosis.

3. A brief history of development of Diagnosis of CM

The following doctors and their writings have contributed greatly to the development of diagnosis of CM and their contributions should be well appreciated and understood.

Table 1-1 Important contributions in the history of diagnosis of CM

Dynasty	Physician's name	Books	Contributions
Spring and Autumn Period (770-476 BC) *Warring States Period* (475-221 BC)		*Yellow Emperor's Inner Classic* (Huáng Dì Nèi Jīng, 黄帝内经)	As the summary of theories and clinical experiences from *Spring and Autumn*, the *Warring States Period, Qin* and *Han* dynasties, this book set up a foundation for the four diagnostic methods and identification of patterns and diseases.
West *Han* 206BC-25AD	Chun Yu-yi 淳于意	*Case Records* (Zhěn Jí, 诊籍)	The first case records in history
East *Han* 25-220	Zhang Zhong-jing 张仲景	*Treatise on Cold Damage and Miscellaneous Diseases* (Shāng Hán Zá Bìng Lùn, 伤寒杂病论)	The classic on pattern identification, which includes the analysis of warm (febrile) diseases using the six channels with miscellaneous diseases by *zang-fu* organ.
	Hua Tuo 华佗	*Central Treasury Classic* (Zhōng Zàng Jīng, 中藏经)	The methods for identifying cold, heat, deficiency, excess of the *zang-fu* organs and determining prognosis
West *Jin* 265-420	Wang Shu-he 王叔和	*The Pulse Classic* (Mài Jīng, 脉经)	The first monograph about sphygmology which summarised the achievements of all previous stages
Sui 581-618	Chao Yuan-fang 巢元方	*Treatise on the Origins and Manifestations of Various Diseases* (Zhū Bìng Yuán Hòu Lùn, 诸病源候论)	The first classic about the aetiology and diagnosis of patterns in the history of Chinese medicine
Song 960-1270	Chen Yan 陈言	*Treatise on Diseases, Patterns, and Formulas Related to the Unification of the Three Aetiologies* (Sān Yīn Jí Yī Bìng Zhèng Fāng Lùn, 三因极一病证方论)	A comprehensive work about aetiology, differentiation, principles and methods in treatment, which created theories on three categories of aetiological factors
Yuan 1206-1368	Hua Shou 滑寿	*Pivot for Diagnosis* (Zhěn Jiā Shū Yào, 诊家枢要)	Taking floating, deep, slow, rapid, slippery, unsmooth pulses as the six fundamental pulses
	Wei Yi-lin 危亦林	*Effective Formulas from Generations of Physicians* (Shì Yī Dé Xiào Fāng, 世医得效方)	Discussing ten moribund pulses which manifest in serious and dangerous diseases
Ming 1368-1644	Li Shi-zhen 李时珍	*[Li] Bin-hu's Teachings on Pulse Diagnosis* (Bīn Hú Mài Xué, 濒湖脉学)	Classifying twenty-eight pulse images by integrating extracts of various school's teachings on pulse reading

Continued

Dynasty	Physician's name	Books	Contributions
Ming 1368-1644	Zhang Jing-yue 张景岳	The Complete Works of [Zhang] Jing-yue (Jǐng Yuè Quán Shū, 景岳全书)	Determining the importance of the eight principles pattern differentiation; regarding yin and yang as the two keys of the eight-principles while exterior, interior, cold, heat, deficiency and excess are six derivatives
Qing 1644-1911	Li Yan-gang 李延罡	The Assemble of Knack in Sphygmology (Mài Jué Huì Biàn, 脉诀汇辨)	Taking floating, deep, slow, rapid, feeble, excess pulse as six fundamental pulses
	Ye Tian-shi 叶天士	Externally-Contracted Warm-Heat Diseases (Wài Gǎn Wēn Rè Piān, 外感温热篇)	Creating wei (defensive)-qi-ying (nutrient)-blood pattern differentiation in warm diseases
	Wu Ju-tong 吴鞠通	Systematic Differentiation of Warm Diseases (Wēn Bìng Tiáo Biàn, 温病条辨)	Creating the san jiao pattern differentiation in warm diseases

In modern times, *Manuals of Colour Graph about Glossoscopy* (彩图辨舌指南) authored by Cao Bing-zhang (曹炳章) is a very important work about tongue diagnosis since the book included a discussion about tongue diagnosis from various dynasties. *Investigation of Glossoscopy* (舌诊研究) by Chen Ze-lin (陈泽霖); *Differential Diagnosis of Symptoms in TCM* (中医症状鉴别诊断学), *Differential Diagnosis of Patterns in TCM* (中医证候鉴别诊断学) by Zhao Jin-duo (赵金铎); in addition successive editions of the *Diagnosis of TCM* (中医诊断学) make the contents of the diagnosis of CM more systematical, comprehensive and accurate.

CHAPTER 2
Inspection Examination

The inspection or looking examination is the method by which the practitioner can understand the pathogenic condition through observation. The practitioner observes the change of the patient's spirit, colour, body shape and postures, as well as the various parts of the body, including the tongue and the colour and quality of the excreta.

The content of an inspection examination includes five parts: the inspection of the circumstances of the entire body; inspection of the circumstances of various parts of the body; inspection of the tongue; inspection of excreta and inspection of infants' and children's hands.

Contents of the Inspection Examination
- Inspection of the circumstances of the entire body
    - Inspection of the spirit or *shen* (神)
    - Inspection of the colour
    - Inspection of the body shape
    - Inspection of the posture
- Inspection of the circumstances of various parts of the body
    - Inspection of the head, face and complexion
    - Inspection of the five sense organs
    - Inspection of the body
    - Inspection of the four limbs
    - Inspection of the genitals and anus
    - Inspection of the skin and nails
- Tongue examination
- Inspection of excreta
    - Inspection of the phlegm-drool
    - Inspection of the vomit
    - Inspection of the stool and urine
- Inspection of infants' and children's hands
    - Inspection of the infant's index finger veins
    - Inspection of the collaterals of the thenar eminence and nails

Section 1
Inspection of the Circumstances of the Entire Body

Inspection of the circumstances of the entire body is a primary diagnostic method. When the practitioner examines a patient, inspection of the spirit (vitality/*shen*), colour, body shape and posture is the first important procedure in the general understanding of any disease. These factors are the outward manifestation of the vital activities of the body, and can allow the practitioner to obtain not only a whole overall impression of the state and characteristics of the illness, but also a deep basic knowledge of the disease.

Inspection of the *Shen* (Spirit)

Concept:

The *shen* is a generic name for the human body's vital movement and it is the summation of all the human body's vital phenomena. The *shen* can be divided into a generalised spirit and the specific sense of spirit (Fig. 2-1). Inspection of the *shen* refers to diagnosis of disease by observing the manifestations of life activities.

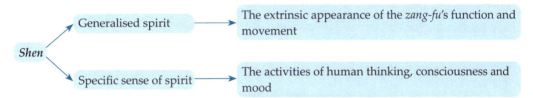

Fig. 2-1 Schematic diagram of the concept of *shen*

Principle:

The material base of *shen* is the prenatal essence-qi, postnatal essence, qi, blood, and body fluids, which transform into each other (Fig. 2-2).

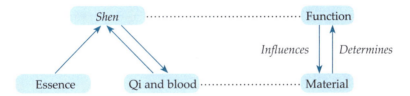

Fig. 2-2 Relationships between *shen*, essence, qi and blood

The relationship between the *shen* and essence qi: If the essence qi is adequate then the body is healthy, the *shen* is prosperous and resistance against any disease is strong. If the essence qi is frail then the body is feeble, the *shen* is debilitated and therefore the ability to resist disease is weak.

Clinical significance:

By inspecting the *shen* it enables one to realise if the essence qi of the *zang-fu* organs is exuberant or deficient. Such an inspection is important for analysing the disease, to help decide whether it is mild or severe, benign or malignant and if the prognosis is good or poor.

Points of note:

During inspection of the *shen*, the expression of the eyes; facial expression; facial complexion; mental status, and movement of the body should all be inspected, but the most important of these is the expression of the eyes.

Judgments that can be made on the *shen* and the manifestations of the spirit include: being spirited (having presence of spirit), lack of spirit, being spiritless (loss of spirit) and false spirit (Table 2-1).

Table 2-1 Differentiation of being spirited, lacking spirit, loss of spirit, false spirit

	Mind, speech	Eyes	Respiration	Complexion, physique	Action, reaction	Appetite and thirst
Spirited	Mental consciousness, energetic/ normal speech	Sparkling eyes	Smooth breathing	Ruddy complexion/ strong build with strong muscles	Natural movements/ reasonable reaction to the environment	Normal and healthy
Lack of spirit	No desire to speak	Dull eyes	Shortness of breath	Pale complexion / Tired and weak body, soft and emaciated muscles	Slow movements, lethargy	Lack of appetite
Loss of spirit	Listlessness, Mental confusion, delirium, or sudden coma/ abnormal speech	Dull eyes, and slow eye movements	Weak breath and possible dyspnoea	Dark and gloomy face, thin and weak body, emaciation	Difficulty in movement, sluggish response, rigidity of hands and lock jaw	No desire to eat or drink
False spirit	Sudden mental improvement, talkative without much sense, desire to see family members	Sudden sparkling of eyes		Pale complexion, flushed cheeks as if wearing make-up	Occurs for short time only	Sudden desire to eat

Spirited ☯: means having *shen*, or good spirit; indicating sufficient *zheng* (healthy) qi, normal functioning of the organs and indicates a favourable prognosis.

Lack of spirit ☯: this is commonly seen in patients with a deficiency pattern; particularly deficiency of qi and blood.

Spiritless (loss of spirit) ☯: this can mean poor spirit and damage of essence, which is due to insufficient *zheng* qi, deficiency of essence qi, and indicates serious disease and unfavourable prognosis. It also includes exuberance of pathogens with mental disorder, which is due to heat disturbing the mental activity, or inward invasion of the pericardium by a pathogen, or liver wind with phlegm confusing the seven orifices, all indicating serious disease.

False spirit ☯: indicates exhaustion of essential qi, separation of yin from yang, escape of *zheng* qi, floating of yang due to exhaustion of yin to control yang. Here the patient is on the verge of death, in a critical state.

Mental disorders ☯: includes irritability, coma, delirium, mania, depression, epilepsy, hysteria, etc.

Panic and **hysteria** often appear as anxiety and fear, which mostly belong to deficiency patterns.

Manic disease and **external heat disease** ☯ present as madness, irritability and restlessness, and belong to yang patterns (*kuáng* 狂).

Mania and **dementia** ☯ present as apathy, vacancy and feeble mindedness, and belong to yin patterns (diān 癫).

Epilepsy appears as sudden coma, convulsion of the limbs, drooling and unconsciousness, after which the person returns to normal (xián 痫).

Inspection of Colour

The inspection of colour mainly includes observation of changes in the colour and lustre of the facial complexion and body skin.

1. Concept, principle and significance

Inspection of colour involves both the colour and lustre.

Colour refers to changes of the skin colour; it is the external manifestation of blood colour and skin colour together. Skin colour reflects the blood and yin and it reveals the different natures of diseases and patterns of different *zang-fu*.

Lustre refers to the sheen of the skin and relates to changes of brightness or radiance. Lustre reflects the quality of the qi and yang; it reveals the exuberance and debilitation of the *zang-fu*'s essential qi, and allows for a judgment of the severity of a condition and its prognosis.

The relationship between colour and lustre is that colour (especially on the face) may be varied so, whatever the colour, the lustre of the skin is always a better reflection of the body's condition. If the complexion is moist and lustrous it indicates that the *zang-fu* organs are normal, the *zheng* qi is adequate and prognosis is favourable. If the complexion is dry and dull it indicates insufficiency of *zang-fu* essence and implies serious illness.

2. Facial areas and their relationship to the *zang-fu* organs

A. The method to divide the face according to the *zang-fu* organs given in the *Basic Questions - Needling the Febrile Disease* (Sù Wèn - Cì Rè, 素问·刺热).

	Forehead-heart	
Right cheek-lung	Nose-spleen	Left cheek-liver
	Chin-kidney	

B. Dividing method of the *The Spiritual Pivot-Five Colours* (Líng Shū-Wǔ Sè, 灵枢·五色). *The Spiritual Pivot - Five Colours* divides the areas of the face into five parts as below (Fig. 2-3).

Nose —— Bright Hall (míng táng, 明堂)
Between the eyebrows —— Gate tower (què, 阙)
Forehead —— Courtyard (tíng, 庭)
Region anterior to the ear and below the cheekbone —— Borderland (fān, 藩)
Tragus of the ear —— Cloud or Shelter (bì, 蔽) (Fig. 2-3)

See Fig. 2-4, for the dividing method of the *zang-fu* organs by *The Spiritual Pivot-Five Colours*.

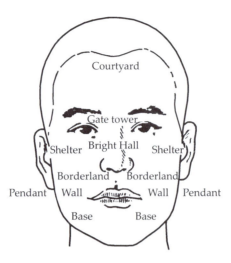

Fig. 2-3 The Bright Hall, Borderland and Shelter

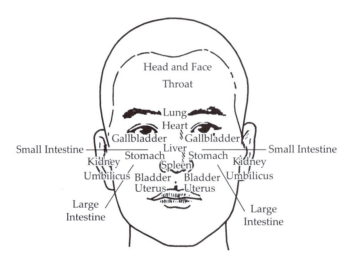

Fig. 2-4 Facial areas and their relationship to the zang-fu organs

3. Ten methods for observing colour

The Classic to Obey for Inspection Diagnosis (*Wàng Zhěn Zūn Jīng*, 望诊遵经) points out ten methods of viewing colour, which was written by Wang Hong (王宏, 1875) in the *Qing* Dynasty. They include: superficial and deep (浮沉); clear and turbid (清浊); faint and extreme (微甚); scattered and conglomerate (散抟); sheen and perishing (泽夭) (Table 2-2).

Briefly, the 'Ten-methods' can distinguish exterior and interior; yin and yang; deficiency and excess; acute and chronic; favourable and unfavourable.

4. Normal colour and morbid colour

Normal colour is divided into the governing colour and the guest colour. Morbid colour is divided into the benign colour and malignant colour.

(1) Normal colour

The normal colour should be the natural colour of the person's race/ethnicity and

Table 2-2 Brief table of the ten methods for observing colour

Ten methods	Characteristic	Pattern	Course
Superficial (浮)	Visible on the skin	Exterior Pattern	Superficial → deep: pathogen moves from exterior to interior
Deep (沉)	Hidden inside the skin	Interior Pattern	Deep → superficial: pathogen moves from interior to exterior
Clear (清)	Clear and distinct transparent	Yang Pattern	Clear → turbid: disease changes from yang to yin
Turbid (浊)	Dark and turbid, dull or dim	Yin Pattern	Turbid → clear: disease changes from yin to yang
Faint (微)	Shallow and light	Deficiency Pattern	Faint → extreme: pattern of deficiency turning into excess
Extreme (甚)	Deep and thick	Excess Pattern	Extreme → faint: pattern of excess turning into deficiency
Scattered (散)	Dispersed and scanty, like powdered medicine over the surface	New Onset Illness	Scattered → conglomerate: gradual gathering of the pathogen
Conglomerate (抟)	Accumulation and obstruction, like small balls of clay	Enduring Illness	Conglomerate → scattered: illness is getting better
Sheen (泽)	Moist and nourished, with lustre	Mild Illness	Sheen → perishing: gradual decline in the essence
Perishing (夭)	Weak and withered	Serious Illness	Perishing → sheen: gradual recovery of the essence

should be moist and with a bright sheen (pinkish-white for white people, and brown-black for black people, slightly yellow-red for Chinese, etc.). However, the characteristics related to being moist with a bright sheen more significantly implies a healthy disposition than the actual colour and this healthy complexion is often described as a blooming or glowing complexion. Thus firstly, the complexion being moist with a bright sheen is a manifestation of engorged essence. Secondly, the complexion colour implied in the skin and not the natural pigmentation of the skin, is the manifestation of essence unable to discharge outward. It is described as the lustrous and moist facial colour with hidden redness (redness should always be seen in combination with whatever the innate colour of the patient is).

The governing colour is the colour, which basically does not change from the time of birth. The guest colour ☯ is the normal changes of complexion due to the different seasons and climates.

(2) Morbid colour

Morbid colour is the change in complexion due to disease; its characteristics are dark and it appears as if exposed on the surface. Firstly, the complexion, which is dull and dry, reflects a decline of essence. Secondly, the complexion, which is obviously abnormal, is a manifestation of critical diseases.

Benign colour is the complexion that is moist and with a bright sheen, which indicates normal condition of the essence and stomach qi, new-onset, mild disease or a yang pattern.

Malignant colour is the complexion that is dull and dry, which indicates insufficient essence and stomach qi, prolonged or serious disease or a yin pattern.

Table 2-3 Differentiation of the normal colour, benign colour, and malignant colour

Five colours	Normal colour	Benign colour (Mild-disease colour)	Malignant colour (Serious-disease colour)
Blue-green	Like dark green jade	Like a kingfisher's feathers	Like the dying stalks of a plant
Red	Like cinnabar (vermilion colour) wrapped in white silk	Like a cock's comb	Like static blood
Yellow	Like realgar (an orange/red mineral) wrapped in white silk	Like a crab's abdomen	Like the colour of unripe oranges
White	Like a swan's feathers	Like pig's fat	Like desiccated bones
Black	Like heavy lacquer	Like crow's feathers	Like soot

5. Major manifestations and significances of the five colours (Table 2-4)

Table 2-4 Pathologies governed by the five colours

Five colours	Five phases	Five zang-organs	Diseases governed and pathology	Features
Blue-green	Wood	Liver	*Governs wind:* the liver failing to govern the free flow of qi and blockage of qi and blood. *Governs pain:* obstruction of qi passage; lack of flow causing pain. *Governs cold:* cold leads to contraction; spasm of channels; blockage of blood movement. *Governs stasis:* stasis blocking the channels and vessels.	Blue-green-grey Blue-green-white Dusky blue green Blue-green with purple
Red	Fire	Heart	*Governs heat:* heat causes quick flow of blood, blood engorged in the collaterals. A. Excess heat B. Deficiency heat (yin deficiency with empty heat) C. Floating yang pattern: deficient yang floating upwards	A. Redness of the whole face. B. Tidal reddening of the cheeks only. C. Red colour like wearing make-up.

Continued

Five colours	Five phases	Five zang-organs	Diseases governed and pathology	Features
Yellow	Earth	Spleen	Governs dampness: A. Dampness syndrome: repression of dampness, blockage of the qi and blood B. Jaundice: damp depression i) Yang jaundice ii) Yin jaundice Governs deficiency: spleen deficiency A. The source of qi and blood production is insufficient with deficiency of *ying*-blood B. Fluid-damp not transforming with blockage of qi and blood	-A. Yellow face as if dirty -B. Yellow face, eyes, body i) Yellow like an orange ii) Yellow like smoke -A. Light yellow colour and emaciated -B. Light yellow colour with oedema
White	Metal	Lung	Governs deficiency: A. Lack of strength, deficiency of qi and blood i) Yang deficiency ii) Qi deficiency B. Blood deficiency: i) *Ying*- blood deficiency ii) Governs loss of blood: blood not filling vessels	-A. White i) Bright white ii) Pale white -B. i) Pale white with yellow and emaciated ii) White without sheen
Black	Water	Kidney	Governs cold: Governs kidney deficiency: A. Kidney yang deficiency: failure to warm the body and blockage of blood B. Kidney yin deficiency: internal deficient heat injuring the yin fluids	-A. Dark black complexion -B. Black, dry complexion
			Governs water-rheum: water flooding due to kidney deficiency causing blockage of qi and blood	-Black eye sockets
			Governs blood stasis: stasis obstructing the channels and network	-Purple black complexion

    A. White:

White may indicate deficiency; cold; desertion of blood or sudden collapse of yang qi.

        a. Complexion is pale without lustre —— Blood deficiency pattern; pattern of blood loss.

        b. White dull complexion and facial oedema —— Pattern of yang deficiency and water floating oedema.

        c. Complexion is pale —— Sudden loss of yang qi and exuberant internal yin-cold.

    B. Yellow:

Yellow may indicate deficiency of the spleen and dampness patterns.

        a. Withered yellow complexion —— Qi deficiency of the spleen and stomach.

b. Yellowish complexion with facial oedema 🔵 —— Deficiency of the spleen and accumulation of dampness.
c. Face, eyes and body all yellow 🔵 —— Jaundice.

C. Red 🔵:

Red may indicate heat patterns and floating yang patterns.
a. Redness of the whole face 🔵 —— Excess-heat pattern.
b. Malar flush - tidal redness only in the cheeks 🔵 —— Yin deficiency.
c. Pale face with occasional migratory bright-red, like the patient is wearing make-up 🔵 —— Floating yang pattern.

D. Blue-green 🔵:

Blue-green may indicate cold; pain; qi stagnation; blood stasis and convulsions in children.
a. Complexion is light blue-green or dark blue-green 🔵 —— Excess of cold, intense pain.
b. Complexion and lips are blue-green and purple 🔵 —— Debilitation of heart qi and heart yang with blood stasis.
c. Complexion is blue-green and yellow 🔵 —— Liver stagnation and deficiency of the spleen.
d. In children, the area between the eyebrows, the nose bridge, and around the lips becomes blue-green 🔵 —— usually associated with convulsions.

E. Black 🔵:

Black may indicate kidney deficiency; cold; water-rheum and blood stasis.
a. Dark black without lustre —— Kidney yang deficiency.
b. Dry and black complexion —— Kidney yin deficiency.
c. Black rim around the eyes —— Retention of fluid due to kidney deficiency or leucorrhoea due to cold-dampness.
d. Blackish complexion with scaly skin —— Prolonged blood stasis.

Inspection of the Form of the Body

Inspection of the form of the body primarily means to observe whether the patient is strong or weak, fat or thin. Inspection of the form of the body considers aspects of the constitution, shape and bearing and whether there is any physical abnormality.

Principle

① Form of the body has a close correlation with the *zang-fu* organs. Body constitution is associated with the *zang-fu* organs, whilst the function and condition of the *zang-fu* organs may be reflected by the body.

② Different forms of the body reflect different conditions of relative exuberance or debilitation of the yin and yang, and this reflects the likelihood of affliction by disease and the expected prognosis of a disease.

Significance

Inspection of the form of the body may help practitioners to examine the deficiency or excess of the *zang-fu* organs, exuberance or decline of the qi and blood, strength or weakness of the disease resistance and prognosis of some diseases.

Content

(1) Inspection of the form of the body

The content of the inspection of the form of the body includes: strong, weak, fat, and thin.

Body Mass Index (BMI) is the index which is commonly used for determining fatness or thinness of the body mass:

BMI=body weight (kg)/ body height (m)^2		
	Western Adults	Asian adults
The normal range of BMI	18.5~25	18.5~22.9
Below the normal range or underweight	<18.5 kg	<18.5 kg
Overweight	25~30	≥23
Start of obesity	25~30	23~25.1
Obesity grade I	30~35	25~29.9
Obesity grade II	35~40	≥30
Morbidly obese	>40	>40

Character and significance of the form of the body:

A. Strong:

Character: big and strong bones, broad and thick chest, well-developed muscles, moist and lustrous skin.

Clinical significance: powerful function of the *zang-fu*; exuberance of qi and blood; strong resistance against pathogenic invasion.

B. Weak:

Character: weak and small bones, narrow chest, thin muscles, withered skin.

Clinical significance: weak function of the *zang-fu*; shortage of the qi and blood; weak resistance against pathogenic invasion.

C. Fatness:

Character: fat and overeating; solid muscles, prosperous and powerful.

Clinical significance: surplus of qi; sufficient essence; healthy body.

Character: fat but eats only small amounts; flabby muscles and skin, mental fatigue.

Clinical significance: obese build and deficient qi; shortage of yang qi; excessive phlegm and dampness.

D. Thinness:

Character: thin body and red cheeks, scorched and dry skin.

Clinical significance: yin deficiency; shortage of yin-blood; internal deficiency fire.

Character: chronic disease and lying in bed, thin as a rake.

Clinical significance: insufficiency of *zang-fu* essence; excessive shortage of qi and fluid; often being critically ill.

(2) *Character and significance of the form of the constitution*

The recognition of the constitution of the human body can be traced back to the *Yellow Emperor's Inner Classic*. Initially there were the five human forms (*The Spiritual Pivot-Yin and Yang Twenty-five People Types*, 灵枢·阴阳二十五人) and "strong constitution" (*The Spiritual Pivot-Treatise on Reversal*, 灵枢·厥论). *Important Formulas Worth a Thousand Gold Pieces for Emergency* (*Bèi Jí Qiān Jīn Yào Fāng*, 备急千金要方) and *Comprehensive Treatise on*

Protecting Children's Lives (*Xiǎo Ér Wèi Shēng Zǒng Wēi Fāng Lùn,* 小儿卫生总微方论) called it "constitution" in the *Tang* Dynasty. Zhang Jie-bin also called it "constitution" in the *Ming* Dynasty. People accepted and recognised it as such gradually in the late-*Ming* Dynasty and the beginning of the *Qing* Dynasty.

The constitution reflects the relative exuberance or debilitation of the yin, yang, qi, blood etc. of the different physical features. Thus, inspecting the type of constitution helps the practitioner to understand the exuberance or debilitation of the yin, yang, qi, blood etc. and the prognosis of the disease.

Characteristic and significance of the form of the constitution:

A. A yin *zang* person:

Character: short and fat body type; round head and thick neck; broad shoulder and thick chest. The pose of the body is usually still.

Clinical significance: yang deficiency and yin excess; cold forming with yin.

B. A yang *zang* person:

Character: thin and tall body type; long head and thin neck; narrow shoulders and flat chest; bowed posture.

Clinical significance: yin deficiency and yang excess; heat forming with yang.

C. A yin and yang harmonised person:

Character: type of the body somewhere between the yin and yang person discussed above.

Clinical significance: harmony of yin and yang, sufficient qi and blood.

Inspection of Posture and Movement

Inspection of posture and movement means to examine the patient's posture in passive and active states as well as look for any abnormal movements.

Principle

① The posture of the patient is closely related to the conditions of yin and yang of the body, as well as the nature of the illness, like being cold or hot or suffering from deficiency or excess.

② Patterns of yang, heat, and excess mostly appear as restlessness; patterns of yin, cold, and deficiency mostly appear as a liking for quietness and dislike of movement.

The abnormal movements of the limbs have a definite relationship with disease.

Significance

Inspection of posture is helpful for deciding the nature of yin, yang, cold, heat, deficiency, and excess in pathological conditions as well as the degree of pathological changes in the *zang-fu* organs. Movement, strength, lifting the head and stretching the body are ascribed to yang, heat and excess patterns; on the contrary, tranquillity or quietness, weakness, bending the head forward and curving the body are ascribed to yin, cold and deficiency patterns.

Contents

Inspection of posture includes examining for abnormal posture, abnormal movements and deficient and exhausted postures (Table 2-5).

Table 2-5 Contents, manifestations and clinical significance of the inspection of posture

Contents	Main manifestations	Clinical significance
Abnormal posture	Sitting with the head raised, wheezing asthma and excessive phlegm	Lung excess and qi counter-flow
	Sitting with the head bent down, shortage of qi and laziness in speaking	Lung deficiency and weak body
	Lying on the bed, facing upwards and out towards the room. Restlessness, with a tendency to turn the body freely	Yang, heat and excess pattern
	Lying on the bed facing downwards or facing the wall, away from the room. Quietness, without turning or moving much	Yin, cold and deficiency pattern
	Lying in a supine position with extension of the limbs and refusal to cover with a quilt or put on clothes	Excess heat pattern
	Huddled up when lying in the bed with a preference to put on more clothes	Deficiency-cold pattern
	Sitting up with inability to lie flat on the bed, lying down causes qi counter-flow	Lung distension, or retention of fluid in the chest and abdomen; cough and asthma
	Lying on the bed with inability to sit up, sitting up causes dizziness	Extreme deficiency of qi and blood or qi and blood exhaustion
Deficient and exhausted posture	Head bent down, depressed eyes with lack of lustre	Exhaustion of essence and spirit
	Dorsal curvature, drooped shoulders	Exhaustion of the heart and lung with *zong* (gathering) qi (宗气) deficiency.
	Soreness and pain of the lumbar region, and inability to move	Exhaustion of the kidney essence
	Dislike of flexing or stretching of the limbs, moving with a bent body and leaning on objects	Exhaustion of the tendons
	Unable to stand for a long time, unstable walking	Exhaustion of bones
Abnormal movements	Tremor of the eyelids, lips, fingers and toes	Sign of convulsions, or shortage of qi and blood with malnutrition of the channels
	Spasm of the limbs; opisthotonus	Internal disturbance of liver wind
	Sudden cloudiness with fainting and collapse with a loss of consciousness, one-sided paralysis, drooping of the angle of the mouth	Wind stroke in the *zang*

Contents	Main manifestations	Clinical significance
Abnormal movements	If the mind is clear, only hemi-paralysis or deviation of the eyes and mouth	Wind stroke in the channels or the sequellae of wind stroke
	A sudden fall, unconsciousness, open mouth, flaccid hands, and urinary incontinence	Wind stroke desertion pattern (flaccid type)
	A sudden fall, locked jaw, clenched hands and tonic movements	Wind stroke block pattern (spastic type)
	Shaking chills	Cold attack leading to shivering, sweating or malaria
	A sudden fall, red face and extreme sweating in the summer	Summer-heat stroke
	Constitutionally weak, a sudden fall, a pale complexion, weak breath, profuse sweating	Qi collapse
	Major blood loss and then a sudden fall, pale complexion, blood pressure drops	Blood collapse
	Great anger and then a sudden fall, with breath holding or excess breath, closed eyes, stiff body or irregular thrashing and waving of the limbs, consciousness, physical symptoms change or disappear if psychological intervention is applied	Qi syncope
	Sudden fall, failure to recognise people, convulsions of the limbs, foaming at the mouth, a shocking cry out loud, coming around after a short while and then a return to normal	Epilepsy
	Flaccid muscles and tendons, lack of strength, loss of function, flaccidity leading to muscular atrophy after a long time	Wěi patterns (痿病) (Atrophy-flaccidity illnesses)
	Joint pain or swelling, distortion, disturbance of activity	Bì patterns (痹病) illnesses due to block or obstruction
	Frowning and holding the bowed head in the hands	Headache
	Palpitations of the heart, closed eyes and loss of speech	Severe palpitations due to deficiency of the heart
	Protecting the breast with both hands and fear of touch	Mammary pain
	Protecting the abdomen with hands, bending from the waist	Abdominal pain
	Supporting the lumbus and unable to turn	Lumbar pain

Continued

Section 2
Inspection of the Circumstances of Various Parts of the Body

Based on the inspection of the circumstances of the entire body, inspection of the circumstances of various parts of the body is used to closely examine some regional areas to obtain necessary clinical data, according to the pathological conditions in the patient. It can increase the understanding of the pathogenic condition more deeply and intimately and can also fill any gaps left in the inspection of the circumstances of the entire body.

Inspection of the Head and Face

Inspection of the Head

Inspection of the head includes the shape of the head, fontanel, mobility of the head and condition of the hair. By observing the head one can understand the state of the kidney and brain as well as the excess or deficiency of the *zang-fu* essence.

The head is the dwelling place of the essence-spirit, or the head is the place where the brain and marrow are housed. The brain is the sea of the marrow and marrow is developed from the essence, which is stored in the kidney. The hair is the outward manifestation of the kidney and an extension of blood. The head is the meeting place of all the yang channels. Three yang channels of the hand and foot and *du mai* all extend to the head. The liver channel of the foot *jueyin* and the *ren mai* also nourish the head. The *yangming* channels and *ren mai* extend to the front of the head, the *taiyang* channels and *du mai* extend to both sides of the head, and the liver channels of the foot *jueyin* have connections up to the eyes and top of the head. The essence of all *zang-fu* organs comes up to nourish the head. Therefore, inspection of the head will help to examine the state of the kidney, brain and the condition of the *zang-fu* essence.

The changes of the head circumference in developing stages: a newborn's head is about 36 cm, at six months is 43 cm, at one year is 46 cm, at two years is 49 cm, and at three years is 50 cm. The head circumference then adds 1.5 cm from four to ten years and then will reach 56 cm at eighteen years; after this there is nearly no change. If it obviously exceeds this range, it is called a big head; if on the contrary, it is less than this, it is called a small head. It does not matter if the head is big or small, if the person has a normal intelligence and development, it usually has no pathological significance.

1. Shape of the head

Big head: A bigger head with smaller face, low intelligence and late closure of cranial sutures in children, is usually caused by innate deficiency, deficiency of the kidney yang and fluid retention in the brain.

Small head: If a child has a small head with a round top, early closure of the fontanel and is mentally of low intelligence, it is a sign of insufficiency of kidney essence and maldevelopment of the skull.

Square-formed head: Protrusion of the forehead with a flat top and square-formed head in children often results from insufficiency of kidney essence or weakness of the spleen and stomach and mal-development of the skull; this anomaly is usually seen in rickets or congenital syphilis.

2. Fontanel

The fontanel is the space between the skull bones of infants, due to the loose-fitting joints of the skull. It includes the anterior fontanel and posterior fontanel. The posterior fontanel is shown as a triangle and is closed by the postnatal period at two to four months. The anterior fontanel is diamond-shaped and is closed at twelve to eighteen months after birth. These two fontanels are the main regions in the clinical examination of the head.

Protrusion of the fontanel: If the fontanel protrudes out, it is called a bulging fontanel. A bulging fontanel relates to an excess pattern and may be caused by a heat pathogen of warm disease attacking upward, malnutrition of marrow or fluid retention in the skull. It may be seen in hydrocephalus, where there is an increase in the volume of cerebrospinal-fluid in the skull. However, when an infant is crying, the temporary protrusion of the fontanel is normal.

Sunken fontanel: A sunken fontanel relates to a deficiency pattern and is seen in children with vomiting and diarrhoea leading to consumption of body fluids; in shortage of qi and blood and insufficiency of congenital essence or marrow. However, if a sunken fontanel is found in infants younger than six months then this is considered normal.

Retarded closure of the fontanel: This is commonly a manifestation of a shortage of kidney qi and mal-development and usually seen in children with rickets. Here it often involves five kinds of flaccidity (head, neck, hands and feet, muscles, mouth), five kinds of retardation (standing, walking, hair, teeth, speech) as well as other manifestations. Retarded closure of the fontanel may also be seen with other causes e.g. hydrocephalus.

3. Mobility of the head

Involuntary shaking of the head or tremor in both children and adults indicates internal stirring of liver wind or deficiency of qi and blood and under-nourishment of the spirit-essence.

4. Hair

The growth of the hair is closely related to the exuberance or deficiency of kidney qi and conditions of the essence and blood. Consequently, the inspection of the hair can help to understand the state of kidney qi or the exuberance or insufficiency of essence and blood. The normal person has strong black, brown, red or blonde, luxuriant and lustrous hair; this is a sign of sufficient kidney qi and adequate essence and blood.

Dry, thin, grey-yellow or white hair with loss of hair may indicate shortage of the essence and blood and can be seen in patients after a chronic and serious disease.

Sudden patchy or elliptical loss of hair is known as alopaecia, which is caused by blood deficiency or wind attack.

Thin hair in young people along with signs of dizziness, forgetfulness, aching of the lumbar region and knee joints may result from kidney deficiency. Greasy hair with pruritus (unpleasant sensation causing desire to scratch) and desquamation on the scalp is usually caused by dryness, which results from heat in the blood.

White hair in young people accompanied by symptoms of kidney deficiency may signify kidney deficiency. White hair with symptoms such as insomnia and forgetfulness are often caused by exhaustion of blood and essence.

Very thin hair in children (or no hair for a long time after birth), accompanied by growth retardation, results from congenital deficiency and damage of kidney-essence.

In children, sparse, brittle and thin hair, which is not luxuriant, is often due to malnutrition.

Inspection of the Face

The facial inspection includes observation of the whole face including the forehead. The face is the outward manifestation of the heart; it is also the location of the ascending glory of the *zang-fu*'s essential qi. According to inspection of the face, we can understand excess or debilitation of the *zang-fu*'s essential qi and related pathological changes.

1. Facial swelling

A. Facial puffy swelling is often seen in water-swelling illnesses or it can be a part of generalised oedema. Yang oedema, which firstly arises around the eyelids and face and has a rapid onset, often results from external contraction of a wind pathogen, which causes impairment in the descending and dispersing functions of the lung. A white face with slow onset oedema indicates yin oedema, which is typically caused by spleen and kidney yang deficiency leading to overflowing of water-damp. Swollen purple blue-green face and lips, palpitations and hasty breathing, indicate heart and kidney yang deficiency, and blood stasis with pathogenic fluid attacking the heart.

B. Facial swelling with hot pain, where colour fades when pressed and the eyes are nearly closed could be facial erysipelas (acute infectious inflammation). If the head is extremely swollen like a pot, it is called swollen-head infection; mostly this is due to inner heat, exuberance of blood heat, epidemic infection, upper fire toxin, or inward invasion of toxin.

2. Cheek swelling

A. Swelling in one or both cheeks below the ear-lobes without a clear borderline and, when pressed, there is a sensation like kneading dough and/or pain, is mumps. This is a warm toxin caused by an exogenous pathogenic factor, which is often seen in children.

B. If there is a red skin swelling in front of the ear, under the zygomatic bone but above the jaw bones, with fever, chills, and pain, this will be suppurative parotitis, which results from upward attack in the *yangming* by a heat pathogen.

3. Emaciated face with high cheek bones

If the patient has an emaciated face with high cheek bones, hollow eye sockets, often accompanied by withering of the major bones and wasting and sagging of the major masses of flesh, it is caused by debilitation of qi and blood, essential qi exhaustion and belongs to the critical stage of chronic diseases.

4. Deviation of the face and mouth

A. If there is deviation of the face and mouth to one side but no half-body paralysis, demonstrating relaxed muscles of the injured side of the face, disappearance of the forehead wrinkles, inability to close the eyes and/or ptosis (drooping of the upper eyelid), a shallow naso-labial groove, change of mouth angle with lips at an inclined angle, this will be damage to the collaterals caused by the wind-pathogen.

B. If there is an inclined mouth angle accompanied by half-body paralysis, it will be wind-stroke due to ascendant hyperactivity of liver yang and blockage of the channels by wind-phlegm.

5. Unusual facial expressions

A. Frightened and fearful face: the patient's emotional facial expression is contorted, frightened and fearful, which is often seen with convulsions in children; rabies; goitre; tumour, etc.

B. Sardonic smile: is due to facial spasm, which is seen in umbilical wind or tetanus, etc.

C. Leonine (lion-like) face: is usually seen in leprosy, which also manifests as thickening of the skin, and disfiguring skin nodules (lumps and bumps).

Inspection of the Five Sense Organs

1. Inspection of the eyes

Significance:

The eyes are the orifices related to the liver and the emissary of the heart. All the essence-qi of the *zang-fu* organs rises upwards into the eyes. Thus, inspection of the eyes may help one understand excess or decline of the *shen*/spirit and essence-qi.

Theory of the five wheels (rings):
- The pupil pertains to the kidney, and is called the water wheel (or ring);
- The brown, green or blue part of the eye (iris) pertains to the liver, and is called the wind wheel;
- The white part (sclera) pertains to the lung, and is called the qi wheel;
- The inner and outer canthus pertain to the heart, and is called the blood wheel;
- The eyelid pertains to the spleen, and is called the muscle wheel (Fig. 2-5).

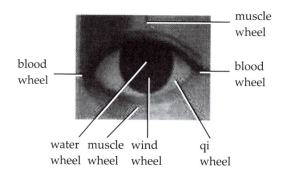

Fig. 2-5 Areas of the eyes related to *zang-fu* organs

Contents:

In inspecting the eyes, attention should be paid to the *shen* of the eyes, colour of the eyes, shape of the eyes and movements of the eyes.

(1) *Spirit of the eye*

A. With spirit: The eyes are bright, shiny and have sufficient lubrication. Eyes with spirit are clear and sparkling and the coloured and white parts of the eyes are clearly demarcated. This condition shows that the disease is mild and easily cured.

B. Without spirit: Dull and inflexible eyes, loss of brilliance, blurred vision, and insufficient lubrication; this situation shows that the disease will be difficult to treat.

(2) Colour of the eye

In normal conditions the veins of the conjunctiva and canthus are ruddy, the sclera is white as porcelain, the colour of the iris is vibrant and the cornea is transparent and without colour.

A. Red, swollen and painful eyes belong to an excess heat pattern.
B. A red canthus indicates excessive heart-fire.
C. Redness of the white part of the eye indicates lung fire.
D. A yellow colour indicates jaundice.
E. Red and swollen eyelids with ulceration are due to spleen fire.
F. Redness and swelling in the entire eye is due to liver fire or wind-heat in the liver channel.
G. A pale canthus indicates blood deficiency.
H. If above and below the eyelids is bright this indicates phlegm-rheum disease.
I. Dark eyelids reflect kidney deficiency.
J. If the cornea is muddy with grey and white colouring it is called a nebula, which indicates an invasion by toxin in the black (pupil) part of the eyes, excessive fire of liver and gallbladder attacking upward, damp-heat sweltering or yin deficiency resulting in vigourous fire, etc.
K. When the medial angle of the eye appears to have a light-yellow plaque in the elderly, it is fat pigmentation, which is caused by damp-heat brewing internally or excessive drinking.
L. If there is a grey-white turbid circle around the cornea, it is called an old circle, which is often seen in the elderly and is caused by liver and kidney deficiency.

(3) Form of the eye

A. Swelling in the eye and eyelid:

Puffy swelling in the eye and eyelid just like when first getting up in the morning and puffy face are the beginnings of oedema. The swelling of eyelids may be due to spleen deficiency and heat. If there is acute swelling of the eyelids and the eyelids are red, this is due to heat in the spleen; if the onset is slow and the eyelids are not red but soft, it is caused by spleen deficiency.

B. Sunken eye socket:

Sunken eye socket is often due to exhaustion of the *zang-fu's* essence, and this is a serious sign.

C. Membranous screen or opacity of the eye (nebula):

A spotted screen generated in the pupil and obstructed vision is usually due to heat toxin, damp-heat or phlegm-heat; it also may develop from the six pathogenic factors, stagnation of the seven emotions and deficiency of the *zang* essence or injury. Typically, if there is a visual disorder but the shape of eye is normal, it will be an internal eye disease which is usually due to seven-emotion internal damage, deficiency of qi and blood, shortage of liver and kidney or yin deficiency with exuberant fire. Generally speaking, external disorders mostly are of an excess type and internal disorders are of a deficiency type.

D. Bulging of the eye:

Bulging of the eyes accompanied by panting breath is lung distension, which is caused by turbid phlegm obstructing the lung, lung failing to diffuse and govern descent. Swelling of the neck (front part) and eye bulging is goitre, caused by wood constraint transforming into fire, binding of phlegm and qi. A single eye bulging indicates a critical disease.

E. Canthus outcrop creeping over the eye (pterygium):

When red vessels and the canthus outcrop creep horizontally from the white part of the eye toward the pupil, this is usually due to wind-heat obstructing the lung and heart channels, stasis of channels or collaterals, steaming of damp-heat or kidney yin deficiency with heart fire flaring-up.

F. Sty and cinnabar (red) eye:

A sty refers to the generation of a small boil like a wheat kernel at the side of the eye, with a little redness, swelling and slight pain. If the red swelling of the eyelid is more severe, this is called "cinnabar eye".

(4) *Movements of the eyes*

The shape of the pupil in healthy people is round. Its diameter is about 2~5 mm in the natural light. It is sensitive to light and the eyeballs can move freely. In inspecting the movements of the eyes, one should pay attention to the pupil, eyeball and eyelid.

A. Miosis:

Miosis is a medical term for constriction of the pupil. In this condition the diameter of the pupil is below two millimetres. It is usually due to exuberant heat of the liver and gallbladder. It is also caused by poisonous substances, such as *chuān wū* (Radix Aconiti), *cǎo wū* (Radix Aconiti Kusnezoffii), toadstools and other wild mushroom that are often poisonous, organo-phosphate pesticides, etc.

B. Mydriasis:

Mydriasis is a dilated condition of the pupil of the eye. In this condition the diameter of the pupil is greater than five millimetres. It is caused by exhaustion of the kidney essential qi, and usually refers to a critical illness. If both pupils become completely dilated, this is one of the indications for clinical death. If just one pupil is dilated, it can be due to wind-stroke, craniocerebral trauma, or glaucoma; it can also indicate other serious illnesses.

C. Staring straight ahead:

Staring straight ahead is a sign of unconsciousness, which can be due to exhaustion of the *zang-fu* essential qi and usually occurs in the critical stage of the disease.

D. Upward staring:

This condition refers to upward staring with failure of the eyes to move, rigidity and spasm of the neck, and arched-back rigidity, indicating a fatal sign of *taiyang* channel disease.

E. Strabismus:

This means abnormal alignment of the eyes, and is due to internal stirring of liver wind, since the eyes are related to the liver channel of the foot *jueyin*.

F. Disorder of closing eyes:

Bilateral disorder of the eyes closing is often caused by goitre tumour. However, one-sided disorder of an eye closing is often caused by wind-strike involving the collaterals.

G. Sleeping with eyes open:

This is due to deficiency of the spleen and stomach and shortage of qi and blood. Deficiency of the spleen leads to failure of the clear yang to ascend and then it can cause a lack of nourishment for the eyelids and the eyes are unable to open or close.

H. Drooping of the upper eyelid (blepharoptosis, also referred to as ptosis):

This is often caused by inherent deficiency, usually spleen and kidney deficiency. Single ptosis is usually due to deficiency of the spleen qi or external injury.

2. Inspection of the ears

The ears are associated with the kidneys and are the place where many meridians converge. Many disorders in the *zang-fu* organs, channels and body forms can be reflected on the ears. Inspection of the ears is particularly helpful for diagnosis of kidney essence disorders and pathological changes of the *shaoyang* channel (Table 2-13).

For a healthy person, the helix (auricle) is red and moist with lustre, which is a sign of sufficiency of qi and blood.

Abnormal ears:

(1) Colour and texture

A. A pale auricle is ascribed to deficiency of qi and blood.

B. A red swollen auricle accompanied by running of purulent fluid from the ear is usually due to damp-heat of the liver and gallbladder or an upward attack of a heat-pathogen.

C. A blue-black ear is a sign of exuberant internal yin-cold or an acute pain pattern.

D. A scorching dry-black ear signifies extreme loss of kidney essence and exhaustion of kidney yin; it is a critical sign of a severe disease.

E. At the beginning of childhood measles, there is a cold feeling at the auricle, and small red spots at the back of the ear.

(2) Form and movement

A. A thin, dry and withered auricle indicates shortage of congenital kidney essence.

B. A scorched dry and withered ear signifies exhaustion of kidney essence and refers to a critical disease.

C. During a prolonged illness, blood stasis may cause a dry and chapped auricle.

(3) Pathological changes in the ears

A. Running of purulent fluid from the ear (otopyorrhoea) indicates liver-gallbladder damp-heat fuming and steaming. In the later stage, it often belongs to kidney yin deficiency and deficiency fire flaming upward.

B. If there are small neoplastic lumps in the external auditory canal, this may be caused by ascending counter-flow of damp-heat and phlegm-fire with qi and blood stagnation.

C. Redness, swelling and pain in the external auditory canal indicates binding constraint of pathogenic heat.

3. Inspection of the nose

The nose is the opening of the lung and the passageway of inhalation and exhalation. The bridge of the nose relates to the liver, the tip of the nose corresponds to the spleen, the wings of the nose reflect the stomach, and the stomach channels of the foot *yangming* are distributed over the sides of the nose. The nose itself is related to the *zang-fu* organs, particularly to the lung, spleen and stomach. Accordingly, inspection of the nose is helpful to examine the pathological changes of the lung, spleen and stomach, and to understand the excess or deficiency of the stomach qi.

The normal colour of the nose is yellow-red and moist, with a bright shining glow, which means sufficient stomach qi.

Abnormal noses:

(1) Colour of the nose

A. A light yellow and moist appearance on the tip of the nose indicates a failure of the stomach qi or the stomach qi returning again.

B. A sombre and withered nose indicates stomach qi failure and belongs to the dangerously ill.

C. A white colour on the tip of the nose indicates deficiency of qi or blood, or loss of blood.

D. A red colour on the tip of the nose means heat in the lung and spleen channels.

E. A green-blue nose suggests deficiency cold or abdominal pain.

F. If the tip of the nose is dark and dry, it may be due to deficiency of the stomach qi and indicates a critical disease.

G. A black nose indicates kidney deficiency or extreme yin-cold.

(2) Form and movement of the nose

A. Red swelling and pain of the nose is usually caused by stomach heat or heat in the blood.

B. A red nose with acne-like pustules on the tip of the nose is called rosacea, which is mostly caused by accumulation of heat in the lung and stomach.

C. Collapse of the nose is often seen in syphilis.

D. Collapse of the nose (saddle nose deformity) with the loss of eyebrows is usually a critical condition in leprosy.

E. Flaring nares (nostrils or nasal passages) is due to obstruction of the lung by heat or asthma. If the onset is slow with asthmatic breathing, it is a sign of depletion of lung qi functions of dispersing and descending.

(3) Pathological changes in the nose

A. Stuffy nose with running of clear nasal discharge indicates wind-cold.

B. Stuffy nose with running of turbid nasal discharge indicates wind-heat.

C. Stuffy nose with the smell of fish and turbid nasal discharge is called sinusitis, which is caused by externally-contracted wind-heat or upward attack of a stagnated gallbladder channel.

D. Bleeding in the nose (epistaxis) mostly relates to the lung and stomach brewing into heat and then burning the nasal vessels.

E. Soft, translucent, smooth small lumps in the nares, which are blocking the nares, and so hindering the breath, are called nasal polyps and are caused by damp-heat blockage in the nose.

4. Inspection of the mouth and lips

The spleen opens into the mouth and manifests in the lips. The *yangming* channels of the hand and foot encircle the mouth and lips. Consequently, inspection of the mouth and lips can aid diagnosis of pathological changes of the spleen and stomach.

Normal lips are red and moist, which indicates sufficiency of stomach qi, qi and blood harmony. In health, the mouth and lips can open and close freely with concordant movement.

Abnormal mouth and lips:

(1) Colour of the lips
　A. Light white ☯: blood deficiency or loss of blood.
　B. Deep red ☯: excessive heat.
　C. Red, swelling and dry ☯: extreme heat.
　D. Cherry colour: gas poisoning.
　E. Blue-green and purple: blood stasis pattern.
　F. Blue-green and black ☯: excessive cold or extreme pain.

(2) Form of the mouth and lips
　A. Dry and fissured or chapped lips: damage of body fluid.
　B. Mouth and lips ulcers ☯: steaming of accumulated heat in the spleen and stomach.
　C. Angle of mouth drooling: deficient spleen and exuberant dampness in infants; wind-strike in adults.
　D. Flat philtrum, mouth and lips rolling and unable to cover the teeth: spleen qi exhausted, dangerously ill.
　E. Grey-white small ulcers inside the lips and on the mucous membranes of the mouth with a red flush around them, fire pain, or erosion all over the mouth which are both called aphthae ☯: blocked heat of the heart and spleen steaming upward.
　F. White patches like snowflakes in the mouth and on the tongue of infants ☯: thrush, foul turbid qi steaming upward to the mouth.

(3) Movement of the mouth and lips
　A. Open (the mouth opens but does not close): a deficiency pattern.
　B. Clenched jaw (the mouth closes but there is difficulty in opening): an excess pattern. This can also be seen in convulsive disease, infant's convulsions, tetanus, etc.
　C. Pursed (the upper and lower lips pursed-together): struggle of pathogenic qi and *zheng* (healthy) qi. This can also be seen in umbilical wind or tetanus.
　D. Deviated (one side of the mouth relaxed and inclined): wind-phlegm obstructing the collaterals. This can be seen in wind-strike.
　E. Shaking (cold shudders and chattering jaws, tense rocking and shaking): yang decline and cold exuberance or severe struggle of pathogenic qi and *zheng* qi. This can be seen in the shiver sweating of cold damage or malaria breaking out.
　F. Stirring (frequent and involuntary mouth opening and closing): the manifestation of stomach-qi weakness.

5. Inspection of the teeth and gums

The teeth are the surplus of bones and the bones are governed by the kidney. The gums are the places where the *yangming* channels of the hand and foot are distributed; therefore, observation of the teeth and gums can help to examine the pathological changes of the stomach and kidney and alterations of the fluid. This observation has an important significance for pattern identification.

The normal teeth appear as white, moist and strong, which is the manifestation of sufficient kidney qi and body fluid. If the gums are light-red and moist; it is the manifestation of sufficient stomach qi, qi and blood in harmony.

Abnormal teeth and gums:
(1) Teeth
  A. Dry teeth: damaged stomach yin.
  B. Teeth are bright and dry like stone: extreme heat of the *yangming*, damage of body fluid.
  C. Teeth are like withered bone: exhaustion of the kidney yin, essence not nourishing upward.
  D. Teeth are sparse, loosening, exposure of the roots of the teeth: kidney deficiency or deficiency fire flaming upward.
  E. Teeth are dry, yellow and fall out: exhausted bone; associated with being critically ill.
  F. Parched teeth with sordes (dark brown or nearly black crusts): extreme heat of the stomach and kidney but qi and fluid not exhausted.
  G. Parched teeth with no sordes: extreme heat of the stomach and kidney, qi and fluid exhausted.
  H. Clenched jaw: wind-phlegm blocked collaterals or extreme heat generating wind.
  I. Grinding of the teeth: extreme heat generating wind, this will be seen as part of a convulsive disease.
  J. Grinding of the teeth in sleep: stomach heat or parasite accumulation.

(2) Gums
  A. Pale gums: blood deficiency or loss of blood.
  B. Red, swollen and painful gums with bleeding: exuberance of stomach fire or stomach fire flaming upward.
  C. Pale and receding gums: kidney deficiency or insufficiency of stomach yin.
  D. Light swollen and bleeding gums without redness and pain: spleen deficiency, blood failing to be secured and contained; or kidney deficiency, deficient fire flaming upward.
  E. Gums are inflamed, discharge of fetid pus, even the lips are corroded, and the teeth are falling out: serious pattern of ulcerative gingivitis, mostly caused by externally contracted pestilence and the accumulated toxin attacking upward.

6. Inspection of the throat

The pharynx is distinct from the larynx. The pharynx is divided into three parts:
- Nasopharynx (above the palatal plane, back of the nasal cavity);
- Oropharynx (extending from the oral cavity and soft palate, under the palatal plane, on the superior border of the pharynx);
- Laryngopharynx also called laryngeal pharynx, (under the oropharynx, in front, it connects to the laryngeal cavity, and the inferior part connects to the oesophagus).

The soft palate extends downward and forms two layers of mucous membrane, respectively called the anterior palatine arch and posterior palatine arch. The tonsils are located in the gap, which is located between the palatine arches. The rear of the posterior palatine arch is called the posterior wall of the pharynx. The larynx is located under the laryngopharynx and connects to the windpipe. The throat is the passage of the lung and stomach and the passageway of breathing and eating; the kidney channel also connects with the throat. Therefore, by inspection of the throat one may understand the pathological changes of the lung, stomach and kidney.

A normal throat is light-red, moist, not painful, no swelling, has unobstructed breathing, normal pronunciation, and smooth swallowing.

Abnormal throat:

(1) Red and swollen throat
 A. Deep red, obvious swelling and pain ☯: extreme heat.
 B. Tender red, mild swelling and pain ☯: deficiency of kidney yin and deficient fire flaming upward.
 C. Pale red, diffuse swelling: collection of phlegm-damp.
 D. One or both sides of the throat are red, swollen and painful, accompanied by yellow white purulent spots, which are easily cleaned off: tonsillitis, mostly caused by extreme heat of the lung and stomach, steaming by fire toxin.
 E. The throat is red, swollen, with abnormal protrusion of the tonsils, severe pain, cold and heat: throat abscess, caused by accumulated heat of the *zang-fu* and external pathogens, heat toxin settling in the throat.

(2) Purulent throat
 A. The throat is deep red and swollen, abnormal protrusion of the tonsils, persistent high fever: the pus has emerged.
 B. The throat is light red, diffuse swelling with unclear boundaries, which mitigates the pain until the pus emerges, thus there is indistinct pain: the pus has not emerged.

(3) Ragged throat
 A. Superficial and dispersed ulcers: slight heat of the lung and stomach or deficient fire flaming upward.
 B. Flaky or hollow ulcers: extreme heat of the lung and stomach.
 C. Chronic ulcers red or pale in colour: a deficiency pattern.

(4) Pseudomembrane
 A. The surface of the throat and ulcers are covered with a layer of yellow-white or pale membrane. It is loose and thick, easily cleaned off, and will not arise again after being cleaned off: stomach heat, mild pathogenic condition.
 B. A grey-white pseudo-membrane on the throat that is difficult to remove, bleeding appears when it is removed and it will recur: white throat (diphtheria), heat toxin of the lung and stomach has damaged yin.

Inspection of the Body

Inspection of the body includes the inspection of the neck, chest and hypochondrium, abdomen, waist and back.

Normally the neck should be erect and symmetrical with active movements and the trachea located in the middle. The laryngeal protuberance is prominent in the male (Adam's apple) but not visible in the female. The carotid artery pulse is not easily seen at rest.

The thoracic cavity is made up of the breast, sternum, ribs and spinal column. The heart and lung are located within the thoracic cavity, which relates to the upper *jiao*, and it is the place of *zong* (gathering) qi. The breasts are located on the front of the thorax and relate to the stomach channel, but the nipples relate to the liver channel. The area from the armpit down to the twelfth rib, the rib-sides, is the place where the liver and gallbladder circulate. Inspection of the chest and hypochondrium may help one understand the pathological changes of the heart, or lung as well as the excess or decline of the *zōng* qi and various breast diseases.

The thorax is an oval-shape, and left to right diameter is greater than the anteroposterior diameter (about 1.5:1). The normal breathing is relaxed and the rhythm is regular, about 16~18 breaths in one minute.

The abdomen means the place below the xiphoid process and above the pubis on the frontal side of the body. It belongs to the middle and lower *jiao*, and the liver, spleen, kidneys, gallbladder, stomach, large intestine, small intestine, bladder and uterus are located within it. This is a place where all channels circulate, for this reason the inspection of the abdomen may help one examine the pathological changes of the internal *zang-fu* organs and excess or deficiency of the qi and blood.

The back of the trunk is the spinal column. The back is the house of the heart and lung. The waist is the house of the kidneys. The *du mai* passes through the spine in the midline. The bladder channel of the foot *taiyang* travels on both sides of the waist, and the back-*shu* points of the *zang-fu* organs are located along it. The *dai mai* (belt vessel) runs around the waist and abdomen and bundles all the channels of the yin and yang. A normal waist and back are symmetrical and are able to bend and turn actively. The spine is in the middle when holding a straight posture, cervical and lumbar segments are slightly curved forward and thoracic and sacral segments slightly curved backward; but there is no lateral curvature. Inspection of the waist and back is helpful for understanding the pathological changes of the *zang-fu* channels.

1. Neck and nape

(1) Unilateral or bilateral lumps like a tumour below the laryngeal protuberance, large or small, one or both sides, moving upward or downward accompanied by swallowing: goitre, stagnation of liver qi and retention of phlegm.

(2) Cervical cluster nodules like beans or like a rosary: (scrofula), yin deficiency of the lung and kidney; deficient fire flaring, the fluid forming the superficial nodules; wind, fire or seasonal pathogens causing accumulation and stagnation of qi and blood forming nodules in the neck and nape.

(3) Contracted or stiff neck (neck rigidity)

A. Tight and strained neck, uncomfortable, aversion to cold with fever: wind-cold attacking the *taiyang* channel, disturbance of channel qi.

B. Stiff neck and inability to bend, high fever, loss of consciousness and convulsions: fire pathogen of warm disease attacking upward or cerebrospinal damage.

C. Stiff neck accompanied by dizziness: yin deficiency and yang hyperactivity or disturbance of channel qi.

D. Stiff neck with pain after sleeping: crick in the neck, mostly due to incorrect posture during sleep, stagnation of channels and collaterals qi.

(4) Softness of the neck, and no strength for raising the head

A. In children: inherent deficiency, deficiency of kidney essence, or acquired constitution deprived of nourishment. Dysplasis (abnormal tissue development) can be seen in children with rickets.

B. Softness of the neck after a long term or serious illness, nutation (nodding habitually and involuntarily), deep hollowing of the eye sockets: exhaustion of the *zang-fu*'s essence, which belongs to a critical illness.

(5) Pulsation of the neck artery

A. Clearly visible at rest: liver-kidney yin deficiency, ascendant hyperactivity of liver yang.

B. Visible in semi-reclining or sitting position, especially in lying down: oedema or abdominal distension.

2. Chest and hypochondrium
(1) Form
A. Flat chest 🔵: yin deficiency of the lung, qi and yin deficiency, or weakness.
B. Barrel chest 🔵: lung distension, cough with asthma, lung-kidney qi deficiency.
C. Pigeon breast, funnel chest: inherent deficiency, acquired constitution deprived of nourishment, insufficiency of kidney qi, dysplasis.
D. Asymmetry of both sides of the bony thorax:
    a. One side of the bony thorax is sunken: sequellae of lung atrophy, pleural rheum or surgery on the lung.
    b. One side of the bony thorax is uplifted: pleural rheum or pneumothorax, etc.
E. Breasts are red, swollen, warm and painful, inhibited lactation, possibly even with ulceration and pus, aversion of cold and heat: acute mastitis, mostly due to stagnation of liver qi and stomach heat or external pathogens.

(2) Breath
A. Prolonged inspiratory phase: hard inspiration due to acute throat disorder, diphtheria, etc.
B. Prolonged expiratory phase: expiratory dyspnoea, asthma, lung distension, etc.
C. Shortness of breath, thorax moves up and down noticeably: excessive heat pattern.
D. Weak breathing, thorax moves up and down, but not noticeably: deficient-cold pattern.
E. Irregular rhythm of breath: lung qi deficiency, critical stage of illness.

3. Abdomen
(1) Abdominal distension 🔵
A. Abdominal distension with emaciation of the limbs: tympanites (gases in the abdomen), stagnation of the liver qi, obstruction by dampness and blood stasis.
B. Abdominal distension with general oedema: oedema, disturbances of the lung, spleen, kidney, water and dampness flowing over the skin.
C. Local abdominal distension: accumulations and gatherings.

(2) Abdominal retraction
A. Emaciation of the body: spleen and stomach deficiency, insufficiency of qi and blood.
B. Scaly, thin skin of the abdominal wall, scaphoid (sunken) abdomen: exhaustion of essential qi, critical stage of illness.

(3) Exposure of blue tendons over the abdominal wall: drum distension, stagnation of the liver qi and blood stasis.

(4) Blue or black navel of the newborn, local hardness: critical pattern of umbilical wind.

(5) Red, swelling, erosion or suppuration in the navel of the infants: umbilical sores, mostly caused by not cleaning the umbilicus which gives rise to damp-heat accumulation.

(6) Acromphalus (abnormal protrusion of the navel) with oedema and drum distension: deficiency of spleen and kidney, critical illness.

4. Waist and back
(1) Humpback or tortoise back: deficiency of the kidney qi, mal-development, or vertebral

illness, old age.

(2) *Bending back and flagging shoulders:* debilitation of *zang-fu*'s essential qi.

(3) *Contraction and pain of the lumbar region, limitation of movements:* invasion of cold-damp; or tumbling down and sudden sprain or contusion.

(4) *Arched-back rigidity accompanied by rigidity of the neck and nape, convulsion of the limbs:* internal stirring of liver wind, tension of the sinews, can be seen in tetanus.

(5) *Skeletisation, extreme emaciation causing the spine to protrude like a saw:* spinal malnutrition, a manifestation of the damage of the *zang-fu* essence, chronic and intractable diseases.

Inspection of the Four Limbs

The four limbs include the shoulders, elbows, wrists, palms, fingers of the upper limbs and the thighs, knees, ankles, metatarsus and toes of the lower limbs. The relationship between the four limbs and *zang-fu* are:
- The lung governs skin and body hair,
- The heart governs blood and vessels,
- The liver governs tendons,
- The kidney governs bones,
- The spleen governs muscles and four limbs.

All of the five *zang* organs have relationships with the four limbs, especially the spleen. According to the relationship of the four limbs and channels and collaterals: the three yin and three yang channels of the hands circulate in the upper limbs, and the three yin and three yang channels of the feet flow in the lower limbs. Therefore, inspection of the four limbs may help one understand the pathological changes of the channels and *zang-fu* organs.

1. Form

(1) *Muscle dystrophy:* flaccidity, hemi-paralysis due to wind-stroke, etc. Muscle weakness mostly caused by deficiency of qi and blood or blockage of the channels and collaterals, when the four limbs are deprived of nourishment.

(2) *Four limbs oedema:* oedematous disease.

(3) *Knees swelling*

A. Knees are red, swollen, and painful with inhibited bending and stretching: heat *bì*, wind-damp transforming into heat.

B. Knees are swollen and tibias are emaciated, just like the knees of the crane (a type of bird): crane's-knee wind caused by persistent cold-damp, deficiency of qi and blood.

C. Knees are dark purple, with diffuse swelling, and are painful: external injury, damage of the knee-caps or joints.

(4) *Exposure of blue vessels on the legs:* internal invasion of cold-dampness, blood stasis in the channels.

(5) *Malformation of the lower limbs*

Knees: genu varum ('O') or bow legs; genu valgum ('X') or knock knees; feet: pes varus or deviation outward; pes valgus or deviation inward: insufficiency of earlier congenital constitution, deficiency of kidney qi or acquired constitutional deprivation of nourishment, dysplasia (abnormal development of tissue due to any number of many possible causes).

(6) Deformity of the fingers

A. Shuttle shape of the finger joints, activities are limited: accumulation of wind-dampness, contracture of the tendons and channels.

B. Clubbing of the fingers: qi deficiency of the heart and lung, blood stasis and obstruction by dampness.

2. Movements

(1) *Limbs paralysis:* flaccidity disease, wind stroke, paraplegia, etc.

(2) *Convulsive spasms of the four limbs:* internal stirring of liver wind, spasms of the sinews and vessels.

(3) *Contracture of the hands and feet:* stagnation of the cold-pathogen, or qi and blood deficiency unable to nourish tendons and channels.

(4) *Trembling of the hands and feet:* blood deficiency unable to nourish tendons and channels, or excessive intake of alcohol, or forewarning of stirring wind.

(5) *Wriggling of the hands and feet:* qi deficiency of the spleen and stomach, unnourished tendons and channels, or yin deficiency generating wind.

(6) *Restlessness of the hands and feet:* exuberance of internal heat, heat harassing the heart spirit.

(7) *Touching the bedclothes, feeling and smoothing the bed, groping in the air and pulling invisible strings:* the manifestation of the loss of vitality, a sign of critical illness.

Inspection of the Anterior and Posterior Yin (Genitals and Anus)

The anterior yin is the yin organ or the genitals and the posterior yin is the anus. Inspection of the anterior yin in males includes observation of the penis, scrotum and testes for disorders such as indurations, swelling, ulcers and any abnormality in form and colour. Inspection in females should be of the external genitalia. Any intimate examination should have a definite indication and the examination should be carried out with suitable respect, an additional professional person should always be present to safeguard both the patient and the practitioner.

1. Anterior yin

(1) *Swelling of the scrotum or vagina (swelling of the vulva)*

A.
- a. Swelling of the scrotum which is transparent is called water *shàn* (hydrocele);
- b. Swelling of the scrotum, which is not transparent and is hard is due to the small intestine falling into the scrotum; it is called fox *shàn* (severe inguinal hernia): Hernias are usually caused by stagnation of the liver qi, exertion of standing for a long time, or invasion of cold-damp.

B. Superficial swelling of anterior yin: oedema.

C. Redness, swelling and pain of the scrotum or vagina: damp-heat pouring down via the liver channel.

(2) *Contraction of the anterior yin:* retracted genitals, cold congealing in the liver channel, spasms and contraction.

(3) *Eczema on the anterior yin:* eczema on the scrotum or labia vulvae, pruritus and

burning pain, moist or effusing fluid: scrotal wind, pudendal eczema, caused by damp-heat pouring down via the liver channel, external attacking of a wind pathogen.

(4) *Sores on the anterior yin*

A. Sores on the anterior yin or stiff and with diabrosis (ulcerative perforation), rotten smell, effusing ichor (acrid, watery discharge) or blood: pudendal sores, mostly caused by damp-heat pouring down via the liver channel or syphilis.

B. Sores on the anterior yin, which is stiff and looks like a cauliflower, bad smell: Cancer, difficult to cure.

(5) *Protrusion of the female yin, just like a pear:* vaginal protrusion, spleen deficiency and sinking of the middle jiao qi, or resuming work immediately after delivery.

(6) *Abnormal testis: small testis or tender testicles in small boys:* dysplasia (abnormal development of tissue) or sequellae of mumps.

2. Posterior yin

(1) *Anal abscess:* redness, swelling, pain, diabrosis (perforated ulcer) and effusing ichor (acrid, watery discharge) around the anus. This is caused by damp-heat pouring down, or an external pathogen blocked around the anus.

(2) *Haemorrhoids:* soft lumps inside or out of the anus, mostly caused by damp-heat accumulated and obstructed in the intestines, blood heat or blood stagnating around the anus.

(3) *Anal fissure:* elongated and lacerated ulcer on the mucous membrane of the anal canal accompanied by small ulcers. This is painful, with bleeding on defaecation and may be caused by heat in the blood and dry intestines, dry stool, with injury during difficult defaecation.

(4) *Anal fistula:* an abnormal, narrow, tunnel-like passageway that connects the remains of an old anal abscess to the surface of the skin. The reasons are the same as those for anal abscesses and haemorrhoids.

(5) *Proctoptosis:* prolapse of the rectum or the mucus membrane of the rectum from the anus, commonly due to deficiency and sinking of middle *jiao* qi.

Inspection of the Skin

Skin is distributed over the surface of the body, and connected to the lung. Skin is the defending barrier of the body and nourished by the qi and blood of the *zang-fu* organs through the channels. Therefore, the invasion of external pathogens or disorders of the viscera can be reflected by the skin. Thus, observation of the changes of the colour, lustre and form of the skin has an important significance in diagnosis.

1. Abnormal colour of the skin

Normal skin is moist and lustre, it is the manifestation of sufficient essential qi and body fluid.

(1) *Red skin*

If the skin suddenly turns red as if covered in cinnabar (vermilion in colour), this is called erysipelas. Red wandering toxin developing all over the body, firstly like a red cloud, then usually transmigrating or floating over the body along with swelling and pain, is mostly caused by hyperactivity of heart fire, attack of wind-heat, or carbuncles of children. If it develops from the leg, it is called 'leg erysipelas'; if from the head, it is called 'head erysipelas'. Redness and swelling of the lower limbs is usually caused by internal accumulation of the kidney fire, or damp-heat pouring down.

(2) *Yellow skin*

Yellow colouration on the skin, face, eyes and nails, indicates jaundice. Jaundice can be divided into yang jaundice and yin jaundice.

A. In yang jaundice, the yellow colour is fresh and bright like an orange and it accompanies dark yellow sweat and urine, with thirst and the skin has a yellowish greasy coating. It is usually caused by damp-heat in the liver and gallbladder, or in damp-heat spleen and stomach pathologies.

B. In yin jaundice, the yellow colour is dusky like ashes and it accompanies chills, tastelessness in the mouth and a white greasy coating. It is usually caused by cold-damp of the spleen and stomach.

(3) *Purple-black skin*

The skin is yellow with a dusky blackness; it is called black jaundice or jaundice due to sexual intemperance, it is mostly caused by overexertion damaging the kidney.

(4) *Vitiligo*

White spots appear on the skin of the limbs, face, etc. They are large or small with a clear boundary and have a chronic course of development. It is called white patch wind and caused by invasion of wind-damp, qi and blood disharmony, and blood not nourishing the skin.

2. Abnormal form of the skin

(1) *Dry skin*

The skin is dry and lustreless, even chapping and scaling. This is due to damage of yin fluids or deficiency of *ying* blood not nourishing the skin.

(2) *Dry, scaly skin*

The skin is dry and rough just like the scales of a fish; it is commonly due to blood stasis not nourishing the skin.

(3) *Sclerotic skin*

The skin is rough, thick, and sclerotic, with swelling, loss of elasticity, inability to move easily and loss of activity. It may be caused by exterior pathogens, or deficiency of yang and blood with lack of nourishment of the skin, which is caused by the emotions, inappropriate eating, blood stasis, etc.

3. Inspection of maculopapular eruptions or rashes

Maculopapular eruptions are the skin signs of systemic diseases. A macule and a papule are different.

Maculae refer to crimson or blue-green purple patches spreading underneath the skin, which cannot be felt by the hand; when one rubs them, they are stable (will not become paler) even after pressing. Maculae can be divided into yang maculae and yin maculae.

Papulae are red, and their shape is small like a pine-kernel and they are slightly raised on the skin, which can be felt by the hand when stroked, and they will fade when pressed. Papulae can be divided into measles, wind papulae and concealed papulae. At the same time as using the appearance of rashes to assist in diagnosis it is important to pay attention to the favourable or unfavourable indications of maculae and papulae.

(1) *Maculae*

A. Yang maculae:

The yang maculae are reddish or purplish, like silk in texture or clouds across the skin. They are accompanied by fever, dysphoria (ill at ease, restlessness, fidgety behaviour), fast pulse and manifestations of an excessive heat pattern. They are caused by invasion of an external warm-heat pathogen, with exuberant heat driving into the *ying* (nutritive) and blood levels e.g. meningitis.

B. Yin maculae:

The yin maculae are blue-green purple in colour, developing without a determined location and are accompanied by a white complexion, cold limbs, deficient pulse, cold feelings, etc. They are due to spleen deficiency failing to govern blood or yang failure causing cold to accumulate in the qi and blood.

(2) *Papulae*

A. Measles:

The measles papulae are pink in colour and have the appearance and size of hemp seeds, appearing first over the hairline and face, gradually extending to the trunk and four limbs and disappearing after full eruption. Firstly there is a cough; sneezing; snivelling; tearing of the eyes; cold ears, and red threads appearing behind the ears. After three or four days papule dots appear. This is a common contagious disease in children; mostly due to the exterior wind-heat pathogen.

B. Wind papulae:

The wind papulae are a light red colour, small in size, with a sparse distribution; there is itchy skin and mild symptoms, with slight fever or no fever. It is caused by seasonal wind-heat pathogen.

C. Concealed papulae:

These are a light red or white colour, they range in size from hemp seeds to sesame seeds but feel more like blossom petals, protruding suddenly on the skin, with clear borders, sometimes concealed and sometimes visible; itching occurs and patches appear after being scratched. This is often caused by a wind pathogen striking or hypersensitiveness.

(3) *Favourable or unfavourable indications of the maculae and papulae*

A. Maculopapular eruptions:

a. Mild and favourable pattern:

There is fever; red rashes appear firstly on the chest and abdomen gradually extending to the four limbs. Spirit-orientation is clear and fresh after abatement of fever. This indicates the positive likelihood of the pathogens being dispelled.

b. Severe and unfavourable pattern:

There are thick, deep red or purplish black rashes, appearing firstly on the four limbs and extending to the chest and abdomen with incessant high fever and even coma. This is caused by pathogens prevailing over *zheng* (healthy) qi and internal sinking of pathogenic qi.

c. Dangerous pattern:

The maculopapular eruptions are black, dark, and withered rashes.

B. Measles:
  a. Favourable pattern:
    There is fever, slight sweat, and exhaustion, red and lustrous rashes, which disappear after abatement of fever.
  b. Unfavourable pattern:
    There is high fever, no sweat, spots unable to erupt, light or dark red or red-purple colour. This is caused by external blockage of wind-cold, internal excess of heat pathogen, deficiency and sinking of the *zheng* qi.
  c. Dangerous pattern:
    When the rash suddenly disappears and there is coma with panting, this is internal sinking of measles toxin.

4. Inspection of skin blisters

Vesicles appear clustered together or scattered over the skin. They can be differentiated as Miliaria Alba, Chickenpox, Pyretic Sores, Eczema, etc.

A. Miliaria alba:
There are small white blisters as small as grains of sand, transparent, protruding on the skin, containing a small amount of watery fluid, often seen on the chest, abdomen or neck and occasionally on the four limbs, not seen on the face. Accompanied by hidden fever. This is due to the internal retention of damp-heat and incomplete perspiration.

B. Chickenpox:
There are pink eruptions on the skin of the infant which soon changes to oval shape blisters or pustules, the tip of the pox is pointed and has no central depression, the root is round and red, a bright, thin shell which is easy to break open, spots are unequal in size, accompanied by slight aversion to cold with fever. This is caused by internal retention of damp-heat and belongs to the common contagious diseases in paediatrics.

C. Pyretic sores:
Around the corner of the mouth, border of the lips and sides of the nose there are clusters of small blisters like millet, they feel scorched and painful. These are often seen as equivalent to cold sores or herpes. These are due to external invasion of wind-heat or accumulation of heat in the lung and stomach.

D. Eczema:
Red spots all over the body frequently changing to papulae and blisters, which have an effusion after rupture and become moist sores dissipated over the surface. This is caused by accumulation and stagnation of damp-heat with wind-pathogen depressing damp in the muscles and skin.

5. Inspection of sores and ulcers

The most common sores and ulcers that can be seen in the skin, muscle, tendon and bone include carbuncles, cellulitis, boils, furuncles, etc.

A. Carbuncles:
The skin has local redness and swelling, which feels hot and painful with tenderness at the root of the eruptions; this belongs to a yang pattern. The characteristic of carbuncles is that the skin is susceptible to ulceration and then healing in different areas, thick pus appears after opening of the sores and it is easily healed. It is mostly caused by

accumulation of damp-heat, stagnation and stasis of qi and blood.

B. Cellulitis:

Inflammation of the soft or connective tissue of the skin in which a thin, watery exudate spreads through the cleavage planes of interstitial tissue spaces; it may lead to ulceration and abscesses, it belongs to a yin pattern. The character is one of difficulty in dispersing with ulcerating and healing alternately, with thin liquid pus; it is difficult to heal. It is caused by deficiency of the qi and blood, accumulation and stagnation of yin-cold.

C. Boils:

The local skin is red, hot and painful, slightly raised on the skin, like a bean, nut kernel or olive pip in size, possibly with a purulent head. Boils are mostly seen on the face, hands and feet; they are full of pathogenic toxin and on the whole easily dispersed. Boils are due to external invasion of a wind pathogen and fire toxin with accumulation of pathogen.

D. Furuncles:

The part of skin affected is small, often a single hair follicle. The furuncle is round in size, red and swollen, has mild heat and pain; healing occurs after ulceration and release of pus. Furuncles belong to the category of minor symptoms and are due to external invasion of a heat-pathogen or accumulation of damp-heat.

SECTION 3
INSPECTION OF EXCRETA

The excreta include secretion, discharge and pathological output. In observation of excreta one should pay attention to the colour, quality, volume and other associated pathological products of the excreta.

Usually whitish, clear and thin excreta indicate deficiency or cold patterns; and yellowish and thick excreta indicate excess or heat patterns.

1. Inspection of phlegm, drool, nasal discharge and saliva

(1) Inspection of phlegm or sputum

Phlegm or sputum is a kind of sticky fluid, excreted from the lung and trachea. Thick and turbid matter is phlegm (*tán*), thin and clear matter is rheum (*yǐn*) and both can often be seen. Phlegm and rheum are produced by disturbance of the fluid metabolism. Fluid metabolism is closely related to the lung, spleen and kidneys, so it is easy to realise why it is said 'the spleen is the source of phlegm; the lung is the container of phlegm and the kidney is the root of phlegm'. Thus, inspection of the phlegm may help one understand the pathological changes of the lung, spleen, and kidneys and distinguish the characteristics of disease.

Abnormal manifestations and clinical significance of phlegm:

A. Cold phlegm: whitish, clear and thin.
B. Heat phlegm: yellowish, sticky and coagulated.
C. Dry phlegm: scanty, sticky and difficult to expectorate.
D. Damp phlegm: whitish, slippery and easily expectorated.
E. Lung abscess: coughing, spitting up phlegm with a fishy smell or with pus or blood.

F. Haemoptysis: phlegm mingled with fresh blood, mostly belongs to lung heat.

(2) Inspection of drool

Drool is related to the spleen. It is excreted in the mouth and helps to moisten the oral cavity, lubricate and digest chewed food; therefore, inspection of the drool can help one examine the pathological changes of the spleen and stomach.

Abnormal manifestations and clinical significance of drool:

A. Clear and abundant drool: deficiency cold of the spleen and stomach.

B. Sticky drool: damp-heat of the spleen and stomach.

C. Salivation from the corners of the mouth and infant's slobbering: deficiency of the spleen, stomach heat and worm accumulation.

D. Salivation in sleeping: stomach heat or food retention, phlegm-heat brewing internally.

(3) Inspection of nasal discharge

Nasal discharge refers to sticky fluid discharged from the nose. Nasal discharge relates to the lung; thus, inspection of nasal discharge is helpful for understanding the pathological changes of the lung.

Abnormal manifestations and clinical significance of nasal discharge:

A. Stuffy nose with clear nasal discharge of recent onset: externally-contracted wind-cold.

B. Stuffy nose with turbid nasal discharge of recent onset: externally-contracted wind-heat.

C. Paroxysmal (convulsive) and continual sneezing with lots of nasal discharge: allergic rhinitis, wind-cold harassing the lung.

D. Persistent discharge of turbid yellowish pus-like nasal discharges with foul smell: sinusitis, damp-heat accumulating and blocking the lung.

(4) Inspection of saliva

Saliva refers to sticky and foamy fluid discharged from the mouth. Saliva is related to the kidney but also related to the stomach; thus, inspection of saliva is helpful for understanding the pathological changes of the kidney and stomach.

Abnormal manifestations and clinical significance of saliva:

A. Abundant saliva escaping from the mouth: cold or accumulated cold, damp-heat or accumulated food in the stomach.

B. Abundant saliva in the mouth: kidney cold or kidney deficiency.

2. Inspection of vomit

Vomiting is caused by counter flow rising of stomach qi. Inspection of vomit is helpful for understanding the pathological changes of the stomach and the nature of the disease.

Abnormal manifestations and clinical significance of vomit:

A. Thin, clear and without foul smell, or water-like vomit: cold vomit.

B. Turbid vomit with sour odour: heat vomit.

C. Vomiting of fresh or purplish blood with clots or food dregs: liver fire invading the stomach, accumulation of heat in the stomach, blood stasis in the stomach.

D. Vomiting of undigested or sour food: food damage/retention.

E. Vomiting of yellowish or green fluid with a bitter taste: accumulated heat or damp-heat in the liver and gallbladder.

3. Inspection of the stool

Stool formation is closely related to the functional conditions of the spleen, stomach and intestines. Stool formation is also influenced directly by purification and descent of the lung, free flow of the liver and the warmth of the *mingmen* fire. So, inspection of the stool may help one examine the pathological changes of the spleen, stomach and intestines and the functional conditions of the lung, liver and kidneys. It also can be useful for distinguishing the nature of the disease.

The normal stool is yellowish and soft with the form of a cylinder or log.

Abnormal manifestations and clinical significance of stool:

A. Clear, water-like stool: cold-damp diarrhoea.

B. Yellowish or brown colour, caustic and fetid stool: damp-heat diarrhoea.

C. Clear, thin, undigested food in the stool or viscous, long and thin like duck stool: diarrhoea due to deficiency of the spleen or kidney.

D. Sticky jelly-like and with pus containing blood inside the stool: dysentery.

E. Fresh blood over the surface of the stool or drops before or after defaecation: distal bleeding, intestinal wind, anal fissures or haemorrhoids.

F. Dark red or purplish black blood, mixed uniformly with the stool: proximal bleeding, excessive heat of the stomach or intestines, which forces the blood to move frenetically or the spleen failing to control blood.

G. Grey and white colour, alternating loose and dry stool: jaundice, liver invading the spleen.

H. Dry and hard to be passed stool: constipation, intestinal dryness and liquid depletion.

4. Inspection of the urine

Urine formation is directly related to the metabolism of the fluid in the body. The metabolism of the fluid is influenced by the functional conditions of the *zang-fu* organs, such as excess or deficiency of yin and yang, qi transformation of the kidneys and bladder, descending function of the lung, transportation and transformation of the spleen and regulation of waterways via the *sanjiao* (triple burner). Hence, inspection of the urine may help one understand not only the pathological changes of the lung, spleen, kidneys and bladder but also aspects of fluid depletion, cold, heat, deficienct and excess nature of diseases.

Normal urine appears clear, slightly yellow in colour and without sediment.

Abnormal manifestations and clinical significance of urine:

A. Copious, clear urine: a deficiency-cold pattern.

B. Scanty, red urine: an excess-heat pattern.

C. Urine mixed with bleeding: haematuria from heart fire, blood *lín* (slow painful urination passed drop by drop), deficiency-consumption of the kidney, tumour in the lower *jiao*, etc.

D. Urine mixed with sediment: stone *lín*: damp-heat burning and condensing impurities in the urine.

E. Turbid urine like rice water or cream: cloudy *lín*: deficiency of the spleen and kidney associated with damp-heat.

Section 4
Inspection of the Superficial Vein of the Index Finger

The superficial vein refers to the medial veins of the infant's index finger. This inspection means to examine the shape and colour of the veins along the palmar margin to detect pathological changes. This method is applicable for the diagnosis of infants under the age of the three. Both index finger veins of the infants and adult *cùn kǒu* pulse belong to the lung channel of the hand *taiyin*. Alterations in the shape or colour of the index finger veins can reflect the changes of the *cùn kǒu* pulse; therefore, inspection of the index finger veins can diagnose the pathological changes in the body, which is similar to inspection of the *cùn kǒu* pulse.

1. Inspecting method
   (1) Three passes
   From the palm to the tip of the finger, the first joint is the wind pass (*fēng guān*), the second is the qi pass (*qì guān*) and the last joint is the life pass (*mìng guān*) (Fig. 2-6).

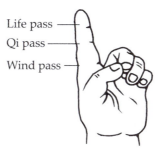

Fig. 2-6 Three passes of the superficial vein on the infant's index finger

(2) Method
The infant must be carried to a place with full light; the practitioner should hold the wrist of the infant with the left hand, and then push lightly on the medial veins of the infant's index finger, several times with the right hand. The pushing should be directed from the tip of the finger (life pass) to the palm (wind pass). The pushing force should be mild and make the vein clearer for observation.

2. Clinical significance
   (1) Significance
   It is helpful for examining the excess or decline of the qi and blood of the *zang-fu* organs, location and nature of the disease and predicting the prognosis.
   (2) Characteristics of the normal index finger vein in infants
   The colour is light red with a yellow tint and dimly revealed in the wind pass; it is not too obvious and not visible at all beyond the wind pass.

(3) Important points

Floating and deep distinguish exterior and interior, the colour of the veins differentiates cold and heat; and pale and dark stagnation determine deficiency and excess. The locality at the three passes indicates severity.

Abnormal manifestations and clinical significance of the superficial vein of the index finger:

A. Colour:
   a. Bright-red: exterior pattern.
   b. Purple-red: interior heat pattern.
   c. Blue-green: convulsions or pain pattern.
   d. Purple-black: obstruction of the blood vessels suggesting a severe case.
   e. Pale-white: deficiency of the spleen or qi and blood, infant's malnutrition with accumulation.

B. Length:
   a. The veins are only visible at the wind pass: pathogenic qi invading the collaterals; mild disease.
   b. Visibility extends to the qi pass: pathogenic qi invading the channels; serious disease.
   c. Visibility extends to the life pass: pathogenic qi invading the *zang-fu* organs; very serious disease.
   d. Visibility extending through all passes toward the nail: A very dangerous and critical sign.

C. Floating and deep:
   a. Floating and visible: exterior pattern.
   b. Deep and indistinct: interior pattern.

D. Paleness and stagnation:
   a. Light colour and no lustre: deficiency pattern.
   b. Deep and dull colour: excess pattern.

E. Thick and thin:
   a. Thick and obvious branch: excess pattern, heat pattern.
   b. Thin and invisible branch: deficiency pattern, cold pattern.

CHAPTER 3
Tongue Examination

Tongue examination is considered today to be an important part of the inspection examination. Holroyde-Downing (2005)[1] outlines the development of tongue diagnosis, from a method to distinguish specific conditions, to how it came to be considered more primary in diagnosis, through epidemic plagues, new methodologies and consistencies with biomedical understanding. This chapter discusses the principles, methods and interpretations of the tongue examination. A practitioner needs to grasp four important perspectives during the study of tongue diagnosis. Firstly, during inspection of the tongue in clinic a practitioner must be able to distinguish between the normal tongue manifestation and pathological tongue manifestation. Also, there are particular changes of the tongue image in severe stages of disease, which should be noticed immediately. Secondly, if the tongue coating quality is not in agreement with the state of the illness, or the tongue coating suddenly changes, the practitioner should inquire about the patient's drinking, eating and living habits; it is essential to differentiate effects caused by specific actions to avoid misdiagnosis, e.g. sucking red sweets can give the tongue a red colour etc. Thirdly, pay attention to the relationship of the tongue body and tongue coating with reference to the changes of each other. Lastly, although tongue diagnosis can be very useful it must always be taken in relation to other diagnostic findings before conclusions are reached.

Contents of the Tongue Examination
- Overview of the tongue examination
    - Principles of the tongue examination
    - Relationship between the tongue manifestation and *zang-fu* organs
    - Normal tongue manifestation
- Inspection of the tongue body
    - Tongue spirit
    - Tongue colour
    - Tongue shape
    - Tongue motility
    - Sublingual veins
- Inspection of the tongue coating
    - Coating texture
    - Coating colour
- General analysis of the tongue body and tongue coating
- Clinical significance of the tongue examination
    - Judging exuberance or failure of the *zheng* qi and pathogen.
    - Distinguishing the nature of the pathogenic factor
    - Analysing the location and tendency of the pattern
    - Estimating the prognosis of the pattern

---

1 Holroyde-Downing, N., (2005) IASTAM. 1 (2):400 www.brill.com

Section 1
Overview of the Tongue Examination

Tongue examination, also called inspection of the tongue, is a diagnostic method carried out through observing the tongue manifestation; tongue manifestation refers to the outer signs of the tongue body and tongue coating. The tongue body is composed of muscle and vessels, which are nourished by the qi and blood of the *zang-fu*. The tongue coating refers to the lichen-like material formed on the surface of the tongue. Chinese medicine believes that tongue coating is created from the rising and evaporation of the stomach qi.

Principles of the Tongue Examination

1. The relationship between the structure of the tongue and tongue manifestation

The tongue is a muscular organ consisting of voluntary muscles. The muscles in the body of the tongue work in all three axes i.e. front to back; side-to-side and top to bottom. In addition, other muscles attach the tongue. This complex muscular structure is what gives the tongue its flexibility and the agility needed for eating and speaking. Plenty of blood vessels and ample blood supply among the muscle bundles give the tongue its light red colour and its brightness. Cast-off cells, food debris, bacteria and mucus fill the gaps and form white moss, which is called the tongue coating.

The top side of the tongue is called the lingual surface or dorsum and the underneath is called the undersurface. The lingual surface of the tongue is covered with a layer of semi-transparent mucous membrane and many papillae. According to their different shapes, these papillae are divided into filiform papillae, fungiform papillae, circumvallate papillae and foliate papillae. Filiform papillae and fungiform papillae are closely related to the form of tongue manifestation, circumvallate papillae and foliate papillae are related to the taste sense.

Filiform papillae are conical milky white, soft projections, their height is about 0.5~2.5 mm and they look like fine threads or when magnified like small tree stumps. Fungiform papillae are few in number. Fungiform papillae are mostly seen on the tip of the tongue and scattered between the filiform papillae; they appear mushroom shaped.

2. The relationships between the forming of the tongue manifestation and the *zang-fu* organs, channels and collaterals

(1) *The five zang organs and six fu organs are related to the tongue through the channels and collaterals*

Heart —— The tongue is the sprout of the heart, the collateral of the heart channel of the hand *shaoyin* flows to the root of the tongue.

Spleen —— The tongue is the external sign of the spleen, and the spleen channel of the foot *taiyin* connects with the root of the tongue and scatters across the undersurface.

Liver —— The liver channel of the foot *jueyin* has a network of vessels in the tongue root.

Kidney —— The kidney channel of the foot *shaoyin* anchors the tongue root.

Other *zang-fu* organs are also related directly or indirectly to the tongue via channels and collaterals. Through inspection of the tongue, the practitioner can understand both the condition of health as well as exuberance and debilitation of the *zang-fu* organs or channels and collaterals.

(2) The relationships between the tongue and heart, spleen and stomach

Amongst the five *zang* organs and six *fu* organs, the relationships between the tongue and the heart, spleen, and stomach are the most intimate. As previously stated, the tongue is the sprout (sometimes called the mirror) of the heart, the external sign of the spleen, and the tongue coating is created from the rising and evaporation of the stomach qi.

In addition, there are plenty of vessels in the tongue and this has a relationship with the heart governing the blood and vessels. Active moving of the tongue can adjust the voice and produces speech and this is related to the heart governing the mind. Consequently, the tongue manifestation can reflect the functional status of the heart. Furthermore, the heart is the great governor of the five *zang* and six *fu*. Accordingly, the functional status of the heart can reflect the functional status of all the *zang-fu*, qi and blood. Therefore, diseases of the *zang-fu* organs or qi and blood can be reflected on the tongue through the heart functions.

The taste sense of the tongue can influence the appetite, as it is related to the spleen governing transportation and transformation, and with the stomach governing reception. The spleen and stomach are the foundation of acquired constitution and the source of qi and blood production; thus, tongue manifestation also reflects exuberance and debilitation of the qi, blood and fluids all over the body.

(3) The relationships between the tongue manifestation and qi, blood and fluids

The shape, texture and colour of the tongue are concerned with exuberance, debilitation and movement of the qi and blood. A moist or dry tongue body and tongue coating are related to the amount or loss of fluids. Body fluids and their generation, transfusion and distribution are closely related to the *zang-fu* organs, such as the kidneys, spleen and stomach, e.g. saliva is the fluid of the kidneys, drool is the fluid of the spleen, they are all types of body fluids. For this reason, inspections of the colour, shape, motility, moistness or dryness of the tongue body and tongue coating are helpful for judging the exuberance or debilitation of qi, blood and body fluids.

(4) The individual reflections of the zang-fu organs on the tongue

The tongue manifestation reflects whole body pathological changes, and there are also symbolic regions on the surface of the tongue, which reflect particular *zang-fu* organs.
- The tip of the tongue reflects the pathological changes of the heart and lung.
- The centre of the tongue reflects the pathological changes of the spleen and stomach.
- The margins of the tongue reflect the pathological changes of the liver and gallbladder.
- The root of the tongue reflects the pathological changes of the kidneys.

Another division: the tip of the tongue can be ascribed to the upper-third portion of the stomach cavity, whilst the centre of the tongue can be ascribed to the middle-third portion of the stomach cavity, and the root of the tongue can be ascribed to the lower-third portion of the stomach cavity.

Method of the Tongue Examination

1. Posture/Position

The patient should be sitting or lying back in a comfortable position, facing the natural light, asked to open the mouth as far as possible, extend the tongue naturally and let it be exposed thoroughly. The tongue body should now be relaxed, unfolded and sufficiently exposed; the tip of the tongue should point downwards.

Note: Excessive tension, curling of the tongue body, only the tip exposed, or extending it out for a long-time, can all affect the validity of the tongue manifestation. The inspection should be rapid, if the practitioner fails to make an assessment, they can repeat the inspection after the patient has rested.

2. Body position
The practitioner should be facing the patient looking straight at them and observe the tongue from above.

3. Sequence
First, examine the colour and lustre, spots, thickness or thinness, roughness or tenderness and dynamic state of the tongue body. Second, observe the condition of the tongue coating, such as thickness, curd-like or greasy, colour, moistness or dryness. Third observe from the perspective of the location of the tongue coating, this is whether it can be seen from the tip of the tongue to the centre, on the margins of the tongue, or on the root of the tongue.

4. Scraping the tongue
By using the border of a disposable tongue depressor with moderate strength, the practitioner should scrape from the root to the tip of the tongue, three to five times. If the tongue coating cannot be scraped, or a dirty coat remains after scraping, this is due to an interior excessive pathogen. If the tongue coating can be scraped easily this indicates that a deficiency pattern is present.

5. Wiping the tongue
By winding sterile absorbent gauze around the forefinger and dipping it in mild sodium chloride, the practitioner should wipe the tongue surface several times.

Scraping the tongue and wiping the tongue can both be used to distinguish if the tongue coating has a root or is rootless, or if it is a stained coating that is being observed.

Summary of the Important Parts of the Tongue Examination

1. Light
It is essential to have sufficient and soft natural light.

2. Stained coating
Drinking and eating often changes the shape and colour of the tongue coating. For example, some foods or medicines can colour the tongue coating; this is called a stained coating. Thus, when inspecting the abnormal colour of the tongue coating, the practitioner should remember to ask the patient about recent eating habits, prior to their visit.

3. Oral cavity
Injured, damaged or infected teeth can make the tongue coating on that side increase

in thickness. Mounting an artificial tooth can make an indentation on the margin of the tongue body. Open mouth breathing can dry and thicken the tongue coating. All of these factors can produce an abnormal tongue manifestation. However, they are not pathological changes of the body, and should be paid attention to and correctly identified.

SECTION 2
NORMAL TONGUE MANIFESTATION AND PHYSIOLOGICAL DIFFERENCES

Normal Tongue Manifestation

The normal tongue manifestation refers to the signs of the tongue body and tongue coating among healthy people.

The characteristics of the normal tongue manifestation: The tongue body is distinguished by being light-red, bright, with moisture and lustre, a suitable size and having softness and flexibility; the tongue coating should be uniform, thin, white, neither dry nor greasy or slippery. The normal tongue manifestation is usually described as "light-reddish tongue with a thin white coating".

The normal tongue manifestation suggests normal functions of the *zang-fu* organs, sufficient qi, blood and body fluids, as well as exuberance of stomach qi.

Physiological Differences of the Tongue Manifestation

The normal tongue manifestation can be influenced by different ages, body constitutions, climates, etc.

1. Seasons and times

The normal tongue manifestation often changes along with the different seasons and times. For example, the tongue coating is mostly thick and/or light yellow, with summer dampness in summer; it is dry and thin in autumn; in winter the tongue is usually moist. The tongue coating tends to be thicker when we wake up, and becomes thinner after eating. The colour of the tongue is more dark and stagnated when getting up in the morning and turns redder after moving about.

2. Ages and body constitutions

The tongue manifestation can change along with the different ages and body constitutions. For example, the tongue body of an elderly person may appear as cracked and the papillae atrophied, which is due to deficiency of qi and blood. The tongue manifestation of the child is light, tender without or with less tongue coating. The tongue manifestation of an overweight person is mostly large and light; on the other hand, the tongue manifestation of an underweight person is thin and reddish.

Section 3
Contents of the Tongue Examination

The tongue examination includes two parts: inspecting the tongue body and inspecting the tongue coating.

Inspecting the tongue body can be divided into four parts: spirit, colour, shape and motility. It is helpful for understanding the deficiency or excess of the *zang-fu* organs, exuberance or debilitation of the qi and blood.

Inspecting the tongue coating is separated into coating texture and coating colour. It is used to analyse the deep or superficial location of the pathogenic qi, exuberance and debilitation of pathogenic qi or *zheng* qi.

Inspection of the Tongue Body

1. Tongue spirit

A. Spirited:

The tongue body is light-red, bright, with moisture, lustre and flexibility. It is called a lustrous tongue and indicates sufficient body fluids, qi and blood, and a vigourous spirit. Even if there is disease it is minor and there is little damage to the *zheng* (healthy) qi and belongs to a favourable manifestation.

B. Spiritless:

The tongue body is dark, dry, inflexible, and short of blood colour. It is called a withered tongue and indicates deficiency of the body fluids, qi and blood, with deterioration of the spirit; it belongs to dangerous illness and is an unfavourable manifestation.

2. Tongue colour

Tongue colour is divided into light red; pale; red; crimson; and blue and purple.

A. Light red:

Light red, moist and lustre of the tongue body indicate harmony of qi and blood of a healthy person or the early onset of exogenous disease. The pathologic condition is mild; no injury has yet occurred to the qi, blood and *zang-fu* organs.

B. Pale:

If the tongue colour is lighter than normal it is called a pale tongue.

   a. If the tongue is white, dry, and has nearly no blood colour; the colour is called dry white tongue. It is due to deficiency of qi, blood and yang. Moreover, dry white tongue corresponds to qi and blood desertion.
   b. If the tongue colour is pale and the tongue body is thin; this indicates deficiency of qi and blood.
   c. If the tongue colour is pale with moisture, the tongue body being fat, tender and with teeth impressions on the sides of the tongue; this indicates yang deficiency and water retention.

C. Red:

Tongue colour redder than normal, even bright red corresponds to a heat pattern and

can be divided into deficiency and excess.
- a. Redness of the whole tongue or only red on the margins and tip of the tongue is invasion of wind-heat and belongs to exterior patterns.
- b. Bright redness of the tongue indicates an excess heat pattern.
- c. The tip of the tongue is red; this is caused by heart fire flaming upward.
- d. The margins of the tongue are red; this is due to excessive heat in the liver channel.
- e. The tongue body is thin and small, reddish, without or with less coating; this corresponds to a deficient heat pattern.

D. Crimson:

The tongue colour is darker than red. It is caused by heat entering the *ying* and blood levels or yin deficiency resulting in vigourous fire. More redness implies more heat. A crimson tongue is hotter than a red tongue.
- a. Crimson with coating indicates a warm febrile disease, heat entering the *ying* and blood levels.
- b. Crimson without coating or with less coating indicates yin deficiency resulting in vigourous fire.

E. Blue-purple:

The whole tongue appears blue or purple and is called a blue and purple tongue. It includes light-purple tongue, purple-red tongue and crimson-purple tongue. It corresponds to inhibited movement of the qi and blood. The range of the blue-purple on the tongue body is related to the degree of the blood stasis in the body.
- a. When the tongue colour is light-purple or blue-purple with moisture, this is due to deficient yang and exuberant yin or stasis of blood and channels.
- b. When the tongue is red-purple, crimson-purple and lacks fluid, this is due to excessive heat damaging fluidss, stagnation of qi and blood.
- c. When there is a light-red tongue with a blue-purple colour, this indicates static blood in the body.
- d. A blue-purple tongue can be seen in congenital heart disease or toxicities from medicines or food.

If only parts of the tongue appear with blue-purple spots, of different sizes, under the surface of the tongue, this is called stasis maculae tongue or stasis spotted tongue. In externally contracted febrile disease, it corresponds to heat entering the *ying* and blood levels, stagnation and stasis of qi and blood, or the forerunner of macular eruption. In internal damage diseases, it is often the sign of blood stasis. Some individuals from ethnicities with darker skin often have blue-purple spots, which do not indicate any pathology and are normal.

3. Tongue shape

The tongue shape indicates the shape and condition of the tongue body. It includes characteristics such as toughness and tenderness, being enlarged or thin, having spots, cracks, teeth-marks, etc.

A. Tough and tender:

Whether a tongue is tough or tender is the crux of distinguishing a deficiency from an excess pattern.

a. Tough tongue: The tongue body is rough and coarse, hard and sturdy. The colour is dark. This corresponds to an excess pattern.
   b. Tender tongue: The tongue body is delicate, weak, slightly swollen and smooth. The colour is light. This corresponds to a deficiency pattern.
  B. Enlarged and thin:
   a. Enlarged tongue: The tongue body is enlarged, flabby and wide and fills the mouth. It is indicative of stagnation of water and dampness.
   If there is an enlarged tongue with light-white colour, it is due to qi and yang deficiency with retention of body fluids.
   If there is an enlarged tongue with red colour, it is due to damp-heat of the spleen and stomach or accumulation of phlegm-heat.
   b. Thin tongue: The tongue body is thin and small. It corresponds to deficiency of qi and blood or yin deficiency resulting in vigourous fire.
   If there is a thin tongue with light colour, it is due to deficiency of qi and blood.
   If there is a thin tongue with red or crimson colour, dry, without or with less coating, it is due to yin deficiency resulting in vigourous fire and damage of body fluids.
   c. Swollen tongue: The tongue body is swollen, fills the mouth, possibly even with difficulty in closing the mouth or retracting the tongue. It corresponds to stagnation of heat or poisoning.
   If the tongue is red-crimson with swelling and pain, it is due to excessive heat of the heart and spleen, heat toxin obstructing upward.
   If the tongue is crimson-purple with swelling, it is due to excessive drinking of alcohol and contracted warm disease, the heat pathogen combined with alcohol obstructing upward.
  C. Spotted:
   a. Spotted tongue: The fungiform papillae are enlarged, increased in number and engorged.
   b. Prickly tongue: The fungiform papillae are enlarged, protruded and forming a spike; it is thorny to the touch.

Spotted and prickly refer to the pathological characteristics of swollen or abnormal protrusion of the fungiform papillae. Spotted and prickly are often seen together, thus can be called a spotted tongue. It indicates excessive heat of the *zang-fu* organs or blood.

According to the colour of the spots and prickles, the conditions of qi, blood and pathological conditions can be judged. A red tongue with prickles is due to excessive heat of qi. A bright red spotted tongue corresponds to internal-exuberance of the blood heat or yin deficiency resulting in vigourous fire. Spots and prickles that are crimson-purple colour indicate heat entering the *ying* and blood levels and stagnation of qi and blood.

According to the position of the spots and prickles, it can be distinguished which *zang* organs the heat resides in. Spots and prickles on the tip of the tongue are due to heart fire hyperactivity. Prickles on the centre of the tongue indicate excessive heat of the stomach and intestines. Spots and prickles on the margins of the tongue indicate excessive fire of the liver and gallbladder.

  D. Cracked:
  There are several shapes of cracks or creases on the dorsum of the tongue. There is

usually no coating found with cracks or creases. Cracks and creases are mostly caused by excessive heat, which damages the yin or spleen deficiency leading to damp encumbrance, but they can also be seen in the healthy person.

    a. Light-white tongue with cracks is indicative of blood deficiency and failure to moisten.

    b. Red-crimson tongue with cracks is indicative of excessive heat damaging fluids or yin deficiency and dried fluid.

    c. Enlarged, tender, light-white tongue with cracks and teeth-marks on the margins is indicative of spleen deficiency leading to damp encumbrance.

    d. If inborn shallow cracks or creases, with coating on their surface, without discomfort, this is called a congenital cracked tongue; it does not belong to an illness manifestation.

E. Teeth-marked:

The margins of the tongue are imprinted with teeth marks and are often seen with an enlarged tongue. This corresponds to spleen deficiency or exuberance of dampness. It is also seen among some healthy people.

    a. A pale, enlarged and moist tongue with teeth marks may indicate cold-dampness congestion or yang deficiency and water retention.

    b. A light-red tongue with teeth marks on the margins may indicate spleen deficiency or qi deficiency.

    c. A red, swollen tongue with teeth marks may indicate stagnation of damp-heat or phlegm-turbidity.

    d. A light-red, tender tongue without being enlarged and with faint teeth marks can be seen in an inborn teeth-marked tongue. Even in illness, it is favourable.

4. Tongue motility

Tongue motility is the active condition of the tongue body. Pathological tongue motility includes abnormal changes such as flaccidity, stiffness, trembling, deviating, protruding, waggling and shortened, etc.

A. Flaccid:

A flaccid tongue is floppy, soft and without strength, unable to extend, curl or turn naturally. It is due to yin damage or deficiency of qi and blood.

    a. A flaccid tongue with a red or crimson colour, without or with less coating, indicates a heat pathogen damaging yin in the late stage of an exogenous heat disease or hyperactivity of fire due to yin deficiency in an interior damage disease.

    b. A flaccid tongue with pale colour and without lustre indicates deficiency of the qi and blood in a prolonged illness.

B. Stiff:

The tongue body becomes stiff and unable to move, extend or retract freely. It can mostly be seen in heat entering the pericardium or fever injuring fluid, or wind-phlegm obstructing the vessels.

    a. A stiff tongue with red-crimson colour, with less fluid indicates an intense heat pathogen.

    b. A stiff tongue with a thick and greasy coating indicates wind-phlegm blocking

the channels.
- c. Sudden onset of a stiff tongue and sluggish speech, accompanied by numbness of the limbs on one side and dizziness, is the forerunner of stroke.

C. Deviated:

When the tongue is extended, it deviates to one side 🌀. This is due to liver wind with phlegm or static blood blocking the channels. This is often a sign of serious underlying pathology.

D. Trembling:

When the tongue is extended, it often quivers without stopping. It is one of the manifestations of generating wind.
- a. A trembling tongue with pale colour indicates deficiency of blood generating wind.
- b. A trembling tongue with red colour and loss of coating indicates yin fluid deficiency generating wind.
- c. A trembling tongue with crimson-purple colour indicates excessive heat generating wind.
- d. A trembling tongue with red-crimson colour, dizziness, and numbness of the limbs indicates liver yang transforming into wind.

E. Protruding and waggling:

A protruding tongue and waggling tongue all correspond to heart and spleen heat.
- a. A protruding tongue: The tongue extends out of the mouth and is unable to be retracted immediately. Critically ill with a protruding tongue is mostly due to expiry of heart qi.
- b. Waggling tongue: The patient sticks out his tongue and licks his lips, and then quickly retracts it. A waggling tongue is mostly due to excessive heat transforming into wind or seen in children with congenital mental deficiency.

F. Shortened:
- a. The tongue becomes shortened and unable to extend beyond the teeth 🌀, this is a critical sign.

  If the shortened tongue is moist with light or blue-purple colour, this may indicate cold congealing in the muscles and vessels, or deficiency of the qi and blood.

  If the shortened tongue has a red-crimson colour and is dry, this is due to heat disease damaging the fluid.

  If the tongue is shortened and enlarged this is caused by wind-phlegm blocking the channels.
- b. Ankyloglossia (Tongue-Tied): This is a congenital anomaly in which the mucous membrane under the tongue is too short, limiting the mobility of the tongue. It has no significance in pattern differentiation.

5. Sublingual veins

Sublingual veins are the veins on the lateral sides of the lingual frenulum.

A. Method:

On curling the tip of the tongue up, either of the sublingual veins can be inspected. Inspection mainly involves assessing the changes of their length, colour, shape, etc.

B. Normal sublingual veins:

Normally the veins are appropriately raised and slender with a light-purple colour, they are not convoluted, do not have branches nor show static spots. The changes of the sublingual veins reflect the flowing conditions of the qi and blood.

C. Abnormal sublingual veins:
- If the sublingual veins are thin, short, and light-red, with obvious small vessels around them and the tongue colour is pale, this is mostly due to insufficiency of qi and blood.
- If the sublingual veins are thick, blue-purple, purple-red, crimson-purple, purple-black, with dark-red or purple net-like small vessels, or bead-like red-purple nodules, all these are signs of blood stasis.

Inspection of the Tongue Coating

Inspection of the tongue coating includes the observation of the texture and colour of the coating.

1. Coating texture

Coating texture means the quality and form of the tongue coating. Inspecting the coating texture includes observing whether it is thick or thin, moist or dry, greasy or curd-like, full or half covered, true or false, etc. By inspecting the coating texture, we can mainly understand the nature of the pathogen and pathogenesis of the disease.

A. Thick or thin:

The standard examination is whether it is possible to see the tongue body surface through the coating. Thick or thin mainly reflects the exuberance or debilitation of the pathogenic qi and *zheng* qi, and the deep or superficial location of the pathogenic qi.

    a. Thin coating: through the tongue coating, one can vaguely see the tongue body. It can be seen in healthy people or in an exterior pattern, or with a mild illness of an interior pattern.

    b. Thick coating: through the tongue coating, one cannot see the tongue body. It corresponds to an interior pattern, such as phlegm-damp, accumulation of food, damp-heat, etc.
- If the tongue coating changes from thin to thick, it indicates gradual exuberance of the pathogenic qi and that the disease is advancing.
- If the tongue coating changes from thick to thin or a new coating is regenerating, it indicates that the *zheng* qi is overcoming the pathogenic qi, and the disease is relieving.

B. Moist or dry:

Moistness or dryness of the tongue coating mainly reflects the exuberance or debilitation and the transfusion or distribution of the body fluids.

    a. Moist coating: the coating has moderate wetness, is not slippery or dry. It is the normal tongue coating or body fluids are not damaged.

    b. Slippery coating: the coating has excess water, which is nearly dropping or dribbling when the tongue is extended. This corresponds to a cold pattern or phlegm-damp pattern.

    c. Dry coating: the coating is dry and without fluid, possibly even cracked. It

indicates consumption of the body fluids, interior blockage of dampness and fluids unable to go upward.
   d. Rough coating: the coating is extremely dry and rough; the coarseness can feel sharp on the roof of the mouth or on the finger if it is touched. This coat is associated with a severe pattern of extreme heat damaging the fluids, or foul turbidity gathering in the middle *jiao*.
      - If the tongue coating turns from moist to dry, it is a serious pattern of extreme heat damaging fluid, and the fluid is unable to transmit and spread.
      - If the tongue coating turns from dry to moist, it may indicate the heat declining and fluid recovering, the water pathogen begins to transform or the heat entering the *ying* and blood levels.
C. Greasy or curd-like:
   a. Greasy coating: the coating has relatively small pellets which are sticky like honey with thick fur in the centre and thin on the sides and does not disappear on being scraped or wiped. It corresponds to damp-turbidity, phlegm rheum and accumulation of food patterns.
      <u>Dirty greasy coating</u>: the tongue coating is greasy and dirty.
      <u>Slippery greasy coating</u>: the tongue coating is greasy, moist and slippery.
      <u>Dry greasy coating</u>: the tongue coating is greasy, dry and with fluid deficiency.
      <u>Sticky greasy coating</u>: the greasy coating is covered with a layer of thick mucus.
      - The thick and greasy coating is mostly due to phlegm-heat, damp-heat, summer febrile disease, damp-warmth, dyspeptic retention, interior accumulation of damp phlegm, or disturbance of *fu* qi, etc.
      - The white and slippery greasy coating is due to dampness or cold-damp obstructing internally, and/or yang qi being obstructed.
      - If the coating is white like powder and thick, greasy but not slippery, it is mostly due to a seasonal pathogen with internal dampness.
      - If the coating is white, greasy but not dry, it is mostly due to deficiency of the spleen and heavy dampness, accumulation of food, and the qi movement being obstructed.
      - If the coating is white, thick, sticky and greasy, it indicates damp-heat of the spleen and stomach with gathering pathogenic qi attacking upward.
   b. Loose coating: tongue coating texture is loose. It often can be seen when the greasy and thick coating is transforming. It indicates that the pathogenic qi of damp-turbidity is being dispelled.
   c. Curd-like coating: the tongue coating is thick and loose, easily scraped off. The coating grains are rough and big like being covered with a residue of soy bean curd. The base of the tongue is smooth and glossy. It corresponds to failure of the stomach qi with damp-turbidity floating upward. This is mostly due to lack of transformation of the accumulated damp-turbidity or food and belongs to the pattern of pathogenic qi in superabundance.
   d. Pus or curd-like coating: there is a layer of coating just like liquid pus. It often can be seen in an interior abscess or binding of a pathogenic toxin. It is the manifestation of exuberance of the pathogenic qi and belongs to a critical illness.
   e. Mouldy bean curd-like coating: there are rotten spots spreading all over the

tongue like milk curds or grains of cooked rice. This is easy to be swabbed away, but regenerates suddenly. After scraping, the tongue body is left without coating. It indicates deficiency of qi and yin or mucky damp-heat pathogen overflowing. It is mostly seen in seriously ill patients or malnourished children.
- If the curd-like coating fades away, and a new thin-white coating grows through, this is the result of the *zheng* (healthy) qi overcoming the pathogenic qi and the pathogenic qi disappearing.
- If the curd-like coating fades away, but without a new coating regenerating, it is due to debilitation of the stomach qi and belongs to rootless tongue coating.

D. Peeled:

Part or full coating peeling off. The peeled area is smooth and glossy without coating. This may indicate shortage of stomach qi, exhaustion of stomach yin or deficiency of qi and blood. It is also a sign of deficiency all over the body.
  a. A peeled-like coating refers to where the peeled area is not smooth, but instead granulation or papillae can still be seen.
  b. A peeled coating is divided into anterior, middle and root peeled coating, patchy peeled coating and mirror-like coating according to the location and range.
  c. A geographic tongue refers to large area of peeled coating. Margins of the peeled area are prominent and the peeled area is able to move.
  d. A red tongue with a peeled coating may indicate deficiency of yin.
  e. A pale tongue with a peeled coating or peeled-like coating may indicate deficiency of blood, or deficiency of qi and blood.
  f. A red tongue with a mirror-like coating may indicate exhaustion of stomach yin.
  g. A bright-white tongue with a mirror-like coating may indicate *ying* and blood depletion, expiring of yang qi.
  h. A greasy and slippery, patchy peeled coating indicates deficiency of *zheng* qi and damp-turbidity unable to transform.

The range of the peeled coating is related to the degree of deficiency of qi and yin or qi and blood. The location of the peeled coating is related to the pathological changes of the *zang-fu* organs. For example, peeled coating on the tip of the tongue indicates shortage of lung yin; peeled on the centre of the tongue indicates shortage of stomach yin; peeled on the root of the tongue indicates exhaustion of kidney yin.

Inspecting the changes of the tongue coating, such as growth and decline, peeled or absence can judge the existence or loss of stomach qi and stomach yin. Changes in the tongue coating also reflect exuberance or debilitation of pathogenic qi and are helpful for judging the prognosis of disease.
- The tongue coating changing from complete coverage to peeled indicates a shortage of stomach qi and yin with a gradual debilitation of *zheng* qi.
- A new thin-white coating growing after the coating has been peeled indicates *zheng* qi dispelling the pathogenic qi or recovery of the stomach qi.

E. Waning or waxing:
  a. Waning: the coating turns from thick to thin. It indicates improvement of *zheng* qi and disease subsiding. But if the whole thick coating suddenly disappears, it reflects severe expiration of the stomach qi.
  b. Waxing: the coating turns from thin to thick, this indicates flourishing of

pathogenic qi, the disease is aggravating; but if the thin coating suddenly turns thicker, it indicates severe expiration of the *zheng* qi and extreme invasion of pathogenic qi.

By inspecting waning or waxing of the tongue coating one can distinguish the prognosis of the disease. If waning or waxing happens suddenly prognosis will be unfavourable.

F. Full or half:
  a. Full coating: the coating spreads over the whole tongue. A full coating indicates scattered pathogenic qi and is seen in phlegm-dampness obstructing the middle *jiao*.
  b. Half coating: the coating only covers some areas of the tongue (anterior, posterior, left, right, middle or edges). This reflects accumulation of the pathogenic qi, which corresponds to the relevant *zang-fu* organs.

G. True or false:

Inspecting the true or false tongue coating has an important significance in the prognosis of the disease and pathogenic conditions.
  a. A true coating or "tongue coating with root": the tongue coating is thick in the centre and thin on the sides, firmly attached to the tongue surface, as if growing on it and hard to scrub off. A true coating appears in the first or second stage of a disease. Thickness indicates stagnation of stomach qi; the disease is deep and critical. Prolonged disease with true coating indicates the presence of stomach qi.
  b. A false coating or "tongue coating without root": the tongue coating is easily scrubbed off and resting on the surface rather than growing out of it. A false coating appears in new (acute) disease, the pathogenic condition is still mild. However, prolonged disease with a false coating indicates deficiency of stomach qi; this belongs to an unfavourable pattern.

2. Coating colour

One can differentiate the nature of a disease by inspecting the colour of the tongue coating. The tongue coating colour includes: White coating, yellow coating and grey coating; they can appear on their own or combined together.

A. White coating:

<u>Thin-white coating:</u> the tongue body can be seen.
<u>Thick-white coating:</u> the tongue body cannot be seen.
<u>Powder-like coating:</u> a spread of white coating like powder over the whole tongue.

A white coating may indicate an exterior pattern or a cold pattern; it can also be seen in the healthy person.
  a. A thin, white and moist coating is the normal tongue coating, the beginning of the exterior pattern, a mild symptom of interior patterns, or an internal cold pattern due to yang deficiency.
  b. A thin, white and dry coating may indicate a wind-heat exterior pattern.
  c. A thin, white and slippery coating may indicate cold-damp due to an exterior invasion, devitalised spleen yang or water-dampness collecting internally.
  d. A white, thick and greasy coating may indicate phlegm-rheum, damp-turbidity, or food accumulation.
  e. A white, thick, greasy and dry coating may indicate damp-turbidity, phlegm-

rheum obstructing in the middle *jiao* with fluids not nourishing upward.
  f. A powder like coating indicates warm patterns, pestilent diseases, turbid-dampness with heat pathogens.
  g. A cracked white coating indicates dry-heat damaging the fluid.

B. Yellow coating:

Yellow coating corresponds to a heat pattern and an interior pattern.

<u>Light yellow coating:</u> a light yellow colour appears steadily over a thin white coating, mostly transformed from a thin-white coating.

<u>Deep yellow coating:</u> the colour is deep yellow.

<u>A scorched yellow coating:</u> grey and brown coatings may be classified under the yellow coating.

  a. The deeper the yellow colour, the more severe the heat. A light yellow suggests a mild heat, a deep yellow suggests severe heat, and a scorched yellow suggests extreme heat.
  b. In an exterior disease, if the coating turns from white to yellow or white mixed with yellow it indicates an exterior pathogen entering the interior and transforming into heat or an interior pattern mixed with an exterior pattern.
  c. A thin, light yellow coating can mostly be seen in an exterior wind-heat pattern or wind-cold transforming into heat.
  d. A yellow and slippery coating can be seen in the body with yang deficiency and cold-dampness or phlegm-rheum accumulating and transforming into heat. It also can be seen in deficiency of qi and blood with further contraction of an external pathogen.
  e. A yellow rough coating, a yellow bloom on the tongue, or a scorched yellow coating, all indicate a heat pathogen damaging the body fluids, dryness accumulation and bowel excess.
  f. A yellow and greasy coating indicates internal accumulation of damp-heat or phlegm-heat or food stagnation becoming putrid.

C. Grey black coating:

<u>Grey coating</u>: the colour of the coating is grey or light black.

<u>Black coating</u>: the colour of the coating is deep grey.

A grey coating and black coating are the same classification, they differ only as to the depth of the tone; thus, they are often both called grey black coating.

A grey black coating corresponds to severe interior heat patterns and interior cold patterns.

The degree of the colour corresponds to the severity of the heat and cold. Moistness or dryness of the coating texture is the key in judging heat or cold of the grey black coating.

A moist grey black coating corresponds to cold. A dry grey black coating corresponds to heat.

Section 4
Main Points for Analysing the Tongue Manifestations

1. Inspecting the spirit and the stomach qi of the tongue
(1) The manifestation of the tongue spirit
This mainly reflects the aspects of tongue colour and tongue body. The main point of pattern differentiation is the degree of redness and brightness of the tongue colour.
(2) Exuberance or debilitation of the stomach qi depends on whether the tongue coating is rooted or not.
   A. A rooted coating is a sign of healthy stomach qi.
   B. A rootless coating is a sign of loss of stomach qi.
In short, the tongue manifestation with spirit and stomach qi indicates a mild condition of disease, sufficient *zheng* qi or a severe condition of disease, but where the prognosis is good. The tongue manifestation without spirit and stomach qi indicates deficiency of the *zheng* qi, a severe condition of disease or a bad prognosis.

2. General analysis of the tongue body and tongue coating
(1) Necessity
Disease is a reflection of the struggle between *zheng* (healthy) qi and pathogenic qi; the tongue coating and tongue body reflect the pathological changes from different angles.
The tongue body reflects the conditions of *zang-fu* organs, qi, blood and body fluids.
The tongue coating is related to the nature of the pathogen and pattern of disease.
(2) Principles
   A. The changes of the tongue coating are in accordance with those of the tongue body, which indicate the same pathological processes. Diagnostically both of these combined together are most significant. For example:
   - A red tongue body with a yellow and dry coating indicates an extreme heat pattern.
   - A pale and tender tongue with a white and moist coating indicates a deficient cold pattern.
   - A red, crimson and cracked tongue with a scorched yellow and dry coating indicates extreme heat damaging fluid.
   - A blue-purple tongue with a white and greasy coating may indicate blood stasis and blockage of qi, phlegm-dampness obstructing in the interior.
   B. The changes of the tongue coating may not be in accordance with those of the tongue body. Therefore this should be analysed according to the aetiological factors, pathogenesis and the relationships between them, and then cross-checking and making an integrated judgement. For example:
   - A pale tongue with a yellow and greasy coating suggests a deficient cold body invaded by damp-heat.
   - A red, crimson tongue with a white, slippery and greasy coating suggests an external

heat pathogen or heat in the *ying* level and dampness in the qi level; or hyperactivity of fire due to yin deficiency; invasion of a cold-damp pathogen or internal food retention.
- A pale tongue with a yellow, greasy coating: The pale tongue body usually indicates deficient cold, but a yellow and greasy coating is the sign of a damp-heat pathogen. This becomes obvious because the tongue body mainly reflects the *zheng* qi and the tongue coating mostly suggests the type of pathogen.
- A red, crimson tongue body with a white, slippery, greasy coating: The red, crimson tongue refers to interior extreme heat, but the white, slippery and greasy coating is often seen in cold-damp accumulation. The tongue coating and tongue body reflect two opposite patterns: a cold pattern and a heat pattern. This may be caused by exterior pathogenic heat, heat in the *ying* level, leading to the redness of the tongue body, and dampness in the qi system, which causes a white, slippery and greasy tongue coating.

Therefore, when the manifestations of the tongue body are not in accordance with those of the tongue coating, it often indicates an occurrence of two or more pathogenic processes in the body. In clinic, if the manifestations of the disease are complex, observation of the tongue will be extremely valuable in conjunction with other signs. Generally one should pay particular attention to distinguish between the root (*běn*) and branch (*biāo*) in analysing a pattern.

3. Dynamic changes of the tongue manifestation

When the tongue manifestation changes follow the pathogenic condition, it is a reflection of the changes of the pathogenic condition.

The tongue manifestation changes that follow the treatment are a reference for the success or failure of treatment, and medication.

In grasping the changes of the tongue manifestation, it is possible to recognise the essence of pathogenic changes sufficiently to assist in diagnosing and treating.

For example, in an exterior disease, the tongue coating changes from thin to thick, this indicates the pathogen is moving from the exterior into the interior; the tongue coating changes from white to yellow, which indicates the pathogen is transforming into heat; when the tongue colour changes into red with a dry coating this indicates a rampant heat toxin, blazing of both qi and *ying*; a red tongue body with a peeled coating indicates heat entering the *ying* and blood levels and deficiency of both qi and yin.

In disease due to internal damage, such as with the tongue manifestation of wind-stroke, the tongue body changes from normal into red, dark-red, crimson, or dark purple with a yellow and greasy, scorched or black coat, or with distended sublingual veins, which indicates wind-phlegm transforming into heat, and/or obstruction of static blood. On the other hand changes in the opposite direction, indicate a mild condition of disease and a good prognosis.

SECTION 5
CLINICAL SIGNIFICANCE OF THE TONGUE EXAMINATION

Judging exuberance or failure of the *zheng* qi and pathogen.
Distinguishing the nature of the pathogenic factor.
Analysing the location and tendency of the pattern.
Estimating the prognosis of the pattern.
For example:
- A **rough** tongue relates to an **excess** pattern.
- A **tender** tongue relates to a **deficient** pattern.
- A **yellow** coating relates to a **heat** pattern.
- A **white** coating relates to a **cold** pattern.
- A **greasy** coating relates to a **damp** pattern.
- A **thin** coating relates to an **exterior** pattern.
- A **thick** coating relates to an **interior** pattern.

A lustrous tongue, where the tongue coating changes from thick to thin, from dry to moist suggests a favourable prognosis, the disease is moving from the interior to the exterior, and fluid is recovering.

A red tongue, where the tongue coating changes from thin to thick, from moist to dry suggests unfavourable prognosis, the disease is moving from the exterior to the interior, and extreme heat is damaging the fluid.

CHAPTER 4
Listening and Smelling Examination

The listening and smelling examination means listening to the patient's sounds and smelling their odours so as to investigate the circumstances of disease. Listening to the sounds means listening and distinguishing various sounds such as speech, breathing, coughing, vomiting, hiccoughing, belching, sighing, sneezing, yawning and intestinal rumbling that occur during the pathological changes of the patient. The smelling examination means smelling the various odours from the patient's body and the abnormal odours of the sickroom including secretions or excreta.

Since sounds as well as odours all come from the physiological activities and pathological changes of the *zang-fu* organs, listening to the sounds and smelling odours are helpful for examining the morbid conditions of the *zang-fu* organs and providing evidence for identifying patterns.

First of all, one should familiarise oneself with the normal sounds and odours of healthy people so as to recognise any change from the norm. Next, it is essential to have sufficient knowledge about sounds and odours in ill health and their clinical significance. Finally, the practitioner needs to combine the identifying of patterns with the contents of the listening and smelling examination and pay attention to its general rules in clinical practice.

Contents of the listening and smelling examination
- Listening to sounds
    - Normal sounds
    - Pathological sounds
- Smelling odours
    - Body odours
    - Sickroom odours

Section 1
Listening to Sounds

The general principle of sound production is qi moving and producing sound. Emitted sounds are concerned not only with vocalisation but also with sounds produced by movement of the internal organs. However, the voice is always significant and is related to the lung, throat, epiglottis, tongue, teeth, lips and nose, etc. The lung governs qi and controls breathing, as the qi moves this causes the sound of the voice, so the lung is the generating power of the sound. The throat is an air passage through which the sound must pass; therefore, the throat has a major action in producing sound. The opening and closing of the epiglottis and adjustment of the tongue, assisted by the lips, teeth and nostrils all influence the creation of the various kinds of sound. Furthermore, the kidney governs inspiration and is the root of qi; the liver governs the free flow of qi; the spleen governs transportation and transformation and is the source of qi and blood production, and the heart governs the mind and is in charge of the speech. Consequently, all of these aspects are related to the production of sounds and are linked to speech.

Listening to sounds means identifying and differentiating high or low pitch, strong or weak volume, clear or husky qualities, slow or acute changes of the speech and breath, as well as the abnormal sounds generating from pathological changes of the *zang-fu* organs such as coughing and vomiting. Through listening to the sounds it can be possible to identify diseases of cold or heat, deficiency or excess. It should also be possible to distinguish shortage of qi from shortness of breath, panting from wheezing and hiccough from belching.

Listening to sounds includes listening to: the patient's voice, speech, breathing, coughing, vomiting, hiccoughing, belching, sighing, sneezing, yawning, intestinal rumblings etc.

Normal Sounds

1. The characteristics of the normal voice and speech are:

Natural pronunciation, harmonious tone, gentle, smooth, consistent and coherent. A normal healthy voice indicates sufficient qi and blood, normal vocal apparatus and regular functioning of the *zang-fu* organs.

2. Factors that can affect these normal sounds:

These factors include sex, age, natural variation and mental capabilities. Typically, men's voices are relatively low and gruff, whilst women's voices are relatively high and clear; children's voices tend to be quite sharp and tuneful, while those of elderly people are lower and deeper.

Pathological Sounds

Pathological sounds refer to the changes of voice and speech, which are a reflection of disease.

1. Listening to the voice

The sound of the voice includes hoarseness, snoring, groaning and howling. General classification: If the voice is loud, sonorous, and strong and has consistency in words this indicates yang patterns, excess patterns and heat patterns. If the voice is low, weak and feeble and the person has a preference for quietness and where the speech is interrupted, this indicates yin patterns, deficiency patterns and cold patterns.

A. Heavy and gruff voice:

A heavy and gruff voice is mostly caused by external wind-cold or blockage of phlegm-damp which both cause the lungs failure to diffuse and lead to obstruction of the nose.

B. Hoarseness and aphonia:

Hoarseness means a harsh voice, while aphonia means complete loss of voice. Hoarseness and aphonia are similar in aetiology and pathomechanism but they are different in severity; if hoarseness becomes very serious, it will develop into aphonia. Hoarseness or aphonia at the onset of disease pertains to an excessive pattern due to externally-contracted wind-cold or wind-warm, or obstruction and accumulation of the phlegm-turbidity; all of which can lead to blockage of the clear orifices due to the lung qi failing to diffuse and purify; such a pathological condition is known as "muffled metal failing to sound".

Hoarseness or aphonia in chronic disease pertains to deficiency patterns due to internal damage of the essential qi, yin deficiency of the lung and kidney or deficient fire scorching the lung, all of which cause insufficiency of fluid and impairment of the lung in producing a normal voice; such a pathological condition is known as "broken metal failing to sound". Hoarseness or aphonia may be caused by shouting with rage, screaming or prolonged raising of the voice, which impairs both qi and yin and deprives the throat of moisture. Hoarseness or aphonia at the advanced stage of pregnancy, which is called "loss of voice during pregnancy", is due to the foetus interfering with the collaterals, which prevents the kidney essence from being transported upwards; it will heal spontaneously after delivery.

C. Snoring:

Snoring means the rattling noise produced by the nose and throat during sleep or coma, which is mostly due to partial obstruction of the respiratory passages. Snoring during sleep is often caused by chronic diseases of the nose or improper posture during sleep. However, it is not always an abnormal state; it can frequently be observed in obese or elderly people. The person in deep slumber with incessant snoring is mostly due to coma and qi dashing out of the respiratory tract; it is often a critical sign as heat is attacking the pericardium or wind-strike entering the *zang* organs.

D. Groaning:

Groaning is an utterance expressing pain or disapproval. The persistent groaning of the patient is often due to pain or a distending sensation that is difficult to bear. The high pitched and strong groan pertains to excessive patterns, whilst the low pitched and weak groan pertains to deficiency patterns. According to the changes in demeanor of a patient seen in clinic it is possible to distinguish the location of the pain. For instance, if the patient is frowning and groaning they may be suffering from a headache; touching the cheek and groaning is mostly due to toothache; protecting the heart or abdomen and groaning will be associated with chest pain or abdominal pain; inability to walk, touching the waist or legs and groaning is mostly due to lumbago or arthritis (*bì zhèng* 痹症).

E. Howling:

Howling is a long, loud, animal like scream with deep emotion, which happens suddenly often accompanied by a scary facial expression. It is mostly caused by acute pain or if terrified. The paroxysmal howl in infants indicates convulsions. Howling, following crying at night, is mostly caused by having eaten excessive cold or uncooked food, resulting in cold of the spleen and abdominal pain. It may also be due to accumulation of food, parasites, or if frightened, etc. The howl in adults usually indicates intense pain. The location of disease may often be in the bones, joints or *zang-fu* organs resulting from blockage of the movement of qi. Howling which sounds like a pig or goat, at the onset of an epileptic attack, results from adverse rising of the liver wind with phlegm.

2. **Listening to the speech**

The speech mainly refers to an analysis of the patient's ability of expression and response and whether or not words are spoken clearly and smoothly. Speech is considered to be the sound of the heart; hence speech is one of the presentations of the mind activity. Consequently, speech problems often have a close relationship with heart patterns. In addition, abnormal speech may help distinguish the excess and deficiency of a disease.

General principles:

Quietness and reluctance to speak, low and weak speech are usually ascribed to deficiency or cold patterns. Vexation and agitation with excessive speaking, high pitched and strong speech are usually ascribed to excessive or heat patterns.

There are some abnormal types of speech described below:

A. Delirious speech:

The mental capacity is not clear and there is strident, strong and incoherent speech. This is due to an excess pattern, which is caused by heat harassing the heart spirit.

B. Muttering and mumbling to oneself:

Muttering and mumbling to oneself means unclear mental capacity with intermittent, low and repeated speech. It belongs to a deficiency pattern, which is mostly seen in exhaustion of heart qi and mental derangement.

Both delirious speech and unconscious muttering and murmuring refer to loss of vitality, which is caused by mental derangement. It should be identified as deficiency or excess in clinic. Delirious speech often appears in the extreme stage of acute heat disease and can be seen in the patterns of heat entering the pericardium, phlegm-heat disturbing the heart, accumulation of heat in the *yangming*, heat invading the blood chamber, inward invasion of a carbuncle, abscess, toxin or furuncle complicated by septicaemia. Delirious speech is usually due to extreme heat disturbing mental activity. Unconscious muttering and murmuring usually appears in the later stage of prolonged disease with deficient *zheng* qi or the yin or yang collapse patterns. It is mostly caused by a scattered heart-mind and extreme deficiency of *zheng* qi.

C. Severe exhaustion of qi:

The voice is gentle, slow, feeble with a desire to speak but unable to do so. It is a sign of extreme deficiency of *zong* (gathering) qi (宗气).

D. Soliloquy:

Soliloquy refers to a dramatic form of speech in which a person talks to himself (herself) or reveals his (her) thoughts without addressing a listener. It is mumbling and muttering to oneself and becoming quiet when coming upon other people. This is due to insufficient heart qi, with failure to nourish the mind or production of phlegm due to qi stagnation misting the heart orifice. Such a condition is usually seen in some kinds of epilepsy and psychotic diseases.

E. Paraphasia:

In paraphasia the patient speaks nonsense while being conscious and may be aware of it afterwards. Paraphasia may be a difficulty finding the correct word despite knowing what it should be. This pattern either belongs to deficiency or excess. Paraphasia is often seen in deficiency of prolonged disease; an elderly person associated with a weak body, deficiency of heart and spleen or failure to nourish the heart-mind. Alternatively, this pattern belongs to excess and is due to the heart orifice being obstructed by phlegm-damp, static blood or qi stagnation.

F. Manic raving:

Manic raving refers to rambling and inconsequential talk as well as shouting nonsense in the street; it is associated with madness and mental disorder. It is often due to qi constraint transforming into fire and phlegm-fire disturbing the heart, which belongs to the pattern of yang, heat and excess. It is often seen in mania or a blood accumulation pattern.

G. Sluggish speech:

Sluggish speech refers to impairment of speech, consisting in lack of coordination and failure to arrange words in their proper order, which is most likely due to a central lesion. In this condition there is clear mind, normal thinking yet unclear speech, also called dysphasia. It is mostly caused by obstruction of the collaterals by wind-phlegm, the forerunner or sequela of wind-strike. However, inherent anomalies of the lingual frenulum or personal habits are also possible causes and should not be considered in this category of cerebral emergency.

H. Somniloquy:

When the patient speaks while sleeping, using unclear words with confused meaning, this is often due to heart fire, gallbladder heat and/or disharmony of stomach qi. Somniloquy can also be caused by prolonged disease with a deficient body and failure of the spirit to keep to its abode.

3. Listening to the respiration

Listening to the respiration refers to examining the speed of respiratory frequency, strength, weakness, roughness or smoothness of the breath, pure or turbid breath sounds, etc. Under normal conditions, the respiration is uniform, smooth, neither quick nor slow. Under movement or agitation, the respiration becomes quick; when sleeping, the respiration becomes slow and deep; these are physiological changes. The respiration is closely related to the lung, kidney, other *zang* organs and *zōng* qi.

Examining the changes of respiration can help identify deficiency or excess of the five *zang* organs and *zong* qi.

General significance:

Normal breath in disease means the physical body-*xing* (形) has illness but qi does not. Abnormal breath in disease means the physical body-*xing* and the qi both have illness.

Rough breath with quick exhalations and inhalations indicates externally contracted pathogenic qi in excess and belongs to heat and excessive patterns. Weak breath with slow exhalations and inhalations indicates internal damage with insufficient *zheng* qi and belongs to deficient and cold patterns.

Rough breath belongs to excess and weak breath belongs to deficiency. However, there is a false excess pattern seen in clinic where prolonged disease belongs to exhausted qi of the lung and kidney but has rough and intermittent breath. There is also a false deficient pattern where there is a warm-heat disease belonging to heat entering the pericardium and there is weak breath and bewilderment.

Main points in examining the respiration:
- uniformity of respiratory rhythm;
- strength, weakness, roughness or smoothness of the breath;
- natural or forced quality of the breath sounds.

The common manifestations of abnormal respiration: panting, wheezing, shortness of breath, weak breathing.

A. Panting (*chuǎn* 喘):

Shortness of breath and irregular respiration with flaring nares (nostrils), open mouth, raised shoulders and difficulty in lying down are the manifestations of panting. There is also obvious difficulty in breathing or dyspnoea; this is related to the lung and kidney and can be divided into deficiency and excess types.

Excess panting: relatively acute onset, rough, rapid and rushed breath with high pitched sound. The chest feels full but with a pleasant feeling on exhalation. The head is lifted up, the eyes bulge and the body is strong, with an excessive and strong pulse. These symptoms mostly belong to wind-cold attacking the lung, excessive heat in the lung or internal retention of phlegm-rheum, when the lung qi fails to purify and govern descent resulting in counterflow of lung qi.

Deficiency panting: slow onset, weak, short and discontinuous breath, low pitched sound, severe panting when moving, with a pleasant feeling on inspiration. Associated with a weak body and a deficient and weak pulse. These symptoms are associated with deficiency or exhaustion of lung qi and kidney qi, failing to contain and receive qi resulting in the qi floating upwards.

B. Wheezing (*xiāo* 哮):

Wheezing is a whistling type of respiratory sound. It often attacks intermittently and is difficult to cure. The sound is caused by phlegm-rheum and retained disease combined with exterior pathogens. Wheezing is also caused by an attack of exterior pathogens with failure to dissipate through the exterior, resulting in binding in the lung channel, counterflow and stagnation of lung qi. Alternatively, it can be induced by long term living in cold and damp rooms or excessive intake of sour, salty, uncooked and cold food.

> **Difference between panting and wheezing:**
> *The Orthodox Tradition of Medicine* (*Yī Xué Zhèng Zhuàn*, 医学正传) indicated clearly "wheezing named for the sound, panting named for the breath. During periods of panting, a sound in the throat, similar to the sound of a frog, is called wheezing". Persistent accelerated breathing with inability to stop is called panting. Wheezing necessarily occurs combined with panting, but panting can occur alone.

C. Shortness of breath (*qì duǎn* 气短):

This refers to rapid and short respiration, insufficient to be useful, discontinuous, no phlegm sounds, like panting but without raising the shoulders, mostly seen in deficiency patterns. However, it can be divided into deficiency and excess types. The deficiency pattern is marked by shortness of breath and weak breathing, usually accompanied by dispiritedness, lassitude and dizziness, which is due to shortage of the lung qi or extreme deficiency of the *yuan* qi (元气). The excess pattern is marked by shortness of breath and husky breathing, usually accompanied by chest oppression, abdominal and chest fullness, which results from phlegm or fluid retention, qi stagnation and obstruction due to stasis.

D. Weak breathing (*shǎo qì* 少气):

This refers to faint and weak respiration, short breaths, feeble voice, and low sounds and is a sign that the qi is insufficient. It usually results from deficiency patterns; it is often part of the manifestation of a deficient body, mostly caused by prolonged disease or deficiency of lung qi and kidney qi.

> **Differentiation of shortness of breath and weak breathing with panting:**
> Weak breathing is more natural and manifests as quietness, it is characterised by insufficient qi to create breath and low sounds, not enough to be heard. Shortness of breath manifests as grudging breath, short, rapid and discontinuous breath. Panting manifests as difficult and rapid breathing, the person even opens the mouth and raises the shoulders and is unable to lie down. Weak breathing belongs to a deficiency pattern, but shortness of breath and panting can be seen either in a deficiency pattern or an excess pattern, which must be distinguished in clinic.

4. Listening to the sound of the cough

The lung corresponds to cough. Cough is the frequent manifestation of failure of the lung qi to disperse and descend resulting in ascending counterflow of lung qi. However, cough is also closely related to the other *zang-fu* organs; so the ancients said "cough is not only due to the lung, but also due to other *zang fu* organs". Cough is usually caused by external pathogens attacking the lung but is also caused by internal damage of the lung or other *zang-fu* organs.

Cough may have sound but be without phlegm, which is called "non-productive cough" (*ké*) or dry cough. Cough may also have phlegm but without sound, which is called "productive cough" (*sòu*). Both phlegm and sound together is called "cough" (*ké sòu*). The sound of cough may be used for pattern identification; however the differentiation of cold or heat, deficiency or excess, depends chiefly on the characteristics of the phlegm such as quality, quantity and colour, as well as time of onset and accompanying symptoms.

Cough with a deep sound, whitish thin phlegm and nasal obstruction is usually caused by invasion of external wind-cold. A deep but quiet cough with thick yellowish phlegm, which is not easy to expectorate, is due to lung heat. Cough that sounds deep and oppressed with excessive phlegm, which is easy to expectorate, generally results from retention and collection of cold-phlegm and damp-turbidity. Dry cough without phlegm or with scanty and sticky phlegm usually results from dryness invading the lung or deficiency of lung yin. Weak cough accompanied by shortness of breath or panting is due to shortage of the lung qi and consequent failure of the dispersing and descending function.

If there is a violent, convulsive cough, returning at longer or shorter intervals and consisting of several expirations, followed by a sonorous inspiration or a whoop sound and accompanied by shortness of breath during an attack, flushed face, tears and nasal discharge, this is called "whooping cough". It is often seen in children and results from a combination of pathogenic wind with latent phlegm, which transforms into heat and obstructs the airway. The cough that is like a dog barking, accompanied by hoarseness and difficulty with inspiration, usually indicates diphtheria that is due to yin deficiency of the lung and kidney or fire pathogen attacking the throat.

5. Listening to the sound of vomiting

Vomiting refers to upward counterflow of stomach qi leading to ejection of gastric contents out through the mouth. When there is a sound but nothing is brought up, it is called retching, while it is called vomiting when some of the gastric contents are regurgitated but no sound is heard. Any disease that impairs the descending action of the

Table 4-1 Clinical significance of the common sounds of the cough

Sound of cough	Accompanying symptoms	Clinical significance
Deep and gruff cough	Whitish thin phlegm	External invasion of wind-cold or collection of phlegm-damp in the lung
Tight and oppressed cough	Plenty of phlegm easily expectorated	Cold-phlegm and damp-turbidity obstructing the lung
Deep and hacking cough	Yellowish thick phlegm difficult to expectorate	Heat attacking the lung
Dry cough	Without phlegm or with scanty phlegm	Dry pathogen attacking the lung or dryness of the lung due to lung yin deficiency
Light, quiet and weak cough	Shortage of qi and panting	Deficiency of the lung qi

stomach qi, leading to upward counterflow of the stomach qi, may cause vomiting. One can distinguish cold or heat, deficiency or excess of vomiting by listening to the sound of vomiting and the characteristics or odours of the vomitus. If the sound of vomiting is weak and vomiting comes slowly and the vomitus appears as clear water, phlegm or fluid retention, it frequently belongs to deficiency or cold patterns. If the sound of vomiting is severe and vomiting comes relatively suddenly and the vomitus appears as thick phlegm and yellowish water, it usually belongs to excess and heat patterns. If heat damages the stomach fluid and the vomiting assumes a spurting character, it is usually due to heat disturbing the mind.

Pattern identification according to vomiting usually needs the addition of the four examinations. For example, if the vomiting occurs after eating, it may be food poisoning. Vomiting and dysentery can result from cholera or cholera like illness. Evening vomiting of materials which have been eaten in the morning, or morning vomiting of that eaten the previous evening are usually due to stomach yang deficiency or deficiency of both spleen and kidney. Dry mouth and desire for drinking, but vomiting after drinking is called water counterflow, which is caused by internal retention of phlegm and fluid or *taiyang* water accumulation pattern. To summarise, vomiting with a sudden onset in serious illness belongs to excess patterns, but vomiting in a long-term illness belongs to deficiency patterns.

6. Other abnormal sounds
A. Hiccough:
Hiccough refers to the upward counterflow of stomach qi through the throat, emitting an uncontrollable pounding sound.
    a. The sound of the hiccough is repetitive, loud, sonorous, short and forceful, which indicates excess patterns and heat patterns.
    b. The sound of hiccough is low, deep and long with weak and forceless breath, which indicates deficient patterns and cold patterns.
    c. Hiccough which appears in a new illness, with a forceful sound, suggests a cold

pathogen or heat pathogen invading the stomach.
   d. Continuous hiccough in a long-term or severe illness, when the sound is low and without force, with shortness of breath, is a dangerous sign of the debilitation of stomach qi.

B. Belching:

Belching refers to the sound of qi transmitting up from the stomach through the throat. The sound of belching is long and slow.
   a. Belching with acid and putrid odour indicates food retention, which belongs to excess patterns.
   b. Continual and loud belching occurring after emotional upsets, is caused by liver qi attacking the stomach and belongs to excess patterns.
   c. The sound of belching that is deep and intermittent, without an acid-putrid odour, but is accompanied by poor appetite and digestion, is caused by stomach deficiency and counterflow of qi. It mostly can be seen in the elderly, weak and in those with long-term illness and belongs to deficient patterns.
   d. Continual belching, without an acid-putrid odour and accompanied by cold and pain of the stomach cavity and abdomen, is due to a cold pathogen settled in the stomach, and belongs to cold patterns.

C. Sighing:

There is the occasional appearance of the sound of a long or short sigh when the patient feels gloomy and inhibited in the chest. It is mostly caused by emotions being suppressed over a long period of time or sudden emotional irritation. Sighing indicates binding constraint of liver qi.

D. Sneezing:

Sneezing refers to lung qi ascending, watery discharge from the nose and emitting a sound.
   a. Sneezing during new-onset illness accompanied by aversion to cold, fever and nasal discharge, is caused by external attack of wind-cold and belongs to external cold patterns.
   b. Sudden sneezing of a person with yang deficiency and long-term illness indicates resurgence of yang qi and the illness taking a turn for the better.

E. Yawning:

Yawning is an involuntary intake of breath through a wide-open mouth with slight sound. If happening all the time there is continuous yawning, which is difficult to stop, this means exuberant yin and reduced yang in a deficient body.

F. Borborygmus:

Borborygmus can be heard as the stomach and intestines peristalsis moves air manifesting as a rumbling or gurgling.
   a. Low, weak and slow borborygmus, often difficult to be heard, indicates a normal process.
   b. Borborygmus in the stomach cavity just like a bag packed with water and giving off a gurgling sound, and the sound reducing as the person stands or massages the stomach, suggests water retention, gathering in the stomach, and obstructing qi movement of the middle *jiao*.
   c. Borborygmus in the stomach cavity and abdomen, which is reduced if warmed

or after eating, and increased in the cold or if hungry; indicates shortage of centre qi or deficiency and cold of the stomach and intestines.

d. Borborygmus sounding like thunder in the abdomen and accompanied by a subjective sensation of a lump in the abdomen and fullness with diarrhoea; suggests wind, cold and damp attacking the stomach and intestines.

e. Slight borborygmus in the abdomen with abdominal distension, low food intake, poor appetite and digestion indicates qi deficiency of the stomach and intestines, and weakening of transmission.

f. Borborygmus disappearing completely and accompanied by abdominal distension, fullness and pain, corresponds to qi stagnation and poor function of the stomach and intestines.

Section 2
Smelling Odours

Smelling odours includes: body odours and sickroom odours.

General significance:

Understanding cold or heat, deficiency or excess of the disease. If the odour is acid-putrid and foul this corresponds to excess heat patterns. It the odour is light or slightly smells of fish, this corresponds to deficiency cold patterns.

Body Odours

Body odours includes breath odours, sweat odours, phlegm and nasal mucus odours, urine and stool odours, menstrual and vaginal discharge odours and vomitus odours.

A. Breath odours:
   a. Bad breath is caused by either by a lack of cleanliness of the oral cavity or dental caries. Alternatively, bad breath results from dyspepsia or constipation.
   b. Sour breath is caused by accumulation and stagnation in the stomach and intestines.
   c. Foul breath is due to stomach heat.
   d. Rancid breath indicates an internal ulcer or abscess.
   e. Foul breath with rotten gingiva indicates ulcerative gingivitis.

B. Sweat odours:
   a. Goatish smell of sweat is due to wind-damp or damp-heat overflowing onto the skin (wind-damp disease, damp warmth disease or heat disease, etc.).
   b. Foul smell of sweat is caused by pestilence, or intense summer-heat, or fire toxin.
   c. Offensive smell like a male goat from sweating in the armpits, indicates internal accumulation of damp-heat

C. Phlegm and nasal mucus odours:
   a. Turbid, purulent phlegm or bloody phlegm with cough and fishy smell is caused by pulmonary abscess.
   b. Yellowish thick phlegm with a fishy smell indicates exuberance of lung heat.

c. Clear and thin phlegm with a salty flavour, without special odours can be seen in a cold pattern.
   d. Turbid nasal mucus with a fishy smell is caused by sinusitis.
   e. Clear nasal mucus without odour indicates an external contraction of wind-cold.
D. Urine and stool odours:
   a. Sour odour of the stool indicates heat stagnation in the intestines.
   b. Sloppy and fishy odour of the stool indicates deficient cold of the spleen and stomach.
   c. Foul smelling diarrhoea like rotten eggs with sour flatus indicates retention of food.
   d. Yellow and red urine with a turbid foul smell suggests damp-heat of the bladder.
   e. Sweat and/or urine with apple odour can be seen in *xiāo kě* (diabetes).
E. Menstrual and vaginal discharge odours:
   a. Foul odour menstruation corresponds to a heat pattern.
   b. Fishy smell menstruation corresponds to a cold pattern.
   c. Yellowish, thick and foul smelling leucorrhoea corresponds to damp-heat.
   d. White, thin and fishy smelling leucorrhoea corresponds to cold-damp.
   e. Cacosmia (putrefactive odours) from flooding and spotting or leucorrhoea mixed with abnormal colours is most often cancer.
F. Vomitus odours:
   a. Clear and thin vomitus without foul odours is caused by stomach cold.
   b. Sour and turbid smell of vomitus indicates stomach heat.
   c. Undigested food in the vomitus and with acid-putrid odour is caused by food accumulation.
   d. Pus and blood in the vomitus and with a fishy smell is due to an internal ulcer.

Sickroom Odours

Sickroom odour frequently comes from the odours of the patient's body or from the patient's discharges.

Table 4-2 Clinical significance of common sickroom odours

Sickroom odours	Significance
Stench	Pestilence
Foul blood smell	Haemorrhage
Rotten smell	Rotten sore or gangrene (sloughing deep-rooted abscess)
Putrefactive odour	Deterioration of the *zang-fu* organs
Smell of urine (smell of ammonia)	Advanced stage of oedema (uraemia), debilitation of the kidneys
Rotten apple odour	*Xiāo kě* (diabetes)
Alliaceous (like garlic) odour	Organo-phosphate poisoning

CHAPTER 5
Inquiry Examination

The inquiry examination is a diagnostic method whereby an interactive verbal exchange or discourse takes place between the patient and the practitioner. The aim is for the practitioner to gain verbal information about the patient's presenting complaint or concern, the onset, progress and past treatment of the disease, and other conditions of the illness.

The data collected by the inquiry examination is the most influential in clinic. In a patient centred diagnosis, feelings such as pain or favourite preferences of the patient himself (herself) are considered to be the most accurate and reliable. Many pathological changes in the body can only be sensed by oneself. Therefore, inquiry is the important step in diagnosis of illness and disease in clinic. By asking about all kinds of subjective symptoms and histories of these, the collected pathological data becomes the chief evidence of diagnosis. The main contents, manifestations and general clinical significance of various kinds of common symptoms are the emphasis in this chapter.

In order to use symptoms for diagnosis, practitioners should not only grasp the clinical manifestation of all kinds of symptoms such as spontaneous sweating, stabbing pain, poor appetite and digestion, dribbling after voiding etc; but should also grasp the general clinical significance of these symptoms such as that spontaneous sweating mostly belongs to yang qi deficiency, stabbing pain is mostly due to blood stasis, etc. In addition, practitioners should be adept at integrating and analysing all kinds of symptoms in order to then discern the disease and/or pattern differentiation correctly.

Contents of the inquiry examination
- Significance and method of the inquiry examination
- Main contents of the inquiry examination
    General information
    Chief complaint (concern)
    Present illness history
    Past medical history
    Individual life history
    Family history
- Inquiry into the presenting symptoms
    Inquiry into cold and heat
    Inquiry into sweat
    Inquiry into pain
    Inquiry into the head, body, chest and abdomen
    Inquiry into ears and eyes
    Inquiry into sleep
    Inquiry into drink, eating habits and taste preferences
    Inquiry into the urine and stool
    Inquiry into menses and vaginal discharge
    Inquiry into children / offspring

Section 1
Significance and Method of the Inquiry Examination

Significance of the Inquiry Examination

The inquiry examination is an important method in understanding the pathological conditions and examining illness and disease; it often takes possession of the most important position in the four examinations. The occurrence, development, changing progress and treatment of the disease, as well as the symptoms of which the person is aware, past medical history, personal life habits, appetite, constitution, etc, are all helpful evidence for diagnosis and treatment. Such information can be acquired only through the inquiry examination.

Method of the Inquiry Examination

If a practitioner wishes to use the inquiry examination effectively in clinic, he (she) should grasp the contents of the inquiry examination and have a sufficient knowledge of theory and plenty of clinical experience, and also should pay attention to the following concepts:

(1) Choose a calm and suitable place in order to avoid interference. When the patient is a child or is unconscious or in a coma and thus unable to speak for themselves to describe the condition, the practitioner should ask the accompanying relatives or persons about the complaints and the history of illness. The practitioner must know clearly the relationship between the teller and the patient in order to get a reliable case history.

(2) The practitioner's attitude should be serious, solemn, courteous and amiable. The practitioner should ask and listen carefully and patiently to the patient who describes the history of the illness. The practitioner should not use pessimistic or frightening words and expressions when encountering a stubborn disease, in order to avoid the loss of the patient's self-confidence and possibly cause the illness to become more serious.

(3) The language should be popular and understandable to the patient and asking questions in medical terms should be avoided.

(4) The practitioner should pay particular attention to collecting comprehensive data concerning the chief complaint or concern of the patient.

(5) Questions should have a purpose and a point and they should be asked in sequence if possible.

(6) For critically ill patients, the inquiry examination should be brief so as not to delay emergency management because one must not hold up urgent treatment by lengthy discourse.

Section 2
Contents of the Inquiry Examination

The inquiry examination includes general information, chief complaints and concerns, present illness history, past medical history, individual life history, family history, etc. (Table 5-1).

Table 5-1 Main contents of the inquiry examination

Main content	Inquiry	Clinical significance	Hints
General Information	Name, sex, age, marital status, place of birth, upbringing, occupation, place of work, address and telephone number, etc.	To follow-up the patient and acquire the data which is related to the disease.	This could be supportive for e.g. diagnosis of endemic disease, contagious disease, occupational disease, and senile diseases.
Chief Complaint or Concern	This refers to the main symptoms and the duration of these sufferings.	The chief complaint or concern is the chief symptom of the illness. According to it, the practitioner can estimate the category of the disease or illness and the severity of the condition.	(1) The chief complaint or concern is the most serious symptom of the patient. The patient emphasises it when examined by the practitioner in the first visit. The practitioner should pay careful attention to this. (2) After firstly confirming the symptoms of the chief complaint or concern, the practitioner further seeks to comprehend the related contents such as the position, nature, degree, time and healing progress. It should not be indiscriminate and obscure.
Present Illness History	The occurrence of the disease	This could be useful for differentiating the cause, location and nature of disease.	Inquiring about the whole course of the onset, development, changes of the illness and the healing progress from its occurrence to the time that the patient visits the practitioner
	The development of the disease	This could be helpful for understanding the struggle between *zheng* (healthy) qi and pathogenic factors, and pathological changes.	
	The procedure of the diagnosis and treatment	This can be taken as a reference for the present diagnosis and treatment.	
	Present symptoms	The main contents of the inquiry examination	

Continued

Main content	Inquiry	Clinical significance	Hints
Past Medical History	The history of past diseases and medical treatments	Finding possible relationships between the previous diseases and the present illness	This can be of benefit in diagnosing the present illness.
Individual Life History	Life history	Screening for endemic or contagious diseases	
	Mental history	Analysing any relation between mental status and present illness. The practitioner can explain to and reassure the patient with emotional disorders.	
	Drinking, eating and activities	This is valuable for analysing the pathogenesis of the disease.	
	Marital status and offspring	This has an important significance in the diagnosis of male diseases and gynaecological disorders.	
Family History	Inquiring about the disease history of close relatives or those who have close contact in daily life	This has important significance in diagnosing certain contagious diseases and hereditary diseases.	This may also have affected the patient emotionally.
	Inquiring about the causes of death of close relatives		

SECTION 3
PRESENT ILLNESS HISTORY

Present illness history, refers to asking about the patient's sufferings and the related condition of the whole body, in detail.

The range of present illness history is very extensive. Zhang Jing-yue wrote a *"Ten Questions Chapter"* on the basis of the inquiry examination. Chen Xiu-yuan modified it and then it became the *"Ten Question Song"* in the *Qing* Dynasty.

First ask hot and cold, second ask sweat,
Third ask head and body; fourth ask stools and urine,
Fifth ask food and drink, sixth ask chest,

Seventh ask hearing, eighth ask thirst,
Ninth ask old diseases, tenth ask cause.
In taking medicines, what changes appear.
Women especially ask the time of menses, slow, fast, block or flood.
For children add experience with measles and chicken pox.

Although the content of the "*Ten Question Song*" is brief and to the point, it still has significance as a guide. But, in practical application, the inquiring should be done with agility, and in succession according to the different conditions of patients; it should not be done mechanically.

Inquiring into Cold and Heat

Inquiring into cold and heat means asking the patient whether he or she has the sensation of fever or aversion to cold. Cold and heat are common symptoms seen in clinic. Inquiring about cold and heat is one of the essential contents of the inquiry examination.

Cold belongs to yin pathogens and exuberance of yin leads to cold. When attacked by cold or with yang deficiency, the patient will feel aversion to cold. Heat belongs to yang pathogens and exuberance of yang leads to heat. When attacked by heat or with yin deficiency, the patient will feel heat.

Cold and heat are important pieces of evidence for distinguishing the pathogenic nature and exuberance or failure of yin and yang.

Classification of cold and heat:

Cold:

① Aversion to wind: this means the patient feels cold in the wind, but this can be relieved by sheltering from the wind.

② Aversion to cold: the patient feels cold that cannot be relieved by wearing more clothes or staying near heat.

③ Shivering: this refers to the severe aversion to cold, which is accompanied by trembling of the whole body.

④ Fear of cold: the patient feels cold, which can be relieved by wearing more clothes and staying by the heat.

Heat:

Heat refers to a body temperature that is higher than usual or the body temperature is normal but the patient has a subjective sensation of general or local fever.

> **The method of inquiring about cold and heat:**
> First, ask the patient whether they feel cold or heat. If any patient says they do, this must be followed up by asking about when, the degree, duration, and related symptoms of the cold or heat.

The symptoms of cold and heat, which are commonly seen in clinic include: aversion to cold with fever, chills without fever, fever without chills, alternating chills and fever.

1. Aversion to cold with fever

Aversion to cold with fever indicates the cold and heat symptoms are appearing at the same time. It is an important piece of evidence for the diagnosis of exterior invasions.

As the external pathogens are attacking the fleshy exterior, *wei* yang is being obstructed and failing to warm the fleshy exterior, and then the patient experiences aversion to cold. On the other hand, as the pathogens are blocking outside then *wei* yang is unable to defend and the *zheng* (healthy) qi and pathogenic qi are struggling, the patient also experiences heat.

The common types of aversion to cold with fever and their clinical significance:

① Severe aversion to cold with low fever:

The combined symptoms are absence of sweating, a heavy body and floating, tight pulse. Severe aversion to cold with low fever is the characteristic of externally-contracted wind-cold and indicates an exterior wind-cold pattern.

② High fever with mild aversion to cold:

The combined symptoms are thirst, red face and floating, rapid pulse. High fever with mild aversion to cold is the characteristic of externally-contracted wind-heat and indicates the exterior wind-heat pattern.

③ Mild fever with aversion to wind:

The combined symptoms are spontaneous sweating and a floating, moderate pulse. Mild fever with aversion to wind is the character of externally-contracted wind and indicates the exterior wind pattern.

The relationship between the strength or weakness of aversion to cold and the *zheng* (healthy) qi:

① Both severe aversion to cold and fever indicates both exuberance of the pathogens and the *zheng* qi.

② Both mild aversion to cold and fever indicates less pathogens and failure of the *zheng* qi.

③ Severe aversion to cold and mild fever indicates exuberance of pathogens and decline of the *zheng* qi.

2. Chills without fever

Chills without fever means that the patient only feels cold but there is no fever.

A. Aversion to cold in new onset disease:

This refers to suddenly feeling cold, chilliness of the four limbs or cold pain in the stomach and abdomen, or cough, panting and wheezing, which belongs to an interior excessive cold pattern. The pathogenesis of this is a severe attack of a cold pathogen, stagnation of yang qi, failure to warm the skin and body hair.

B. Fear of cold in chronic disease:

This refers to cold of the four limbs, which can be relieved by warmth; it is associated with a pale, fat and tender tongue and a deep, slow and weak pulse; which indicates an interior deficient cold pattern. The pathogenesis of this is deficiency of yang qi with consequent failure to warm the body.

3. Fever without chills

Fever without chills refers to when the patient only feels fever but does not feel cold.

A. High fever:

High fever means the body temperature can reach 39℃ and above, no aversion to cold but aversion to heat. The clinical manifestations are thirst and preference for cold water, profuse sweating, a surging and large pulse and a red face. It belongs to an interior excessive heat pattern and mostly can be seen in a *yangming* channel pattern of cold damage or the qi stage of warm disease.

B. Tidal fever:

Tidal fever refers to the fever that comes and goes regularly like the tide, arriving at a definite time every day.

    a. Late afternoon tidal fever:

        Obvious fever in the afternoon (3-5 p.m.), also called *yangming* tidal fever. It can be accompanied by thirst with preference for cold water, abdominal pain, constipation and red tongue with a yellow, dry coating. It can be seen in a *yangming* bowel pattern.

    b. Damp warmth tidal fever:

        Unsurfaced fever (the practitioner does not feel feverishness when he touches the skin, but feels scorching heat after touching for a while; more fever in the afternoon; accompanied by a subjective feeling of a lump in the stomach cavity; *pǐ* (abdominal distension); heavy body, and red tongue with greasy coating. It is mostly seen in damp warmth disease.

    c. Yin-deficiency tidal fever:

        Yin-deficiency tidal fever means low fever in the afternoon or evening, manifesting as vexing heat in the five centres (chest, palms and soles), steaming bone fever (sensation of steaming fever in the bones), red cheeks and night sweat. It is mostly seen in a yin deficiency pattern.

C. Mild fever:

Fever is low; the body temperature is not more than 38°C or there is only a subjective sensation of fever.

The aetiology and pathogenesis are complicated; it is mostly seen in some internal damage disease or the latter stage of warm febrile disease.

    a. Qi deficiency and fever:

        This manifests as long-term mild fever, more severe when tired, accompanied by tiredness, weak breathing, spontaneous sweating, etc.

    b. Qi-constraint fever:

        Mild fever when emotion is suppressed, which is accompanied by chest oppression and irritability.

    c. Summer fever in children:

        The child has long-term mild fever in the summer, which is accompanied by vexation, thirst, increased urination, absence of sweating, etc. It will be cured in the autumn.

4. Alternating chills and fever

This occurs when the cold or heat appears alternately and repeatedly, which is the manifestation of struggle of pathogenic qi and *zheng* (healthy) qi.

A. Irregular alternating chills and fever:

The chills or fever appear alternately and continually, several times in one day and without regular time. This indicates the *shaoyang* disease of cold damage and has the character of the half-exterior and half-interior pattern.

The pathogenesis is that the exterior attack arrives to the stage of the half-exterior and half-interior, struggling between pathogenic qi and *zheng* qi. The predominance of pathogenic qi leads to aversion to cold, while the predominance of the *zheng* qi leads to fever. So aversion to cold and fever alternately break out.

B. Regular alternating chills and fever:

Chills (severe aversion to cold with shivering of the whole body) or fever breaking out alternately, at regular times either once a day or once in two or three days, accompanied by severe headache, thirst and profuse sweating, can be seen in malaria. When malaria invades the body, it stays in the half-external and half-internal region. When it gets inside, there is a struggle with yin and when it gets out, there is a struggle with yang; that is the reason why chills and high fever appear alternately and repeatedly.

Inquiring into Sweating

Sweat is created by means of yang qi transforming and steaming yin fluids, which emerges on the outside of the body from the sweat pores. If the *wei* qi (defensive qi) or yang qi is insufficient, it leads to abnormal opening and closing of the sweat pores and sweat appears spontaneously. It does not matter if there is external invasion or internal damage, if there is only the exuberance or decline of the yin and yang or lapse of *wei* qi, all can lead to abnormal sweating.

The difference between physiological sweating and pathological sweating:

① Physiological sweating:

The normal person sweats when active, eating hot food, in hot weather, wearing thick clothes and as a result of emotional stimulations, etc.

② Pathological sweating:

This is when there is no sweating when there should be sweating. Profuse sweating when there should be no sweating, or where there is just local sweating on the body. Pathological sweating can help in diagnosing the nature of the pathogen and exuberance or decline of yin and yang in the human body.

> **The method of inquiring about sweating:**
> First, asking whether the patient has sweat or not; and then if they do, asking the time, quantity, location and accompanying symptoms of the sweat.

1. Sweating or not

Inquiring about abnormal sweating can differentiate the nature of the pathogenic factors and deficiency or excess of *wei* yang or deficiency of the yin aspect of *ying* qi.

A. External pattern:
   a. Sweating: this mostly belongs to an external deficiency pattern or an external heat pattern in external invasion of wind-heat. Wind tends to open pores, while heat tends to rise and disperse. As the wind-heat is attacking, the muscular interstices become loose and sweat comes out.
   b. Without sweating: this mostly belongs to an external cold pattern in an external invasion of wind-cold. Since cold tends to stagnate and contract, the muscular interstices become tense and the sweat pores are closed up.

B. Internal pattern:
   a. Sweating: this mostly belongs to an internal heat pattern, deficiency of yang qi and insecurity of *wei* (defensive) qi, or yin deficiency with internal heat. Exuberant internal heat drives the body fluid outward or deficiency of yang qi results in insecurity of exterior muscles. Yin deficiency with internal heat steams the fluids outside.
   b. Without sweating: this mostly belongs to yang deficiency in chronic disease or consumption of fluid and blood. Deficient yang qi leads to lack of strength for steaming fluids or consumption of fluid and blood leading to lack of source for transforming into sweat.

2. Special sweating

Special sweating means the pathological sweating that occurs under a particular condition with distinct manifestations and at a special time.

A. Spontaneous sweating:
Spontaneous sweating indicates frequent sweating during the daytime, especially after little physical movement. It usually indicates a qi deficiency pattern or yang deficiency pattern.

B. Night sweat:
Night sweat means sweating after falling asleep but without sweating while awake. It usually indicates deficiency conditions of yin deficiency with an internal heat pattern or deficiency of both qi and yin. However, it may indicate excess conditions of damp obstruction or recent pathogenic invasions.

C. Exhaustion sweating:
This means profuse sweating in the process of a disease, which is a critical sign.
   a. Sweating of yin exhaustion (yin collapse): the manifestations of this are high fever, vexation, warm limbs, extreme thirst, profuse sweating, warm, oily and sticky hands, and thready and rapid pulse.
   b. Sweating of yang exhaustion (yang collapse): the manifestations of this are cold body and limbs, profuse sweat clear sweating, listlessness and chills, faint pulse verging on expiry.

D. Shiver sweating:
Sweating after chills and shivering in a severe stage of disease. This is a reversal point in the development of the disease.
   a. If fever abates, pulse calms down and the body turns cool after sweating, it is a sign that pathogens are being expelled and the heat has gone with the sweat.
   b. If the fever refuses to subside and the symptoms fail to be relieved after sweating, this indicates exuberance of pathogenic qi and decline of *zheng* (healthy) qi. The disease could become serious.

E. Profuse sweating:
Profuse sweating is mostly due to an excessive heat pattern.

F. Yellow sweat:
The colour of sweat is just like the juice of amber cork-tree bark (a yellowy bronze colour) and the sweat sticks on the clothes. This is due to the wind, damp and heat interactive steaming.

3. Local sweating

Local sweating indicates abnormal sweat in some location of the body. It reflects the pathological changes of the body. The patterns of local sweating have the difference of deficiency, excess, cold and heat.

A. Head sweating:

The sweat only appears over the head or neck. This is due to extreme heat in the upper *jiao* driving the sweat outward, or accumulation and stagnation of the damp-heat in the middle *jiao*, then steaming damp-heat and driving the fluid upward. It is also caused by internal exuberance of yin-cold, desertion of *yuan* (original) qi, upward and outward movement of deficient yang and fluid following yang, or just exuberance of yang qi and then heat steaming upward.

B. Hemi-lateral sweating:

Sweating appears only on half of the body, either the left side or the right side, upper or lower half of the body. It can be seen in stroke, flaccidity and paraplegia. It is due to obstruction of the collaterals on the affected side and consequently being unable to circulate qi and blood (the side without sweat). Great care must be taken if this symptom is accompanied by insufficient qi and blood.

C. Sweating of the palms and soles:

More sweating occurs on the palms or soles. This is mostly caused in yin deficiency with internal heat, extreme heat in the *yangming*, or accumulation of damp-heat in the middle *jiao*.

D. Chest sweating:

There is a propensity for sweating easily, or profuse sweating on the chest. This is mostly due to deficiency of the heart and spleen, or failure of the heart and kidney to interact.

Inquiring into Pain

Inquiring into the experience of pain has a great deal of diagnostic significance in Chinese medicine. Main points in inquiring about pain include: Location, nature, degree, time, desire or reluctance for heat, pressure, activity etc.

The forming mechanism of pain:

① Pain caused by excess:

When the person succumbs to an external pathogenic invasion, stagnation of qi and stasis of blood, congealing and stagnating of phlegm, food stagnancy or parasitic worm accumulation, which blocks the channels of the *zang-fu* organs and qi movement and thus prevents the qi and blood from being circulated, they will feel pain due to the stagnation.

② Pain caused by deficiency:

When a person has deficiency of qi and yin essence depletion, which leads to malnutrition of the *zang-fu* organs' channels, he or she will feel pain due to this malnutrition.

1. Inquiring into the nature of pain

By asking the characteristics of pain, the practitioner can differentiate the reason and pathogenesis of pain.

A. Distending pain:

This is a pain with a distending sensation and due to stagnation of qi.

B. Stabbing pain:
This is a sharp pain, like being stabbed by a needle and is caused by stasis of blood.

C. Colicky pain:
This is a pain like a knife being twisted and is often due to blockage of an excessive pathogen or stagnation of qi movement by a cold pathogen.

D. Dull pain:
The pain is bearable but steady, which mostly belongs to a deficiency pattern.

E. Cold pain:
The pain is with a cold sensation and preference for warmth, which is mostly due to congealed cold or yang deficiency.

F. Burning pain:
The pain is with a burning sensation, a preference for cold and aversion to heat, which belongs to a heat pattern but has the differentiation of deficiency or excess.

G. Heavy pain:
This pain is with a heavy sensation and usually due to dampness blocking and stagnating qi movement.

H. Migratory pain:
The area of pain is not fixed; the trend is for it to migrate. It is usually due to stagnation of qi or a *bì* pattern caused by wind-damp.

I. Fixed pain:
The area of pain is fixed, which is usually due to blood stasis or a *bì* pattern caused by cold-damp.

J. Pulling pain:
This pain radiates out to other locations of the body and is due to malnutrition or blockage of the channels, it mostly indicates liver disease.

K. Empty pain:
The pain is with a vacuity sensation and is usually due to deficiency of qi, blood and essence, malnutrition of tissues and organs.

L. Aching pain:
The pain is with an achy sensation and mostly due to a damp pathogen or kidney deficiency.

Differentiation between excessive pain and deficient pain:
① Excessive pain:
Excessive pain mostly belongs to new disease and the pain is severe, persistent, without relief, and aggravated by pressure.

② Deficient pain:
Deficient pain usually belongs to chronic disease and the pain is mild, intermittent, and able to be relieved and alleviated by pressure.

2. Inquiring into the position of pain

Clinical significance of the pain in different locations is a means to distinguish the diseases of the channels of the *zang-fu* organs according to the different locations of the pain.

A. Headache:

There are many reasons for headache; whether there is external invasion or internal damage, deficiency or excess patterns, is irrelevant as all these can lead to headache. By considering the integration of the concrete location of the headache, and the circulating locations in the channels and collaterals, the practitioner can define exactly which channel the headache belongs to.
   a. Headache connects with neck ache; this belongs to the *taiyang* channel headache.
   b. Pain appears on the both sides of the head; this indicates the *shaoyang* channel headache.
   c. Pain appears on the forehead and supra-orbital bone; this is a problem related to the *yangming* channel headache.
   d. Pain appears on the vertex; this indicates the *jueyin* channel headache.
   e. Headache connected to the teeth; this belongs to the *shaoyin* channel headache.
   f. Headache with vertigo and a heavy head, diarrhoea, spontaneous sweating; this belongs to the *taiyin* spleen channel headache.
   g. Headache that connects to the neck and is more severe in the wind; this is a wind-cold headache.
   h. Headache and fear of heat with a red face and eyes; this is a wind-heat headache.
   i. Headache just like the head being wrapped up by a cloth, encumbered and heavy feelings of the four limbs and body; this is a wind-damp headache.
   j. Perpetual headache, which is severe when tired; this is due to qi deficiency.
   k. Headache with dizziness, pale complexion; this is due to blood deficiency.
   l. The head has an empty pain and is accompanied by a weak aching lumbus and knees; this belongs to kidney deficiency.
B. Chest pain:
Chest pain is mostly due to heart and lung diseases.
   a. Precordial pain or the pain that radiates to the medial side of the arm indicates a heart problem - chest *bì*.
   b. Severe chest and back pain accompanied by a blue-grey complexion, cold hands and feet; this is called real heart pain.
   c. Chest pain accompanied by high fever, a red complexion, hasty panting, flaring nostrils; this indicates the pattern of excess heat in the lung.
   d. Chest pain accompanied by tidal fever, night sweats, and small quantities of blood-flecked phlegm; this indicates lung yin deficiency.
   e. Chest pain with fever, purulent and bloody phlegm with a putrid smell; this is called a lung abscess.
   f. Chest distending and scurrying pain with sighing, irascibility, is due to qi stagnation.
C. Hypochondriac pain:
This is usually due to liver and gallbladder diseases.
   a. Hypochondriac distending pain with sighing, irascibility, is due to constraint of liver qi, oppression of emotions.
   b. Hypochondriac burning pain with red complexion and eyes, is caused by excess gallbladder fire.
   c. Hypochondriac distending pain with a yellow body and eyes, is called jaundice.
   d. Hypochondriac stabbing and fixed pain, is due to blood stasis.

e. Hypochondriac pain with the morbid side inter-costal area feeling full, and there is pain with coughing and spitting, is called pleural rheum.

D. Epigastric pain (Upper abdominal pain):

This is usually due to stomach problems.

    a. Alleviation of the pain after eating indicates a deficiency pattern.
    b. Aggravation of the pain after eating indicates an excess pattern.
    c. Epigastric cold pain that is relieved by warming is due to pathogenic cold invading the stomach.
    d. Epigastric burning pain, swift digestion with rapid hunger again soon after eating, halitosis and constipation, is caused by intense stomach fire.
    e. Epigastric distending pain, belching, severe pain after suppressed anger, is due to qi stagnation of the stomach.
    f. Epigastric stabbing and fixed pain, is caused by static blood.
    g. Epigastric dull pain that likes warmth and pressure, vomiting clear water, indicates stomach yang deficiency.
    h. Epigastric burning pain and upset, hunger with no desire to eat, red tongue with lack of coating, indicates stomach yin deficiency.
    i. Severe, unusual and constant epigastric pain may possibly be due to stomach cancer.

E. Abdominal pain:

According to the position of the abdominal pain, the practitioner can examine the pathological changes belonging to different *zang-fu* organs. Combining the nature of pain and accompanying symptoms, the practitioner can understand the reason for the pain and differentiate the deficiency or excess of the disease.

Above the umbilicus is called the greater abdomen, which belongs to the spleen and stomach. Under the umbilicus and above the pubis is called the lower abdomen, which belongs to the kidneys, bladder, large and small intestines, and uterus. The lateral aspects of the lower abdomen are the lesser abdomen, which belongs to the foot *jueyin* liver channel.

    a. Greater abdominal dull pain that likes warmth and pressure, poor appetite and digestion, and loose stool, indicates deficient cold of the spleen and stomach.
    b. Greater abdominal distending pain, and inhibited urination, indicates bladder damp-heat.
    c. Lesser abdominal cold pain and drawing in of the external genitalia is due to cold congealing in the liver channel.
    d. Pain around the umbilicus and accompanied by a bump which moves as it is being pressed, is due to worm accumulation.
    e. Lower abdominal distending or stabbing pain, occurs during the menses, and is mostly due to qi stagnation and blood stasis in the uterus.
    f. Lesser abdominal pain, tenesmus (desire to pass stool) and pain relieved by diarrhoea, is usually caused by qi stagnation in the intestines.

F. Backache:

The foot *taiyang* bladder channel and *du mai* pass through the back. The back of both shoulders have the three yang channels of the hand, so backache is often related with these channels.

    a. Spine pain and inability to bend is usually due to damage of the *du mai*.

    b. Backache connecting to the neck is often caused by wind-cold intruding into the acupuncture points of the *taiyang* channel.
    c. Pain of the shoulders and back are mostly due to obstruction and stagnation of wind, cold and dampness and then channel qi disturbance.
G. Lumbago:
Lumbago belongs to kidney disease.
    a. The lumbar region is often flaccid soft and painful, which is usually due to kidney deficiency.
    b. Lumbar cold and heavy pain indicates cold-damp.
    c. Lumbar and spinal pain connecting downwards to the lower limbs, is due to obstruction and stagnation of the channels and collaterals.
    d. Sudden lumbago, which radiates to the lesser abdomen, plus haematuria, is mostly caused by stagnation of calculus (stones).
    e. Lumbago just like a needle stabbing, fixed and refuses pressure, indicates blood stasis.
    f. Lumbago, which connects to the abdomen, circling the waist like a girdle, is due to damage of the *dai mai* (带脉).
H. Pain of the limbs:
Pain of the limbs is often caused by attacks of wind, cold and dampness, or accumulating and binding of damp and heat, qi and blood obstruction and stagnation, or deficiency and damage of the spleen and stomach.
    a. The pain in the joints and muscles of the four limbs is usually seen in *bì*, this is caused by wind, cold, damp and heat.
    b. Pain of the limbs accompanied by lack of strength is often due to spleen and stomach deficiency-detriment.
    c. Aching pain of the heels or tibias and knees is usually due to kidney deficiency.
I. General pain:
Pain of the head, body, waist, back and four limbs can be caused by excess or deficiency patterns.
    a. General pain in new onset disease is usually due to an excess pattern.
    b. General pain in prolonged disease is often due to a deficiency of both qi and blood, malnutrition of the channels.
Inquiring about the position of the pain can only help the practitioner understand where the pain is located; but inquiring about the nature of the pain can help distinguish cold and heat or deficiency and excess patterns; therefore combining both position and nature can help to analyse and distinguish the pathogenic conditions.

Inquiring into the Head, Body, Chest and Abdomen

The range of queries for inquiring about the head, body, chest and abdomen apart from pain, should also include inquiring about other discomforts, such as vertigo, palpitations, gastric stuffiness, chest distress, hypochondriac distension, abdominal distension, heaviness of the body, numbness, etc.

1. Vertigo
Vertigo means that the patient feels subjectively his (or her) body or the things in view

are swirling. The practitioner should ask about the presence or absence of other symptoms, and also ask about initiating causes, predisposing factors, and aggravating factors connected to the patient's vertigo.

A. Vertigo accompanied by distension, restlessness and irritability, red tongue and rapid wiry pulse. This indicates liver fire flaming upward, which is due to fire and heat attacking the head and eyes along the channel, qi and blood rushing forth into the channels.

B. Vertigo accompanied by distending pain, tinnitus, aching and weakness of the lumbar region and knees, red tongue and lack of coating, thready wiry pulse, inclination to become angry, indicates hyperactivity of liver yang. This is due to yin deficiency of the liver and kidney, liver yang rising and troubling the upper orifices.

C. Vertigo accompanied by a pale face, a tired spirit and body, a pale tongue, thready pulse, intensified when tired, indicates deficiency of qi and blood. This is due to malnutrition of *ying*-blood, or non-ascending of clear yang.

D. Vertigo accompanied by a heavy sensation in the head, which feels like the head is wrapped in a cloth, chest distress and vomiting, white and greasy coating, indicates internal obstruction of phlegm-dampness. This is due to internal obstruction of phlegm-dampness, non-ascending of clear yang.

E. Vertigo accompanied by stabbing pain after external damage, indicates obstruction and stagnation of static blood. This is due to blockage and blood stasis obstructing the brain vessels.

2. Chest distress

Chest distress refers to a subjective sensation of discomfort and fullness in the chest.

This symptom is closely related to the non-smooth flow of the heart and lung qi.

A. Chest distress, hypochondriac distension, sighing, indicate accumulation and stagnation of liver qi.

B. Chest distress, shortness of breath, and palpitations, indicate deficiency of heart qi, devitalised heart yang.

C. Chest distress accompanied by stabbing pain indicate stasis and blockage of heart blood.

D. Chest distress and profuse sputum, indicate the lung is obstructed by phlegm-dampness.

E. Chest distress, high fever, flaring nostrils, indicate a heat pathogen or phlegm-heat obstructing the lung.

F. Chest distress, laboured breathing, fear of the cold and with cold limbs, indicate a cold pathogen intruding into the lung.

G. Chest distress, laboured breathing, shortness of breath, may be due to lung qi deficiency or qi deficiency of the lung and kidney.

3. Palpitations

Palpitations are a symptom, which is experienced as an awareness of, or flustered heartbeat even unable to work independently. Palpitations can include palpitations due to fright and severe palpitations, which usually are a sign of heart or heart-spirit disorders. Usually palpitations due to fright can lead to severe palpitations.

When inquiring into palpitations, the practitioner should pay attention to the degree,

characteristics and accompanying symptoms of the palpitations.
   A. Palpitations due to fright:
   This is caused by fright and accompanied by restlessness and the timing is intermittent, which means a mild condition of the whole body with a good prognosis.
   B. Severe palpitations:
   This has no obvious outside inducement, it just appears as an excessively rapid heartbeat from the chest to the navel and it is of a longer duration. It indicates a serious condition of the whole body with a poor prognosis.

   4. **Hypochondriac distension, stomach cavity pǐ, abdominal distension, heaviness of the body, numbness, lack of strength**
   A. Hypochondriac distension:
   This refers to distension and discomfort over one side or both sides of the hypochondrium, which indicates pathogenic changes of the liver and gallbladder.
      a. Hypochondriac distension with propensity to anger is usually due to emotional upsets and stagnation of the liver.
      b. Hypochondriac distension with bitter taste in the mouth and yellowish greasy tongue coating is usually caused by damp heat in the liver and gallbladder.
      c. Hypochondriac distension with inter-costal fullness, coughing and spitting that induces pain, is mostly due to fluid retention in the chest and hypochondrium.
   B. Stomach cavity pǐ:
   This refers to a feeling of oppression and discomfort in the gastric area, which indicates pathogenic changes of the spleen and stomach.
      a. Stomach cavity pǐ with putrid belching and acid regurgitation is often due to the stomach being damaged by eating.
      b. Stomach cavity pǐ with diminished appetite and loose stool is usually caused by deficiency or weakness of the spleen and stomach.
   C. Abdominal distension:
   This refers to a subjective sensation of distension and discomfort in the abdomen, which usually indicates disturbances of the spleen, stomach, intestines, liver or kidneys.
      a. Abdominal distension with "no pain on pressure" refers to a deficiency pattern, which usually results from deficiency of the spleen and stomach unable to perform transportation and transformation.
      b. Abdominal distension with "pain on pressure" refers to an excess pattern, which usually results from retention of food in the stomach and intestines or internal retention of excessive heat, all of which obstruct the circulation of qi.
      c. Abdominal distension like a drum accompanied by a yellow skin colour and pale bulging veins on the abdominal wall, is a sign of tympanites (swelling of the abdomen with gaseous or liqueous fluids). This is due to malfunction of the liver, spleen and kidney, and then qi, blood and water gathered in the abdomen.
   D. Heaviness of the body:
   This refers to the heavy, aching and lethargic sensation of the patient's body, which is mostly related to dampness attacking or pathogenic changes of the lung, spleen and kidneys.
      a. Heaviness of the body with oedema is usually due to invasion of pathogenic

wind, contention between wind and water.
   b. Heaviness of the body with spiritual lassitude and shortness of breath is usually due to deficiency and weakness of the spleen qi.
E. Numbness:

This refers to partial or total lack of sensation in a part of the body, which usually is due to deficiency of qi and blood, internal disturbance of liver wind or damp-phlegm and static blood obstructing the channels.

F. Lack of strength:

This refers to a sense of fatigued limbs with forceless movement, which is usually seen in deficient patterns of the spleen, stomach, lung or liver, etc.

Inquiring into the Ears and Eyes

Inquiring into the condition of the ears and eyes can help one understand the local changes of the ears and eyes and also the disturbances of *zang-fu* organs such as liver, gallbladder, kidneys and *sanjiao*.

1. Inquiring into the ears

A. Tinnitus:

This refers to an awareness of noise in the ears, such as ringing, buzzing, roaring or clicking, which is without an external stimulus and obstructs the hearing.
   a. Severe and sudden tinnitus like the noise made by a frog or the tide, is unable to be reduced by pressure, mostly belongs to an excess pattern, such as exuberant liver and gallbladder fire disturbing the upper orifices.
   b. Low and gradual tinnitus like the chirping of a cicada, is able to be reduced or stopped by pressure, mostly belongs to a deficiency pattern, such as liver and kidney yin deficiency or insufficiency of the spinal marrow due to kidney essence deficiency.

B. Deafness:

This refers to the lack or loss, complete or partial, of the sense of hearing.
   a. Sudden deafness in new disease mostly belongs to an excess pattern, which is usually caused by liver and gallbladder fire flaring up and congesting the ears or a warm-heat pathogen accumulated in the upper *jiao* and confusing the orifices.
   b. Gradual deafness in chronic disease mostly belongs to a deficiency pattern, which is usually caused by deficiency and failure of the kidney essence qi and thus inability to hear.

C. Hearing impairment:

This means diminution of hearing, unclear hearing or duplicated hearing.
   a. Sudden hearing impairment mostly belongs to an excess pattern, which is usually caused by phlegmatic turbidity or a wind pathogen attacking upward and obstructing the ears.
   b. Gradual hearing impairment mostly belongs to a deficiency pattern, which is usually caused by deficiency and failure of the kidney essence qi, resulting in malnutrition of the ear orifices.

2. Inquiring into the eyes
A. Itchy eyes:
This means an itching sensation in the eyelid, canthus or pupil of the eyes. It can be eased by light rubbing in mild cases, but can be unbearable in severe cases.
   a. Severe itching mostly belongs to an excess pattern.
   b. Mild itching mostly belongs to a deficiency pattern, such as blood deficiency, malnutrition of the eyes.
   c. Itchy eyes just like a worm creeping on it and accompanied by photophobia, dacryorrhoea (excessive tears), and a heat feeling, which is due to wind-fire of the liver channel harassing the upper body.

B. Eye pain:
This means pain in one or both eyes.
   a. Severe eye pain usually belongs to an excess pattern.
   b. Mild eye pain usually belongs to a deficiency pattern.
   c. Unbearable, severe eye pain with red face and eyes, is due to liver fire flaming upward.
   d. Red, swollen and painful eyes with photophobia, lots of eye discharge, is due to wind-heat attacking upward.
   e. Mild pain and redness of the eyes, dryness, occasional pain or not, is caused by vigourous empty fire due to yin deficiency.

C. Dizzy vision:
This is a sensation of unsteadiness or disequilibrium, which is just as if sitting in a boat or car, or having mosquitoes and flies flying in front of the eyes.
   a. Dizzy vision accompanied by a red face, headache, distension of the head, and heaviness of the head, mostly belongs to an excess pattern caused by wind-fire attacking the upper orifices or damp-phlegm confusing the upper orifices.
   b. Dizzy vision accompanied by a tired mind, vertigo, dizziness and tinnitus, mostly belongs to a deficiency pattern caused by sinking of the middle qi and non-ascending of the clear yang or shortage of essence and blood due to deficiency of the liver and kidney.

D. Blurred vision:
This means unclear sight.

E. Sparrow vision (night blindness)
This means the sight is normal in the daylight but unclear in the evening, just like the birds' eyesight.

F. Diplopia:
This appears as the perception of two images of a single object.

The three pathological changes above are different degrees of decreasing eyesight, which have different characteristics but similar aetiology and pathogenesis. They usually are caused by deficiency of the liver and kidneys, shortage of the essence and blood, resulting in malnutrition of the eyes. This progression is commonly seen in prolonged disease or in elderly people.

Inquiring into Sleep

Sleep has a close relation with the circulation of the *wei* (defensive) qi, exuberance or decline of the yin and yang, excess or deficiency of the qi and blood, and functions of the heart and kidney.

The *wei* qi transmits in the yang in the daytime and in the yin at night. When the *wei* qi is transmitting from yang into yin, the person will go to sleep. On the other hand, when it is transmitting from yin into yang, the person will wake up. This is the relationship between sleep and movement of the *wei* qi.

> **Main points of inquiring into sleep:**
> Long or short duration of the time in bed, difficult or ease of falling asleep, whether or not restless sleep, or profuse dreaming and accompanying symptoms, etc.
> By inquiring into sleep, the practitioner can understand exuberance or debilitation of yin, yang, qi and blood, strength or weakness of the foundations of the heart and kidney.

The common abnormal sleep concerns seen in clinic are insomnia and somnolence.

1. Insomnia

This is characterised by difficulty in sleeping, or waking up easily and difficulty in falling asleep again, or shallow sleep, or easily disturbed sleep, or even unable to sleep all night.

The forming mechanism of insomnia is yin deficiency and yang exuberance, failure of yang transmitting into yin and failure of the spirit to keep to its abode.

There are two kinds of aetiology of insomnia. One belongs to a deficiency pattern, which includes deficiency of *ying*-blood, malnutrition of the heart spirit or yin deficiency resulting in vigourous fire, internal harassment of heart spirit or qi deficiency of the heart and gallbladder, a restless heart spirit, etc. The other belongs to an excess pattern, which includes pathogens harassing the interior and results in a restless spirit, such as phlegm-heat harassing the heart spirit upward or food stagnation stomach disharmony leading to restless sleep, and so on.

2. Somnolence

This refers to sleeping in both daytime and night, closing the eyes and sleeping while sitting or lying. It is usually due to internal exuberance of phlegm-heat or deficient yang and exuberant yin, and then yang unable to come out of yin.

There are three kinds of aetiology of somnolence.

A. Somnolence accompanied by lassitude, heaviness of the head, eyes and limbs, oppression and fullness of the chest, which is usually caused by phlegm-dampness disturbing the spleen and failure of clear yang to rise.

B. Postprandial somnolence (somnolence following a meal), which is accompanied by spirit-lassitude, poor appetite and indigestion, is often due to insufficiency of stomach-spleen qi and failure of the spleen to transform and transport.

C. Extreme spirit-lassitude and somnolence as if sleeping but not sleeping due to yang deficiency of the heart and kidneys, internal exuberance of yin cold.

Inquiring into Diet and Partiality

Inquiring into diet and partiality refer to asking the pathological conditions of thirst, drinking, eating, etc.

Inquiring into the quality of the diet can help the practitioner understand the strength or weakness of the spleen and stomach and exuberance or decline of the fluid. Inquiring into the likes or dislikes or of partiality can help the practitioner understand deficiency or excess of the *zang-fu* organs.

1. Thirst and drinking

Thirst means the sensation of dryness in the mouth and being thirsty. Drinking refers to the qualities and quantity of water drunk. Thirst and drinking reflects exuberance or debilitation and transforming or distributing of the internal fluid.

A. Absence of thirst:

Absence of thirst means the body fluid is intact. It appears as absence of thirst and no desire to drink. It is mostly seen in a cold pattern and dampness patterns. It also can be seen in the manifestations of a pattern with no obvious dry-heat symptoms.

B. Thirst:
   a. Thirst with desire to drink water:
      This means consumption of body fluid, often seen in a dryness pattern and a heat pattern.
      ① Dry mouth with mild thirst accompanied by feverishness, slight aversion to wind-cold, swelling and pain of the throat, which can be seen in the initial stage of invasion by external warm-heat, and belongs to mild damage of the body fluid.
      ② Extreme thirst with preference for cold drinks accompanied by a reddish complexion, sweating, a large and rapid pulse, is probably due to excessive internal heat, extreme damage of the body fluid.
      ③ Thirst with much drinking of water, accompanied by polyphagia (a great desire for food), profuse urination and gradual emaciation, which is called *xiāo kě* (wasting-thirst), caused by kidney deficiency, where water fails in converting into body fluids.
      ④ Vomiting and then thirst with a desire to drink water, which is the manifestation of damage to the body fluid and hence the patient drinks water for self-care.
   b. Thirst without desire to drink:
      This is often due to abnormal transformation and distribution of the fluid, water and fluid being unable to be transported upward. It also can be caused by pathogenic heat entering the *ying* (nutrient-blood) and steaming *ying*-yin bearing upward.
      ① Thirst with preference for hot drinks but without much drinking, which may be caused by internal retention of phlegm-rheum or deficiency of yang and failure of the body fluid to flow and spread.
      ② Thirst without a desire to drink accompanied by unsurfaced fever, heaviness of the body and head, epigastric oppression and a yellow greasy coating, which is usually seen in a damp-heat pattern.
      ③ Thirst with a desire to drink water at first, and then vomiting or immediate vomiting after drinking, both of which belong to a water counterflow pattern,

which is due to retention of water in the stomach.
④ Dry mouth with a desire to gargle but without a desire to drink water, which indicates there is blood stasis in the body.
⑤ Reduced thirst and less desire to drink water, which is mostly seen in the pattern of the *ying* (nutrient) stage of warm disease.

2. Appetite and quantity of food

Appetite means an instinctive physical desire for food and an enjoyment sensation of taking food. Quantity of food just refers to the actual quantity of food eaten.

By inquiring about the appetite and quantity of food eaten, the practitioner can judge the function of the spleen and stomach as well as the prognosis of the disease.

A. Decreased appetite:

Decreased appetite includes three aspects, no desire to eat, diminished appetite, poor appetite and digestion.

No desire to eat also is called poor appetite. Diminished appetite means the quantity of food is diminished, it is often due to no desire to eat. Poor appetite and digestion refers to no sense of hunger and refusing the request to take food, even anorexia.

   a. New disease with decreased appetite is often a kind of protective reaction by *zheng* (healthy) qi resisting pathogenic qi. It belongs to mild disease and with good prognosis.
   b. Enduring illness with decreased appetite and accompanied by spiritual lassitude, sallow yellow complexion, pale tongue and weak pulse, this often belongs to deficiency and weakness of the spleen and stomach.
   c. Poor appetite and indigestion accompanied by a heavy sensation of the head and body, distending oppression of the gastric area and abdomen, thick and greasy coating, which is mostly due to exuberant dampness encumbering the spleen or stagnation of food and drink, failure of the spleen to transport.

B. Aversion to food (anorexia):

Anorexia means a patient dislikes food or has an aversion to the smell of food.

   a. Anorexia accompanied by acid regurgitation, distending fullness of the gastric area and abdomen, is mostly due to dietary irregularities, retention of food in the stomach.
   b. Aversion to fatty diet accompanied by chest distress and vomiting, distending fullness of the gastric area and abdomen, which usually belongs to damp-heat of the spleen and stomach.
   c. Aversion to a fatty and rich diet accompanied by distending pain and scorching sensation of the hypochondrium, with body heat trapped inside, which may be caused by damp-heat in the liver and gallbladder.
   d. Anorexia in the gravida (pregnant woman) belongs to a pregnancy reaction; it usually results from physiological changes.

C. Swift digestion with rapid hungering:

This means excessive appetite, hungry not long after eating when a huge quantity of food has been eaten. It is due to intense stomach heat with consequent excessive decomposition of the food.

   a. Swift digestion with rapid hungering, emaciation, polydipsia (excessive thirst),

polyuria, which can be seen in *xiāo kě* (wasting-thirst).
  b. Swift digestion with rapid hungering, sloppy diarrhoea, which belongs to a strong stomach and weak spleen.
D. Hungry but no desire to eat:
This means the patient feels hungry but has no desire to eat or eats less than normal, which may be caused by stomach yin deficiency, deficiency-fire harassing the interior.
E. Pica:
An abnormal craving or appetite for non-food substances such as raw rice, clay, paper, etc. It is usually seen in children, and mostly indicates a worm accumulation pattern.
F. Food predilection:
  a. The patient likes to eat fatty food after which it is easy to produce phlegm.
  b. The patient likes to eat raw and cold foods after which this then easily damages the spleen and stomach.
  c. Excessive consumption of hot-spicy acrid foods easily produces dry-heat in the body.
  d. The gravida (pregnant woman) who likes to eat acidic and spicy foods in the progress of pregnancy; this does not belong to an abnormal state.
G. Eliminated centre:
In a prolonged and serious illness when there is a long period of forcing food or an inability to eat, suddenly the patient has a thought of food, even asking for food or overeating, this is the eliminated centre pattern of the spleen and stomach qi. This kind of sudden temporary improvement, which is not in accordance with the synchronous alleviation of the pathological conditions, is a false manifestation of vitality, indicating that the patient is on the brink of death.
H. Changes in the quantity of food:
  a. The appetite is recovering and the quantity of food increases gradually in the stage of disease. This indicates that the stomach qi is recovering gradually and the disease will be cured.
  b. The appetite is lost and the quantity of food decreased gradually in the later stages of disease. This suggests severe disease, functional failure of the spleen and stomach.

3. Taste

Taste refers to an abnormal taste sensation or smell in the mouth. Abnormal taste reflects disorder of the spleen and stomach function and the pathological changes of other *zang-fu* organs.
A. Bland taste:
The characteristics of this are tastelessness in the mouth and diminished ability of the tongue to taste things. It is usually seen in a cold pattern or qi deficiency of the spleen and stomach.
B. Sweet taste:
This means the patient's awareness of a sweet taste in the mouth. This mostly belongs to damp-heat of the spleen and stomach or spleen deficiency.
C. Sour taste:
The patient has a sour taste in the mouth or there is an acid and putrid decomposing

smell that can be smelled by others. This is usually due to dyspepsia of the spleen and stomach, or liver and stomach disharmony, or impaired harmonious down-bearing of the stomach.

D. Bitter taste:

The patient experiences bitterness in the mouth, which is often seen in vigourous flaring of liver-gallbladder fire or internal accumulation of damp-heat due to upward reverse flow of gallbladder qi.

E. Acerbic taste:

There is an acerbic taste in the mouth just like eating a raw persimmon. This is due to dry-heat damaging the fluid or exuberant yang and heat of the *zang-fu* organs, upward counterflow of qi and fire.

F. Salty taste:

There is a salty taste in the patient's mouth, which means kidney deficiency and cold-water flooding upward.

G. Greasy taste:

The patient feels greasiness and discomfort in the mouth, which is caused by retention and stagnation of damp-turbidity, phlegm-rheum, food stagnation, etc.

Inquiring into the Urine and Stool

The excretion of stool is related to conduction and transmission of the large intestine, transportation and transformation of the spleen and stomach, free flow of qi by the liver, warming of the *mingmen* (gate of vitality), purification and descent of lung qi, etc.

The excretion of urine is related to kidneys and bladder qi transformation, transformation and transfusion of the spleen, purification and descent of the lung, free flow and regulation of the *san jiao*, etc.

Through inquiry as to the condition of the urine and stool, the practitioner can not only understand the function of digestion and water metabolism, but also the important evidence in judging the cold or heat, deficiency or excess of the disease.

On inquiring about urine and stool one should pay attention to their characteristics, colour, smell, time, quantity, frequency, sensation and accompanying symptoms, etc. The colour and smell have been discussed in the inspection method and smelling method. The characteristics, time, quantity and sensation will be introduced in detail below.

1. Stool

The stool of adults generally moves once a day, is shaped and excreted smoothly; it is neither dry nor damp, mostly yellowish, with neither pus nor blood, without mucus or undigested foods, etc.

    A. Abnormal frequency of defaecation:

        a. Constipation:

Desiccated and hard stool accompanied by difficulty in defaecation or long intervals between stool movements (once only in several days). It is usually due to retention of heat in the intestines or deficiency of fluid or insufficiency of yin-blood, or qi deficiency and weakness or yang deficiency and cold congealing.

        b. Diarrhoea:

Diarrhoea refers to loose, watery and frequent discharge of stool. It mostly

belongs to damp-heat in the large intestine or food stagnation in the stomach and intestines, or deficient-cold of the spleen and stomach, or kidney deficiency and decline in the *mingmen* fire.
B. Abnormal texture of stool:
   a. Undigested food in the stool:
      There are often a lot of undigested food remnants in the stool. It is usually due to deficient cold of the spleen and stomach or kidney deficiency and decline in the *mingmen* fire.
   b. Alternating loose and dry stool:
      The intermittent dry and loose stool indicates hyperactive liver qi and spleen deficiency, disharmony between the liver and spleen. If loose stool is followed by dry faeces, it indicates deficiency and weakness of the spleen and stomach.
   c. Purulent stool with blood:
      Stool mingled with pus, blood and mucus, which is usually seen in dysentery.
   d. Stool with blood:
      The blood outflows from the anus, stool with blood includes faeces mixed with blood or bleeding after defaecation, or both (it can be distinguished as distal bleeding and proximal bleeding depending on colour, the darker the colour, the further up the digestive tract, the origin). Stool with blood present is mostly caused by damaged vessels of the stomach and intestines.
C. Abnormal sensation on defaecation:
   a. Scorching sensation at the anus:
      There is a scorching sensation at the anus when defaecating, which can be seen in diarrhoea due to heat or dysentery due to damp-heat.
   b. Tenesmus:
      Abdominal pains with frequent desire to defaecate, a sensation of anal prolapse and obstructed defaecation; which are some of the main symptoms of dysentery.
   c. Sensation of incomplete defaecation:
      This means lack of smoothness of defaecation and has the sensation of being stagnated and difficult to pass.
      ① Difficult and astringent sensation on defaecation accompanied by abdominal pain, yellow and sticky diarrhoea, superficial ulcerations may be the cause of local pain; all of which belong to accumulation and stagnation of damp-heat.
      ② Abdominal pain, diarrhoea, sensation of incomplete defaecation, abdominal distension, flatus, which indicates hyperactive liver qi attacking the spleen.
      ③ A sensation of incomplete defaecation mixed undigested foods with sour and rotten odours, abdominal pain being released after diarrhoea, which is called diarrhoea due to indigestion.
   d. Incontinent diarrhoea:
      Faecal incontinence (inability to control the passage of stool) is due to deficiency and failure of the spleen and kidneys.
   e. Qi prolapse of the anus:
      Sensation of anal prolapse or even actual prolapse of the anus, which is due to deficiency of the spleen and sinking of the middle qi which is itself caused by chronic diarrhoea or prolonged dysentery.

2. Urine

The healthy adult generally urinates three to five times in the daytime and up to once at night. The total quantity of urine is about 1000~2000 ml in twenty-four hours. The frequency and quantity of urine are influenced by factors such as quantity of drinking, air temperature, sweating, age, and so on.

A. Abnormal volume of urine:
   a. Profuse urine:
      This means the frequency and quantity of the urine is obviously more than the normal, which indicates a deficient cold pattern. It also can be seen in *xiāo kě* (wasting-thirst).
   b. Scanty urine:
      This means the frequency and quantity of the urine is obviously less than the normal, which can be seen in all kinds of heat patterns or oedema.

B. Abnormal frequency of urine:
   a. Frequent urination:
      This means the frequency of urinating has increased or the desire to urinate at regular intervals.
      If the frequent urination presents with brownish scanty urine with urgency, this is usually due to damp-heat in the lower *jiao*. If the frequent urination presents with a large volume of clear urine, especially at night, this is usually due to deficiency of kidney yang or failure of kidney qi to control water.
   b. Dribbling urinary block:
      Difficulty in micturition or dripping discharge is known as dysuria; blockage of urine is called anuria; mixed dripping and blockage is called dribbling urinary block.
      The dribbling urinary block which belongs to a deficiency pattern is mostly due to qi deficiency or yang deficiency, disturbance of qi transformation, disturbance of opening and closing.
      The dribbling urinary block which belongs to an excess pattern is mostly due to stagnation of excessive pathogens such as static blood, calculus or damp-heat, leading to disturbance of bladder qi transformation.

C. Abnormal sensation of urination:
   a. Difficult and painful urination:
      This means a lack of smoothness and pain of urination or urination accompanied by a sensation of urgency, scorching heat, etc., which is mostly due to damp-heat pouring downward.
   b. Dribbling urination:
      This means dribbling after voiding.
   c. Urinary incontinence:
      The patient has an inability to control the voiding of urine and involuntary discharge of urine occurs.
   d. Enuresis:
      The adult or child over three years old cannot control the discharge of urine when sleeping.
      All three above usually belong to kidney qi insecurity, deficiency and cold of the

lower *jiao*, and bladder failing to ensure retention.

Inquiring into Menstruation and Vaginal Discharge

The inquiry of women should pay attention to conditions relating to menses, vaginal discharge, pregnancy, childbirth, lactation, etc.

The female patient should be asked about abnormal conditions of menses and vaginal discharge particularly if the disease is not in the stage of pregnancy, childbirth or lactation, which can be used as evidence in diagnosing gynaecological or other diseases. The pregnancy, childbirth and lactation history may already have been covered as general contents of personal life history.

1. Menstruation

Menstruation means organised and intermittent uterine bleeding. It is a permanent cycle once a month. The initial arrival of the menses of a healthy girl is called menarche, usually at about fourteen years old, till about forty-nine years old, when the menses will stop, which is called menopause. The cycle of menses is about twenty-eight days and the menstrual period is three to five days. The menstrual volume is variable, the colour of menses is bright red; the menstrual discharge is neither too thin nor too viscous and there may be small simple blood clots, which do not contain any other matter.

Inquiring about menstruation, should pay attention to understanding the cycle, times of day, quality, colour, properties of the discharge, whether menstrual block and abdominal pain occur during menstruation or not, the ages of menarche and menopause, the last occurrence of the menses, etc. By inquiring about the menses, the practitioner can assist diagnosing the functions of the liver, spleen, kidneys, uterus, *chong mai* and *ren mai* and exuberance or debilitation of qi and blood.

A. Abnormal menstrual cycle:
   a. Early menstruation:
      This means menstruation occurs over seven days in advance, which is due to qi deficiency or blood heat.
   b. Delayed menstruation:
      This means menstruation occurs up to seven days later than usual. If it is a deficiency pattern, it mostly due to *ying*-blood depletion or debilitation of yang. If it is an excess pattern, it is mostly due to qi stagnation and blood stasis or cold congealing and blood stasis.
   c. Irregular menstrual cycle:
      This means menses that arrives at irregular times, sometimes early and sometimes late. If it is a deficiency pattern, it is mostly due to spleen and kidney depletion. If it is an excess pattern, it is mostly due to liver qi stagnation or static blood accumulation and stagnation.
B. Abnormal amount of menstrual flow:
   a. Hypomenorrhoea:
      The menstrual cycle is normal, but there is a diminution of the flow or a shortening of the duration of menstruation. If it is a deficiency pattern, it is caused by shortage of the *ying*-blood, deficiency of kidney qi. If it is an excess pattern it is caused by cold congealing, blood stasis, blockage of phlegm-damp.

b. Amenorrhoea:
   This occurs when the girl, over eighteen years old, has not had menarche or has had an absence or abnormal stoppage of the menses for more than three months without pregnancy or lactation. The stoppage of menses is the physiological manifestation in the gestational period, lactation and menopause. If a girl has stopped menses, every now and then, in the two years of menarche and without other discomfort, it also does not belong to amenorrhoea.
   The deficiency pattern of this is usually due to spleen and kidneys depletion, insufficiency of liver and kidney, deficiency of qi and blood. The excess pattern of this is often due to stagnation of qi and blood stasis, cold congealing and obstruction of phlegm.
c. Hypermenorrhoea:
   The menstrual cycle is normal, but the amount of menstrual flow is obviously more than usual, which is due to blood heat or qi deficiency, blockage of phlegm-damp.
d. Flooding and spotting:
   This refers to the vaginal blood flow during the menstrual period, flooding is with rapid force, large amount of menses, spotting is with slow force and small amount of menses. They are both due to heat damaging the *chong mai* and *ren mai*, blood stasis blocking the *chong mai* and *ren mai*, or qi deficiency of the spleen and kidneys, insufficiency of kidney yin, etc.

C. Abnormal colour and texture of menstrual flow:
  a. Pale and thin menstrual flow indicates blood deficiency.
  b. Brownish and thick menstrual flow suggests exuberant heat in the blood.
  c. Purplish menstrual flow with blood clots indicates cold congealing and blood stasis.

D. Dysmenorrhoea:

This is a condition marked by lower abdominal pain during menstruation or before and after menstruation. It mostly belongs to qi stagnation, blood stasis, cold congealing, yang deficiency, deficiency of qi and blood. The practitioner should identify them through inquiring about the nature of the pain and accompanying symptoms in clinic.

2. Vaginal discharge

Vaginal discharge refers to a woman's vaginal secretions. The normal vaginal discharge is small in volume, white in colour, without foul smell, which has the function of moistening the vagina.

The pathological vaginal discharge means superabundant vaginal secretions, constant dripping wet or with changes of colour and texture or with foul smell.

A little increase of vaginal discharge is normal before or after menstrual period, or in the ovulation period and gestation period.

Inquiring about the vaginal discharge should focus on the quantity, colour, texture and smell of it.

A. White leucorrhoea:

White leucorrhoea is the vaginal discharge with white colour, large quantity, watery, constant dripping wet, which is mostly due to spleen and kidney yang deficiency, cold-damp pouring down.

B. Yellow leucorrhoea:

This refers to the yellowish, sticky and foul vaginal discharge, which is usually due to damp-heat pouring down.

C. Red-white leucorrhoea:

This means white leucorrhoea mixed with blood, which is caused by stagnated heat in the liver channels or damp-heat pouring down.

Inquiring of Children

In paediatrics, when a child is unable to sufficiently or reliably express itself through language, the practitioner can gain the pathological data by inquiring of the accompanying person.

Children have the physiological characteristics such as tender *zang-fu* organs, an ascending source of vitality, and rapid growth. They also have the pathological characteristics of quick onset of disease, plenty of changes, and easily become deficient or excessive. Therefore, for children, one should ask whether the baby was born in normal labour, and also inquire about the events before and after birth, vaccination, history of infectious disease, and whether the child has been exposed to contagious diseases.

1. The conditions before or after birth

A. Neonates (birth to one month):

Neonates should be asked questions with emphasis on the nutrition and healthy conditions of their mothers in the period of pregnancy, childbearing and lactation, as well as previous diseases, overdosed medicines, whether dystocia (abnormal labour) and premature delivery occurred or not, etc.

Through the above, the practitioner can understand the congenital conditions of the newborn because the diseases of the newborn are mostly related to congenital factors or conditions of parturition.

B. Infant (one month to three years):

Inquiry should pay attention to the infant's feeding method and late or early ability to sit, crawl, stand, walk, speak, and times of tooth eruption etc.

From the above, the practitioner can discouer if the infant's congenital nutrition and growth are appropriate. The infant grows quickly and needs more nutrition than adults, it also has weak function of the spleen and stomach; so, unmerited feeding will result in dystrophy, the five retardations (late in standing, walking, hair-growing, teething, and speaking) and the five kinds of flaccidity (located in head, neck, limbs, muscle, and mouth), etc.

2. The histories of prophylactic immunisation and infectious diseases

With children inquiry should be made about the vaccinations such as chickenpox, measles, as well as ailing or contagious infectious diseases.

It is helpful for a definitive diagnosis, because the child can easily be infected by acute infectious diseases such as polio, chickenpox and measles. The prophylactic immunisation can help the child build its acquired immune function and reduce infectious diseases.

However, some infectious diseases such as measles can give lifelong immunity to the child but there is also a risk e.g. chickenpox and hepatopathy are closely related.

3. The conditions under which it is easy to induce infant disease

Children are easily invaded by exterior pathogens and easily damaged by overindulgence in food and drink, and can easily be frightened, etc.

CHAPTER 6
Pulse Examination

The pulse examination is one of the distinctive diagnostic methods in CM. It can help in measuring the pathological location among *zang-fu* organs' patterns, qi patterns and blood patterns, as well as highlight developing conditions.

The pulse examination has important practical value in clinic. There are different methods for feeling the pulse, among which the *Cùn Kŏu* Diagnostic Method is the most commonly used for pulse examination. First of all, it is essential to grasp the characteristics of the normal pulse perfectly; this gives some hints for discriminating abnormal pulse manifestations. It is also essential to grasp the characteristics and diseases associated with the twenty-eight kinds of pathological pulses. Moreover, if the practitioners can distinguish subtle changes of similar pulses, it will be helpful for coming to a definite diagnosis.

The practitioner should draw conclusions with caution in clinic. Initially grasping the basic skills of pulse examination; next combining this with knowledge of the diseases and patterns; correlating this with the other four examinations; and only then discerning the nature of an illness.

Contents of the pulse examination
Influencing factors.
The pulsation of the heart is the driving force of the pulse condition.
The qi and blood, circulating within the vessels, is the material foundation of the pulse condition.
The five *zang* organs work cooperatively to guarantee a normal pulse condition.
- Regions
    Three positions and nine pulse-takings
    Cùn kŏu examination method
    Examination method at ST 9 (*rén yíng*) and *cùn kŏu*
    Three-section examination method of Zhang Zhong-jing
- Methods
- Normal pulse image
    With stomach qi
    With spirit
    With root
- Abnormal pulse images
    Twenty-eight pulses
    True visceral pulse
- Combined pulses
- Pulses of women and children
- Clinical significance and applications of the pulse examination
    To distinguish the conditions of the disease
    To explain pathogenesis
    To guide the treatment
    To estimate the prognosis

Section 1
Overview of the Pulse Examination

Concept: The pulse examination, also called pulse-reading, means the practitioner uses his/her fingers to press on the patient's artery to understand the pathogenic conditions and distinguish patterns and symptoms according to the images of the pulse.

Principles of the Pulse Examination

The pulse manifestation is the variety of images of the pulse beating in response to the fingers, or it can be explained as the fingers feeling the images of the beating pulse.

As stated previously, the production of the pulse image is directly related to the pulsation of the heart, which is the driving force of the pulse condition; the qi and blood, circulating within the vessels, which is the material foundation of the pulse condition; and the five *zang* organs working cooperatively to guarantee normal pulse conditions. So, the heart and vessels are the main organs forming the pulse image; qi and blood are the material foundation forming the pulse image. Therefore, sufficient heart qi, heart blood, heart yang, heart yin, full vessels and smooth transmission of qi and blood, are the necessary factors in forming the normal pulse condition.

The features of how the other organs influence the generation and movement of the qi and blood and participate in forming the normal pulse condition are as follows:

> Firstly, the lung governs qi and unites all vessels.
> Secondly, the spleen and stomach are the source of production of qi and blood.
> Thirdly, the liver can store blood, and is responsible for regulating the volume of blood and dominating free flow, raising the qi, and maintaining the qi dynamic.
> Finally, the kidneys can store essence and are the root of *yuan* qi.

The Positions of Pulse Examination

1. Three positions and nine pulse-takings method

The three positions and nine pulse-takings method is also called the "General Examination Method". According to the *Yellow Emperor's Inner Classic*, it is divided into the upper (head), centre (hands), lower (feet) portions, each of which is divided into heaven (upper), human (middle) and earth (lower) (Fig. 6-1).

A. Upper portion (head):
 a. Heaven:
 The corresponding channels and points are on the bilateral temporal arteries at *tài yáng* (EX-HN5), relating to the foot *shaoyang* channel. The diagnostic significance of these is that they reflect the qi of the frontotemporal area.
 b. Earth:
 The corresponding channels and points are on the bilateral buccal arteries at ST 3 (*jù liáo*), relating to the foot *yangming* channel. The diagnostic significance of this is that they reflect the qi of the mouth and teeth.

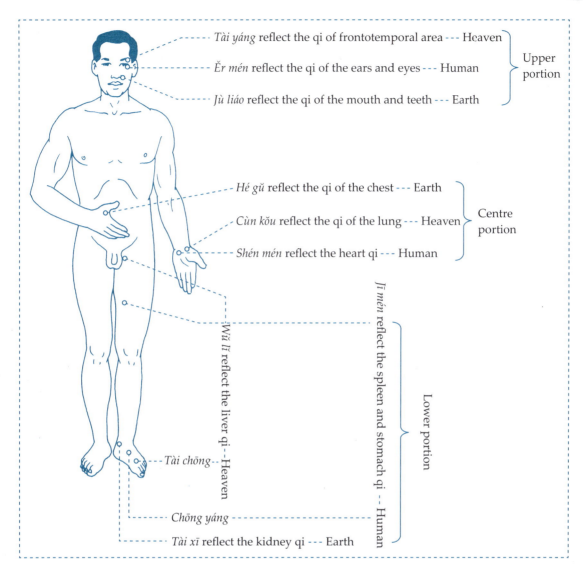

Fig. 6-1 A schematic diagram of the three positions and nine pulse-takings

   c. Human:

   The corresponding channels and points are on the auricular arteries at SJ 21 (*ěr mén*), relating to the hand *shaoyang* channel. The diagnostic significance of this is that they reflect the qi of the ears and eyes.

B. Centre portion (hands):

   a. Heaven:

   The corresponding channels and points are on the radial artery at *cùn kǒu*, relating to the hand *taiyin* channel. The diagnostic significance of this is that they reflect the qi of the lung.

   b. Earth:

   The corresponding channels and points converge at LI 4 (*hé gǔ*), relating to the hand *yangming* channel. The diagnostic significance of this is that they reflect the qi of the chest.

c. Human:
   The corresponding channels and points are on the ulnar artery at HT 7 (*shén mén*), relating to the hand *shaoyin* channel. The diagnostic significance of this is that they reflect the heart qi.
C. Lower portion (feet):
   a. Heaven:
      The corresponding channels and points are on the femoral artery at the LV 10 (*wŭ lĭ*) or LV 3 (*tài chōng*) points, relating to the foot *jueyin* channel. The diagnostic significance of this is that they reflect the liver qi.
   b. Earth:
      The corresponding channels and points are on the medial posterior malleolar artery at KI 3 (*tài xī*), relating to the foot *shaoyin* channel. The diagnostic significance of this is that they reflect the kidney qi.
   c. Human:
      The corresponding channels and points are on the medial femoral artery at the SP 11 (*jī mén*), or ST 42 (*chōng yáng*) points, relating to the foot *taiyin* channel. The diagnostic significance of this is that they reflect the spleen and stomach qi.

2. The *cùn kŏu* examination method
Significances:
A. *Cùn kŏu* — the pulsation of the radial artery on the wrist, also known as the radial pulse or wrist pulse.
B. The *cùn kŏu* examination method refers to palpating for the beat of the radial artery and analysing the physiological and pathological conditions of the body.
C. The *cùn kŏu* pulse is composed of three positions: *cùn*, *guān*, and *chĭ*; each position is divided into three depths: superficial, middle and deep, totally called "three positions and nine pulse-takings". Although it seems like the same name, it is different from the "three positions and nine pulse-takings" mentioned earlier.
   a. *Cùn*:
      The *cùn* in the left hand corresponds to the *zang-fu* organ, the heart; in the right hand it corresponds to the lung. The corresponding location is above the diaphragm and head.
   b. *Guān*:
      The *guān* in the left hand corresponds to the *zang-fu* organs of the liver and gallbladder; in the right hand it corresponds to the spleen and stomach. The corresponding location is below the diaphragm and above the umbilicus.
   c. *Chĭ*:
      The *chĭ* in the left and right hands corresponds to the *zang-fu* organ of the kidneys. The corresponding location is below the umbilicus to the foot.
D. The theoretical basis of the *cùn kŏu* examination method:
   a. The *cùn kŏu* is located at the position of the *yuan*-source point on the lung channel of the hand *taiyin* and is the convergence of all the vessels of the lung. The lung channel originates in the middle *jiao* and reflects the strength or weakness of the spleen and stomach qi.
   b. All vessels converge in the lung, so the changes of the qi and blood of the *zang-fu*

organs reflect in the *cùn kǒu* through the lung channel.
  c. The position of the *cùn kǒu* is fixed and convenient for pulse-taking.

3. Examination method at ST 9 (*rén yíng*) and *cùn kǒu*

The examination method at ST 9 (*rén yíng*) and the *cùn kǒu* is a method whereby ST 9 (*rén yíng*) and *the cùn kǒu* pulses are pressed and cross referenced with each other, and then analysed.

4. Three-section examination method of Zhang Zhong-jing
  A. Palpation of the *cùn kǒu* pulse - reflects *zang-fu* organs.
  B. Palpation of BL 59 (*fū yáng*) pulse - reflects stomach qi.
  C. Palpation of KI 3 (*tài xī*) pulse - reflects kidney qi.

Methods of Pulse-Taking

1. Time of pulse taking

The best time for pulse taking is in the early morning, before getting up or eating. The duration of each pulse taking must be at least fifty beats.

2. Position of the patient's body

The patient should be sitting erect or lying supine, keeping the *cùn kǒu* at the same level as the heart with the arm resting flat, the palm facing upwards.

3. Fingers method
  A. Placement of the practitioner's fingers:

The tips of the three fingers should be aligned. Firstly, press the middle finger on the *guān* region and palpate the pulse using only the pads of the fingers. Attention should be paid to adjust the spacing of the fingers in relation to that of the patient's size.
  B. Manipulation of the fingers:

This includes lifting, palpating, searching, mild pressing and heavy pressing, single pressing and simultaneous pressing.

4. Normal and calm breath

The practitioner's breathing should be natural and quiet. The practitioner should count the number of pulse beats during a full cycle of the patient's expiration and inspiration.
  Points to note:
  ① If the patient has calm qi and blood, and a quiet internal and external environment, this pulse is relatively true.
  ② The practitioner should keep his breath natural and uniform to count the pulse beats of the patient.
  ③ The edge of the boundary of the finger belly, the position between finger-tip and finger pulp is the sensitive region for the sense of touching.

The commonly used manipulating methods of pulse examination include: lifting, palpating, searching, mild pressing, pushing, combined pressing and single pressing.

① Lifting — Place the fingers lightly upon the skin (superficial level).
② Palpating — Palpate the pulse with a heavy force (deep level).
③ Seeking — Press the fingers to the muscles; vary the pressure to look for a more distinct pulse reading.
④ Mild pressing — The fingers moving along the longitudinal direction of the vessel to understand how long (wide) or short a pulse it is and the deficiency or excess nature of the pulse strength.
⑤ Pushing — Pressing the vessel with the belly of the fingers and slight pushing to the left, right, exterior and interior.
⑥ Combined pressing — Three fingers apply palpation and press simultaneously, so the practitioner distinguish the pulse images in total.
⑦ Single pressing — The practitioner uses a single finger to examine a specific portion of the pulse image such as the *cùn, guān,* and *chǐ*.

Elements of the Pulse Image

The ancient records often analyse and sum up pulse images from four aspects: position, rate, shape and dynamic. In modern times, the image can be divided into eight aspects: position, rate, length, breadth, strength, fluency, tension and uniformity.

1. Position
The position is the depth or shallowness of the beat of the pulse, such as with a floating pulse and sinking pulse.

2. Rate
The rate refers to the frequency of the pulse beating, such as a slow pulse and a rapid pulse.

3. Length
The length means the longitudinal range of the pulse beat, such as a long pulse and a short pulse.

4. Breadth
The breadth indicates the range of the pulse as it relates to the thickness or thinness of the beats, such as with a surging pulse and a thready pulse.

5. Strength
The strength means the strength of the pulse beats, such as with a deficient pulse and an excessive pulse.

6. Fluency
The fluency refers to the degree of ease of the approaching pulse, such as with a slippery pulse and a choppy pulse.

7. Tension
The tension indicates the degree of tightness or slackness of the vessel, such as with a

wiry pulse, a tight pulse and a moderate pulse.

8. Uniformity

The uniformity means not only missed pulse beats as with arrhythmia, but also uniformity of the consistency of the pulse, such as with a hasty pulse, a knotted pulse and an intermittent pulse.

Every pulse image can be analysed and described by these eight features of the pulse image. Some pulses describe the change of one feature, for instance a floating pulse; some pulses describe the changes of various features, such as a soggy pulse (deep, thin and soft pulse).

Section 2
A Healthy Pulse Image

A healthy pulse image (also called a balanced pulse) is a reflection of the normal function; it has defined rules and a specific range of changes.

Characteristics of the Normal Pulse Image

The normal pulse can be felt at all sections of the *cùn, guān,* and *chǐ* with four or five beats per breath, neither floating nor deep, neither too large nor too small, moderate, peaceful, powerful and uniform. The normal pulse has three characteristics: with stomach, with spirit and with root.

1. With stomach

It manifests as even, rhythmic, moderate, is calm and fluent, this reflects exuberance of the spleen and stomach's function. It also can be used to judge the prognosis of disease.

2. With spirit

It manifests as soft, forceful and regular, which reflects qi and blood being sufficient and the heart-spirit being prosperous. The pulse with spirit has an inherent stability.

3. With root

It manifests as powerful at the *chǐ* and can be felt by deep palpation, which reflects sufficient kidney qi.

Physiological Variation of the Pulse Image

The pulse image is closely related to the interior and exterior circumstances of the body. It is not only influenced by the age and sex, the build of the body, the person's daily life and psychological factors, and the seasons and the environment, but also results in a range of physiological variations through adapting to these interior and exterior circumstances.

1. Balanced pulse of the four seasons

A normal pulse image has the physiological characteristics of being wiry (taut) in spring, surging in summer, floating in autumn, and deep in winter.

A. In spring, the rising yang is restrained by the remaining cold, and the qi movement is restrained, which manifests as a slightly wiry pulse.

B. In summer, yang is extremely exuberant and the pulse has an energetic coming and going dynamic, which manifests as a slightly surging pulse.

C. In autumn, yang is gradually being restrained, surging and exuberance of the pulse will be decreasing and then the pulse becomes just like feathers in a cloth bag, which is described as a slightly superficial pulse.

D. In winter, yang is hidden; the arrival of the pulse is deep but still palpable, which is described as a slightly deep pulse.

2. The variation of the pulse image due to the changes of the anatomy of the radial artery

A. Oblique flying pulse:

The pulse cannot be felt at the *cùn kǒu* region, but on the dorsum of the hand from the *chǐ* region.

B. Dorsally located radial artery:

The pulse is shifted to the back of the *cùn kǒu* region i.e. dorsally and proximally from the usual position.

SECTION 3
ABNORMAL PULSE IMAGES

Generally speaking, all pulses are considered to be abnormal except those that are due to normal physiological changes and individual physiological characteristics. There are various ways to classify abnormal pulse images, but the most common classification is by the twenty-eight pulse conditions. All kinds of pulse are still subject to the changes and combinations of the four aspects (position, rate, shape and dynamic) and the eight factors.

Common Abnormal Pulses

The characteristics and associated diseases of the common abnormal pulse images have been classified, and should be learnt by heart.

1. Floating pulses

A floating pulse means the pulse is accessible using light pressure.

A. Floating pulse (*fú mài* 浮脉):

The floating pulse is clearly felt using light pressure, but feels weak with heavy pressure, which indicates exterior patterns and deficiency patterns. A floating pulse can be described as bobbing, downy or at the surface. It is due to the pathogen struggling with *zheng* (healthy) qi on the exterior, and vessel qi acting on the exterior surface. It can also be found in a deficient body with long-term disease, where the pulse is mostly floating and powerless.

B. Surging pulse (*hóng mài* 洪脉):

The surging pulse is of generous shape and powerful, just like roaring waves which come vigourously and fade away, this indicates extreme heat patterns. The surging pulse is due to the pathogenic heat filling the vessels, and then the vessels become enlarged with exuberant qi and gushing blood.

C. Soggy pulse (*rú mài* 濡脉):

The soggy pulse is floating, thin and soft, and it indicates deficiency patterns and dampness patterns. The soggy pulse is due to insufficient qi and blood with depleted vessels. It can also be caused by a dampness pathogen blocking the vessels.

D. Scattered pulse (*sǎn mài* 散脉):

The scattered pulse is floating, scattered without root, it disappears on pressure and has an irregular pulse rate; which indicates *yuan* (original) qi dissipation, and *zang* qi exhaustion. The scattered pulse is due to *yuan* qi being dissipated, unconstrained yin and yang, vessel qi being scattered, disordered and loose.

E. Hollow pulse (*kōu mài* 芤脉):

The hollow pulse is floating and large with an empty centre, just like a scallion stalk, this indicates loss of blood and damaged yin. The hollow pulse is due to extreme loss of blood, insufficient *ying* and blood, or extreme damage to body fluids, drained vessels, yin being damaged and yang unable to adhere to it and then becoming scattered on the outside.

F. Drumskin pulse (*gé mài* 革脉):

The drumskin pulse is floating under the finger, has a hollow centre and is hard and leathery outside just like a drum. This type of pulse indicates blood and essence exhaustion, metrorrhagia and metrostaxis. The drumskin pulse is due to extreme consumption of essence and blood, qi floating outside no longer being able to be held.

2. Deep pulses

The deep pulse means it only begins to be obtained using heavy pressure.

A. Deep pulse (*chén mài* 沉脉):

The deep pulse is not evident with light pressure, but is with heavy pressure. The deep pulse indicates interior patterns. A deep and powerful pulse is due to the pathogen stagnating in the interior, qi and blood being blocked, vessel qi being restrained inside. A deep and powerless pulse is due to deficient *zang-fu* organs, yang deficiency and vessel qi unable to be roused.

B. Hidden pulse (*fú mài* 伏脉):

The hidden pulse is only evident with heavy pressure; it is finally obtained when the bone is reached. The hidden pulse indicates interior stagnation of pathogens, syncope (temporary loss of consciousness) and extreme pain. It is caused by internal hidden pathogens; syncope due to counterflow and disorder of qi movement; pain due to qi movement retention or vessel qi lacking in diffusion and free flow.

C. Weak pulse (*ruò mài* 弱脉):

The weak pulse is extremely soft, deep and thin. This pulse indicates insufficiency of qi and blood or deficiency and failure of yang. It is due to blood deficiency, emptiness of vessels, or qi deficiency, pulse movement lacking in power, or yang deficiency, with consequent lack of power.

D. Firm pulse (*láo mài* 牢脉):

The firm pulse is deep, large, powerful, wiry and long, obtained only using heavy pressure. This firm pulse indicates internal accumulation of yin-cold, *shàn qì* and concretions and conglomerations. It is due to internal accumulation of yin-cold and yang deeply hidden.

3. Slow pulses

A slow pulse means that the pulse arrives slowly.

A. Slow pulse (*chí mài* 迟脉):

The slow pulse is less than four beats per respiration, which indicates cold patterns. A slow and powerful pulse is caused by qi stagnation due to congealing cold. Alternatively, a slow and powerless pulse is caused by yang deficiency, qi and blood moving slowly.

B. Moderate pulse (*huǎn mài* 缓脉):

The moderate pulse is four beats in one breath, the pulse arrives leisurely. This moderate pulse indicates spleen deficiency and damp patterns, but can also be found in a healthy person. The moderate pulse, when due to spleen deficiency, reflects insufficiency of qi and blood, with vessels inadequately filled. If associated with damp, the nature of damp is sticky and stagnant, which then blocks and stagnates the movement of qi. It is also the manifestation of abundant spirit in the healthy person.

C. Choppy pulse (*sè mài* 涩脉):

The choppy pulse is one that arrives coarsely, slowly and stagnating, just like a light knife scraping along bamboo. It is sometimes referred to as a rough pulse and can feel hesitant, lacking in smoothness or incomplete. This choppy pulse indicates qi stagnation or blood stasis. A choppy and powerless pulse is due to essence damage or deficiency of blood, with loss of nourishment in the channels and collaterals. A choppy and powerful pulse is due to qi stagnation and blood stasis with the vessels consequently being blocked.

D. Knotted pulse (*jié mài* 结脉):

The knotted pulse or bound pulse is slow with a loss of beats at irregular intervals. The knotted pulse is indicative of exuberant yin and qi stagnation; cold phlegm and static blood; concretions and conglomerations; accumulations and gatherings; deficiency and failure of qi and blood. A knotted and powerful pulse is due to cold pathogens and excess pathogens blocking channels and collaterals, vessel qi is thus unable to flow smoothly. A knotted and powerless pulse is due to deficiency and failure of qi and blood, weakness of yang, and vessel qi unable to flow.

4. Rapid pulses

This means the pulse arrives rapidly, over five beats in one breath.

A. Rapid pulse (*shù mài* 数脉):

The rapid pulse is more than five beats per respiration, which is indicative of heat patterns. A rapid and powerful pulse is due to exuberance of pathogenic heat with accelerated movement of qi and blood. A rapid and powerless pulse is due to a deficient yang pattern.

B. Racing pulse (*jí mài* 疾脉):

The racing pulse is urgent and rapid, seven or eight beats per breath, which indicates excessive heat, yin exhaustion and floating yang, *yuan* qi will be depleted.

C. Hasty pulse (cù mài 促脉)

The hasty or skipping pulse is rapid with irregular intervals. This pulse indicates exuberant yang and excessive heat; stagnation and stasis of qi and blood; accumulation of phlegm and food; or debilitation and failure of *zang* qi. A fast and powerful pulse is due to exuberant yang and binding heat, excessive pathogens blocking and stagnating, and vessel qi unable to flow smoothly. A rapid, thin and soft pulse is due to deficiency and weakness of *zang* qi, failure and insufficiency of yin-blood.

D. Throbbing pulse (dòng mài 动脉):

The throbbing or bouncing pulse jumps like a spinning bean and is slippery, rapid and powerful. This pulse indicates pain and fright. Pain can cause disharmony of yin and yang, and qi stagnated by blood. Fright can cause disorder of qi and blood, restlessness of pulse movement, yin struggling in yang.

5. Deficient (feeble) pulses

This means the pulse reflects against the fingers powerlessly.

A. Deficient pulse (xū mài 虚脉):

The deficient or depleted pulse is forceless and empty in the three depths which indicates a deficiency pattern, mostly qi and blood deficiency. It is due to insufficient qi and blood, all kinds of deficiency of the *zang-fu* organs with depleted vessels.

B. Thready pulse (xì mài 细脉):

The thready pulse is thin like a fine thread, but very distinct and clear. This pulse indicates deficiency of qi and blood, all kinds of deficiency or dampness. If it is due to deficiency of qi and blood then the vessels cannot be filled or moved; likewise if dampness pathogens block the vessels.

C. Faint pulse (wēi mài 微脉):

The faint pulse is extremely thin and soft, hardly palpable by pressure. The faint pulse indicates all kinds of deficiency of yin, yang, qi and blood, as well as dangerous conditions of yang deficiency. It is due to deficient and weak yang acting without power, or extreme deficiency of qi and blood in the vessels unable to fill the vessels and move.

D. Intermittent pulse (dài mài 代脉):

The intermittent pulse is a loss of beats and pausing a little longer at regular intervals. This pulse indicates failure and weakness of *zang* qi, wind patterns, pain patterns, seven emotions, fright, knocks and falls. Failure and weakness of the *zang* qi, deficiency and damage of qi and blood, pulse moving powerlessly, can all prevent the vessel qi from being smooth and rhythmical. It is also caused by excessive pathogens blocking and stagnating vessels with consequent stagnation of qi.

E. Short pulse (duǎn mài 短脉):

The short pulse is short in extent; unable to reach the usual position. The short pulse when powerful indicates qi stagnation; when powerless indicates qi damage. A short and powerless pulse is due to qi deficiency and inability to keep the blood moving. A short and powerful pulse is due to qi stagnation and blood stasis, both of which block the vessels.

6. Excess (forceful) pulses

This means the pulse acts with powerful beating acting against the fingers.

A. Excess pulse (shí mài 实脉):

The excess pulse is vigourous and forceful when using light or heavy pressure. This pulse indicates excess patterns; it also can be seen in healthy people. It is due to exuberant *zheng* qi and excessive pathogens, *zheng* qi struggling with a pathogen, congestion and exuberance of qi and blood, fullness of the vessels.

B. Slippery pulse (*huá mài* 滑脉):

The slippery pulse is round and smooth like a bead rolling on a plate. The slippery pulse indicates phlegm retention, food accumulation or excessive heat; it also can be seen in young people and pregnant women. It is due to internal exuberance of excess pathogens, excess qi and blood, and the pulse moving smoothly. A slippery pulse in healthy people or pregnant women is the manifestation of sufficient and harmonised qi and blood.

C. Wiry pulse (*xián mài* 弦脉):

The wiry pulse or bow-string pulse is taut and long, like pressing over the string of a musical instrument. The wiry pulse indicates liver or gallbladder diseases, pain patterns, phlegm-rheum retention and malaria, it can also be seen in the elderly, and the pulse is usually slightly wiry in spring. When pathogens are stagnating in the liver channel, liver qi loses its gentleness, qi movement is stagnated or phlegm-rheum is blocking inside, channels and collaterals are inhibited, the vessel qi will be tense and will appear as a wiry pulse. An elderly person has insufficient yin-blood, vessels lose their softness, and then the pulse appears wiry.

D. Tight pulse (*jĭn mài* 紧脉):

The tight pulse is one that arrives tight and forcefully, like a stretched and twisted rope. The tight pulse is so tense it is almost vibrating. This pulse indicates cold, pain and food retention. The tight pulse is due to excessive pathogens struggling rigourously with the *zheng* qi.

E. Long pulse (*cháng mài* 长脉):

The long pulse is with long extent, longer than its basic position. The long pulse indicates that yang is in superabundance, heat patterns exist or it belongs to a healthy person. A long and powerful pulse is due to yang hyperactivity and exuberant heat; phlegm-fire accumulated internally with fullness of vessel qi. A long pulse indicates sufficient qi and blood in a healthy person.

F. Large pulse (*dà mài* 大脉):

The large pulse has a wide (broad) form but is without turbulent force. The large pulse can be seen in healthy people or indicates development of disease. The healthy person has sufficient qi and blood, so the pulse is large. When the disease is long term and has developed severely, the body is full of pathogens; the pulse here may also appear as large.

Differentiation of the Pulse Images

The pulse images are varied with tiny changes, some of them are very similar and can cause confusion. Therefore, in order to enhance the comprehension and differentiation of the pulse images, they can be categorised and compared with each other.

1. Categorisation of pulses

The same category pulses are a group of pulse images, which are similar in one aspect, such as position, rate, form, etc.

A. Category of the position: floating pulses and deep pulses.
B. Category of the rate: slow pulses and rapid pulses.
C. Category of the breadth:
   a. Wide and large pulses:
      ① Large pulse: the body of the pulse is broad and several times larger than normal.
      ② Surging pulse: the surging pulse is floating, large and powerful, exuberant in coming and failing in going.
      ③ Excess pulse: the excess pulse is large and powerful, irrelevant of whether it is floating or deep.
      ④ Hollow pulse: the hollow pulse is floating, large and hollow in the middle.
      ⑤ Firm pulse: the firm pulse is excessive, large, deep, and wiry.
   b. Thready pulses:
      ① Thready pulse: the pulse is like a thread and still palpable.
      ② Faint pulse: the faint pulse is extremely thin and soft, sometimes present, sometimes not.
      ③ Soggy pulse: the soggy pulse is floating, thready and soft.
      ④ Weak pulse: the weak pulse is deep, thready and soft.
D. Category of the length:
   a. Long pulses:
      ① Long pulse: the long pulse is palpable and large, extending beyond the three portions.
      ② Wiry pulse: the wiry pulse is straight and long, like the string of a musical instrument.
      ③ The firm pulse, surging pulse, and excess pulse all have the characteristics of the long pulse.
   b. Short pulses:
      ① Short pulse: the short pulse is palpable and of short extent, not filling the three portions.
      ② Throbbing pulse: the throbbing pulse is short, slippery and rapid.
E. Category of the strength:
   a. Deficiency pulses:
      ① Deficiency pulse: a deficient pulse has a powerless beat or is without root when pressed.
      ② Soggy pulse: a soggy pulse is floating, thready and powerless.
      ③ Weak pulse: a weak pulse is deep, thready and powerless.
      ④ Faint pulse: a faint pulse is extremely thin and powerless with obscure beating.
      ⑤ Scattered pulse: a scattered pulse is floating, scattered and without root.
      ⑥ Hollow pulse: a hollow pulse is floating, large and hollow in the middle.
      ⑦ Drumskin pulse: a drumskin pulse is floating, wiry and hollow in the middle.
   b. Excess pulses:
      ① Excess pulse: an excess pulse is forceful with light pressure and also with more pressure in all three depths.
      ② Surging pulse: a surging pulse is floating, large and powerful, exuberant in

coming and failing in going.
③ Long pulse: the length of the pulse extends beyond the three portions, the strength of the pulse is less than the surging pulse and the excess pulse.
④ Wiry pulse: the form of the pulse is straight and long, and has tense beats. The strength of the pulse is less than the surging pulse and excess pulse.

F. Category of the fluency:
  a. Fluent pulses:
    ① Slippery pulse: the slippery pulse arrives and departs smoothly, like pearls rolling on a plate.
    ② Throbbing pulse: the throbbing pulse is short, slippery and rapid.
  b. Rough pulses:
    ① Choppy pulse: the pulse arrives very roughly and its departure is also not smooth.
    ② Knotted pulse and intermittent pulse: These are slow and lack smoothness, they are intermittent.

G. Category of the tension:
  a. Tense pulses:
    ① Wiry pulse: a wiry pulse is like pressing the string of a musical instrument.
    ② Tight pulse: the tension is higher than the wiry pulse.
    ③ Drumskin pulse: a drumskin pulse is floating, wiry and hollow in the middle.
    ④ Firm pulse: a firm pulse is deep, wiry, excessive, long and large.
  b. Low tension pulses:
    The common points of the soggy pulse, weak pulse, faint pulse, scattered pulse and moderate pulse are that they are soft and powerless, but for differentiation, make reference to the aspects of the strength.

H. Category of the uniformity:
  a. Knotted pulse: the pulse arrives moderate to slow, sometimes there is a stop, and stops are irregular.
  b. Intermittent pulse: sometimes there is a pause in the pulse, pauses are regular.
  c. Hasty pulse: the pulse arrives rapidly, sometimes there is a pause, and pauses are irregular.
  d. Scattered pulse: a scattered pulse is floating and without root, scattered and in disarray.

2. Opposite pulses

Opposite pulses means the pulse images are completely opposite in one aspect of the position, rate, form or strength.

A. Floating pulse and deep pulse:
Contrast in the shallowness or depth.
  a. A floating pulse is floating superficially, indicating an exterior and yang pattern.
  b. A deep pulse is deep within, indicating an interior and yin pattern.

B. Slow pulse and rapid pulse:
Contrast in the rate.
  a. A slow pulse is less than four times per breath, indicating cold patterns.
  b. A rapid pulse is more than five times per breath, indicating heat patterns.

C. Deficient pulse and excess pulse:
Contrast in the power of the beat.
   a. An excess pulse is fullness of the vessel; the three portions are all powerful.
   b. A deficient pulse is emptiness of the vessel, with powerless beating.
D. Slippery pulse and choppy pulse:
Contrast in the slipperiness or roughness of the movement.
   a. A slippery pulse indicates exuberance of the blood and qi, it arrives smoothly.
   b. A choppy pulse indicates shortage of blood and stagnation of qi, it arrives in a rough and non-uniform manner.
E. Surging pulse and thready pulse:
Contrast in the size of the shape.
   a. A surging pulse, like roaring waves, which come vigourously and then fade away, indicates an extreme heat pattern.
   b. A thready pulse is thin like a thread, mostly soft, weak and powerless, but with obvious beating.
F. Tight pulse and moderate pulse:
Contrast in the tautness of the shape.
   a. A tight pulse is tight and powerful, like a twisted rope.
   b. A moderate pulse is a little slack and the pulse arrives leisurely.
G. Long pulse and short pulse:
Contrast in the extent of the pulse.
   a. A long pulse extends through the three portions and crosses the *chǐ* portion.
   b. A short pulse has only the *cùn* beating obviously on pressing.

3. Combined pulses

The development of illness is usually complicated and may be caused by various pathogenic factors or different natures. In the course of an illness, because of the different conditions of the body resistance in the injured organs, there may be more than two pathogenic factors, and also the struggle between the pathogenic factors and *zheng* qi constantly changes in the course of the illness, and the nature and position of the illness may also be changing along with the illness. Therefore, usually two or more pathological pulses appear at the same time. A pulse with two, or more than two, single pulses is called a combined pulse or a compound pulse.

Within the twenty-eight abnormal pulses, some of the pulses indicate a single pulse quality, such as floating, deep, slow, rapid, long, short, large, thready, etc. However, some pulses themselves are in fact combination pulses; for instance, a weak pulse is deep, fine, and soft; a soggy pulse is floating, thready and soft; a bouncing pulse is slippery, rapid and short; a firm pulse is deep, excessive, long, and wiry.

The illnesses of the combined pulse are usually the total sum of the indications of the pulses, which make up the combined pulse. For example:
   ① A floating pulse indicates exterior patterns and a rapid pulse signifies heat patterns, so if these two pulses are combined they indicate exterior heat patterns;
   ② A floating pulse indicates exterior patterns and a slow pulse signifies cold patterns, so combined they indicate exterior cold patterns.
   ③ A floating, rapid and powerless pulse indicates exterior deficient heat

④ A deep, slow and forceful pulse indicates interior excessive cold, etc.

4. Visceral exhaustion pulses

Visceral exhaustion pulses are the pulse images that exist in the critical stage of an illness, when life processes have already been interrupted. The characteristics of the visceral exhaustion pulses are: without stomach, without spirit and without root. It is a sign of severe illness, exhausted *yuan* qi, and failure of the stomach qi, and can also be called "vanquished pulses", "exhausted pulses", "dead pulses", or "unusual pulses". Visceral exhaustion pulses are usually divided into three groups: without stomach, without root, without spirit.

A. Without stomach:

This pulse has hard beats but without rushing and is mild. The clinical significance is exuberance of the pathogen and failure of the *zheng* qi, without stomach, single appearance of the qi of the heart, liver, kidney, and an indicator of the critical condition of the illness.

   a. Upturned knife pulse (*yǎn dāo mài*, 偃刀脉): this arrives string-like and tense, like spinning the knife blade.
   b. Bean-rolling pulse (*zhuàn dòu mài*, 转豆脉): this is short, tense and beats strongly like spinning coix seeds (also known as Job's Tears, a grain slightly bigger than pearl barley) or like rolling pearls.
   c. Flicking stone pulse (*tán shí mài*, 弹石脉): this is hasty and hard, like tapping on stone. Comes slow and leaves fast.

B. Without root:

The pulses are deficient, without root or weak, and not obvious.

   a. Bubble-rising pulse (*fǔ fèi mài*, 釜沸脉): this is extremely floating and rapid, with countless beats, like water seething in a cauldron, floating, rootless. It is due to extreme heat in the three yang with exhausted yin.
   b. Fish-swimming pulse (*yú xiáng mài*, 鱼翔脉): the pulse is on the surface (skin), with a fixed head and swimming tail, sometimes present and sometimes not, like a fish swimming in water.
   c. Shrimp-darting pulse (*xiā yóu mài*, 虾游脉): the pulse is on the skin or surface, faint and weak, is countless, like a darting shrimp, coming and then suddenly disappearing,

Both of these (b. and c.) are due to extreme cold in the three yin with exhaustion of yang on the outside, floating of deficient yang, it is extremely critical, and a sign that indicates death.

C. Without spirit:

The rate of the pulse has no sequence; the form of the pulse is scattered and chaotic.

This is due to the expiry of the spleen and stomach qi and kidney yang qi, which indicates collapse of the spirit, imminent death.

   a. Sparrow-pecking pulse (*què zhuó mài*, 雀啄脉): the pulse is extremely rapid with irregular rhythm, suddenly stopping and restarting its beat, like a bird pecking its food at irregular intervals.
   b. Roof-leaking pulse (*wū lòu mài*, 屋漏脉): this is extremely slow, like water leaking through a roof, one drop at a time.

c. Untwining rope pulse (*jiě suǒ mài*, 解索脉): this is sometimes rapid, sometimes slow, like a rope that has been twisted becoming unravelled.

SECTION 4
EXAMINATION OF THE PULSES OF WOMEN AND CHILDREN

The Pulse in Women

1. Menstrual pulse

The pulse at the left *guān* and *chǐ* portions is fuller and larger than on the right, there is a lack of bitter taste in the mouth, no fever, abdomen is not distended. This pulse means that the menses will arrive soon; pre-menstrual tension (PMT).

2. Pulse of pregnancy

This appears with sudden loss of periods, and then the pulse arrives slippery, rapid, rushing and harmonious, or the pulse at the *chǐ* portion is slippery and rapid.

3. Parturition pulse (birthing pulses) (anomalous pulse)

The *chǐ* pulse becomes tense, like a taut rope or rolling bead, or the pulse beats are found on the sides of the distal phalange of the middle finger.

The Pulse in Children

In examining the pulse of a child, only yin and yang, exterior or interior, cold or heat, excess and deficiency should be regarded.

1. Only one finger feels all three regions

A. Three years old and under:
The thumb is placed above the styloid process and the child's pulse is not divided into three portions.

B. Four years old and over:
The midline of the styloid is regarded as the *guān*, then the pulse can be felt by moving the thumb along from the *guān* region.

C. At seven or eight years old:
The thumb can be shifted to feel the three regions.

D. Nine or ten years old and over:
Press in order: *cùn*, *guān*, and *chǐ*.

E. Fifteen years old and over:
The three regions can be felt as for adults.

2. Just by examining floating, deep, slow, rapid, strong, weak, moderate, tight, the practitioner can distinguish yin or yang, exterior or interior, cold or heat, exuberance or debilitation of pathogen and zheng qi.

A. Under three years old: seven or eight beats per breath is normal.

At five or six years old: six beats per breath is normal.
B. A rapid pulse indicates heat.
A slow pulse indicates cold.
A floating and rapid pulse relates to yang.
A deep and slow pulse relates to yin.
C. Strength or weakness differentiates deficiency or excess.
D. Moderate and tight differentiate the pathogen and the *zheng* qi.
Tight indicates cold.
Moderate indicates dampness.
Changes in beats mean food retention.

Section 5
Clinical Application and Significance of the Pulse Examination

Clinical Application of the Pulse Examination

The internal relationship of the pulse images and illness governed by pulse images are very complex. In pulse examination, one should pay attention to several items when analysing the different aspects of the illness reflected by the pulse image, then one should be able to distinguish the different pulse images that appear in diseases.

1. Disease governed by a single abnormal pulse image in the *cùn*, *guān*, and *chǐ* regions
Single abnormal pulse image:
A. Single position:
One kind of pulse image only, is felt in one region.
For example, a wiry pulse in left *guān* indicates stagnation of the liver.
B. Single *zang* qi:
Some pulse images are often seen in diseases corresponding to the *zang-fu* organs. For example, a knotted pulse, intermittent pulse and a hasty pulse are all the manifestations of heart disease.
C. Single pulse shape:
This means the sudden appearance of one kind of pulse image during the disease, and then the indicated pattern is obvious. For example, a tight pulse indicates cold-damage patterns and pain patterns.

2. Identification of the diseases indicated by the pulse should not be limited
There are normal and abnormal conditions for pathological pulses.
A. Normal:
Floating indicates exterior, deep indicates interior.
Rapid usually indicates heat, slow usually indicates cold.
Wiry and large indicates excess, thready and faint iindicates deficiency.
B. Abnormal:

Floating indicates deficiency, deep indicates excess.
Rapid may indicate deficiency, slow may indicate heat.
Floating and surging indicate loss of yang; thready and moderate indicate stagnation of damp.

3. Favourable and unfavourable pulses and the priority of the pulse or the signs

Favourable or unfavourable pulses and signs refer to whether the pulse and the signs are in agreement or not. If the pulse and signs all reflect the nature of the disease, it is called a favourable pattern. If the pulse and the signs are not in agreement, or are opposite, it is called an unfavourable pattern. There are priorities for abandoning the pulse and signs. If the signs are true and the pulse is false, the practitioner should prioritise the signs over the pulse. If the pulse is true and the signs are false, the practitioner should prioritise the pulse over the signs.

On the whole, diagnosis involves correlating all four examinations and connecting the pulse with the signs. For example:

A. Favourable or unfavourable prognosis:
- At the onset of a new disease or a sudden illness, a floating, surging, rapid and excess pulse is auspicious and reflects exuberance of *zheng* qi and resistance against the pathogen.
- In prolonged disease, if the pulse arrives deep, faint, thready or weak, this is auspicious and indicates shortage of the *zheng* qi but without exuberance of the pathogen.
- In a new disease, if the pulse is deep, thready, faint, and weak, this is unfavourable and indicates deficiency and failure of the *zheng* qi.
- In prolonged disease, the pulse is floating, surging, rapid, and excessive which is unfavourable and indicates failure of the *zheng* qi and exuberance of the pathogen.

B. Priority of the pulse or the signs:

When assessing a disease, one should investigate the root (*běn*) of the disease. If a sign is not in agreement or a pulse is inconsistent, one should not follow the conventional procedures. A weak pulse may be seen in an excess pattern, or an excess pulse may be seen in a deficiency pattern; firstly one should decide whether the pulse is favourable or unfavourable. For example, distension and fullness of the abdomen, but with a faint and weak pulse is due to deficiency and weakness of the spleen and stomach (priority of the pulse); or no distension, fullness and pain, but with a wiry and strong pulse, which is not an excess pattern (priority of the signs); or the chest and abdomen is not scorching, but there is a surging and large pulse, which is not caused by a fire-pathogen.

Significance of the Pulse Examination

① To distinguish the conditions of the disease
② To analyse the pathogenesis of the disease
③ To guide the management of the disease
④ To estimate the prognosis of the disease

CHAPTER 7
Palpatory Examination

Palpating is a diagnostic method by which the practitioner uses his (or her) hand to touch or press specific parts of the body to obtain an accurate understanding of abnormal changes and to find the location, nature, and pathological conditions of the disease.

The palpatory examination is an important part of the diagnostic process and plays an important role in pattern identification; it cannot be ignored, as it is an essential part of the four examinations. The manipulations of palpating and the theory of palpating the chest and abdomen should be the main points of emphasis to be grasped in the palpatory examination. The practice and theory of palpating the skin, the hands and feet, and the transport points should also be familiar to the practitioner.

Contents of the palpating examination
- Manipulations
    - Feeling
    - Palpating
    - Pressing
    - Tapping
- Areas for examination by palpation
    - Palpating the chest and hypochondrium
    - Palpating the stomach cavity and abdomen
    - Palpating the skin
    - Palpating the hands and feet
    - Palpating the transport points

The chest and abdomen are the home of the *zang-fu* organs. In addition, the chest and abdomen are not only the origins of the *wei* qi and *ying*-blood, but also the residing place of pathogenic factors. Palpating the chest and abdomen can distinguish excess and deficiency of the *zang-fu* organs and the characteristics of any pathogenic factors. The thoracic and abdominal palpation should be combined with tongue and pulse manifestations, and with all the other signs, for comprehensive analysis of the data based on the four examinations; subsequently pattern identification should become clearer.

SECTION 1
CONTENTS OF THE PALPATORY EXAMINATION INCLUDING METHODS AND SIGNIFICANCE

1. The main positions that the patients should take when having a palpatory examination are sitting and lying supine

2. Manipulations of the palpatory examination include: feeling, palpating, pressing and tapping

A. Feeling:

Touching the local skin lightly by using fingers or palms, such as the skin of the frontal region, four limbs, chest and abdomen is the first stage of this examination.

Touching the skin lightly and investigating whether it is cold or feverish and moist or dry (temperature, moisture), so as to distinguish external contraction or internal damage and exuberance or debilitation of the body fluids.

B. Palpating (superficial palpation):

Searching and feeling the regions with a little force by the fingers, such as the areas of chest, abdomen, acupuncture channels, swellings, etc.

Feel the muscular layer; probe the regions to feel the size, shape and any swelling, so as to distinguish the position of disease and deficiency or excess.

C. Pressing (deep palpation):

Pressing deeply is done next in the examination. This deep palpation is done using the fingers in regions such as the chest, abdomen, acupuncture points and any swelling.

Heavy pressing can be carried out on the bones and muscles or deep parts of the abdominal area to examine shape, texture, size or bulk, range of motion, tenderness, and swelling, so as to distinguish deficiency or excess of *zang-fu* organs and the conditions of pathogenic qi.

D. Tapping (percussion):

Tapping can be performed on some regions of the body by using the hands; thus diagnosing the condition of the underlying parts or internal organs by the sound or the resonance obtained.

3. General order of a palpatory examination

A. Methods:

Feeling, palpating, pressing, tapping (direct tapping, indirect tapping).

B. Force:

From slight degree (light pressure) to heavy degree (heavy pressure).

C. Location:

From superficial to deep.

From distal to proximal area.

From upper to lower.

4. Main points of tapping examination

A. Direct tapping:

Tapping the superficial parts with the fingers directly.

For example, when tapping the abdominal area in patients with drum distension: resonance like a drum sound is simple distension, but resonance with a dull, muffled sound is ascites (accumulation of fluid in the peritoneal cavity).

B. Indirect tapping:

The practitioner puts his left palm over the surface of the body and uses his right fingers to tap the dorsum of his left hand.

For example this is used for those who have the feeling of lumbago (pain in patients' lumbar region), which may indicate bone diseases or kidney diseases.

5. Hints for carrying out the palpatory examination
   A. Select the appropriate body position and methods according to the condition being assessed.
   B. Keep manner steady and calm, with a serious and polite attitude.
   C. Keep manipulation delicate and soft; avoid too heavy force or palpating with cold hands.
   D. Get the exact reflection of feeling back from the patient.
   E. When palpating pay attention to the changes in the patient's facial expression.

6. Significance of the palpatory examination
   The palpatory examination is an obligatory part of the physical examination in the clinic. The palpatory examination can help not only to understand the location, nature and severity of the disease, but also to diagnose some manifestations of diseases. It is a method used to further detect the location and the nature of the disease on the basis of inspection, listening, smelling and interrogation or inquiry.

Section 2
Areas for Palpatory Examination

The areas that are suitably included in the palpatory examination include palpating the chest and hypochondrium, abdominal area, skin, hands, feet, and acupuncture points particularly the transport points, etc.

1. Palpating the chest and hypochondrium
   The chest refers to the area from the supraclavicular fossa to the bottom of the ribs. The hypochondrium is also called the rib-side, and relates to the area on both sides of the chest, from the armpit to below the eleventh or twelfth ribs.
   Palpating the chest and hypochondrium is mostly used to examine the pathological changes of the heart, lung, liver and gallbladder.
   (1) Palpating the chest
   Palpating the chest can help to understand the changes of the heart, lung and to assess the throbbing of the left ventricle of the heart or apical pulse (*xū lǐ*).
   A. Protruding or bulging of the chest walls with clear sound when tapped indicates lung distension or pneumothorax.
   B. Distending pain after palpating the chest, with dull sound, suggests retention of fluid in the chest or phlegm-heat obstructing the lung.
   C. Protruding or bulging chest with possible barrel-chested appearance, deep breathing, irregular and rapid pulse, is the forerunner of heart and lung qi exhaustion.
   D. Local tenderness, swelling, and an aversion to pressure indicate thoracic injury.
   Palpating *xū lǐ* (apical pulse):
   A. Location:

Below the left nipple, between the fourth and fifth ribs is the apex point (heart apex).

B. Physiologic characteristics:

Pulsation is palpable but not strong, range of fluctuation about 2~2.5 cm, beating smoothly, moderately and rhythmically.

C. Clinical significance:

Detecting whether the *zong* qi is strong or weak, the disease is deficient or excessive or if the prognosis is favourable or unfavourable.

D. Method:

The patient lies on their back; the practitioner stands beside the patient's right side and touches his apical pulse gently with the right hand.

Clinical significance of abnormal changes of the apical pulse:

① Weak beats mean deficiency of the *zōng* qi.

② Strong beating and vibrating of the clothes indicates outburst of *zōng* qi.

③ Occasional and intermittent fast beats suggests failure of middle qi to keep in its place.

④ Slow and feeble beats or fast beats, because of weakness due to chronic diseases, governs insufficiency of heart yang.

⑤ Protruding or bulging chest with dyspnoea and scattered and fast beats, indicates exhaustion of the heart and lung qi.

⑥ Weak beating, with no fatal symptoms, is mostly due to phlegm-retention.

Attention: The factors, other than pathogenic factors that influence the apical pulse beating include: fright, great anger or violent thoughts, exercise, and obesity.

(2) Palpating the hypochondrium

Palpation of the hypochondrium can help detect pathological changes in the liver and gallbladder.

A. Distending pain on both sides, involving the lesser abdomen, indicates constraint of liver qi.

B. Distending pain in the right rib region and heat sensation, which the patient is reluctant to have pressed, are signs of a liver abscess.

C. Hypochondriac pain, which the person likes to have pressed and demonstrates vacuity and weakness when being pressed, indicates liver deficiency.

D. Hypochondriac lumps with stabbing pain and dislike of pressure, indicates blood stasis.

E. Right hypochondriac lumps, which are hard and uneven, is possibly liver cancer.

F. Persistent malaria with lumps in the hypochondrium, is called malaria with splenomegaly.

2. Palpating the area below heart

Through feeling and palpating the stomach cavity and abdomen, the physician can understand the conditions of cold or heat, softness or hardness, distension or fullness, swelling, nature of pain, etc. This is a diagnostic method to distinguish different *zang-fu* organs' patterns and their nature.

(1) Common divisions of the abdomen

A. The area below the heart:

From the lower edge of the xiphoid process to the umbilicus.

B. Stomach cavity:
Epigastric zone.
C. Upper abdomen:
Above the umbilicus.
D. Lower abdomen:
From the umbilicus to the superior border of the pubis.
E. The lesser abdomen:
Both sides of the lower abdomen.
F. The umbilical region:
Around the navel.

(2) Contents of palpating the area below heart

A. Stomach cavity:
The stomach cavity governs the stomach patterns.
    a. Pǐ-with fullness and distension: the patient experiences gastric fullness like a mass or stuffiness below the heart. If the stomach cavity is pǐ but has more fullness like a mass, and if pressed is hard and painful; this is mostly due to an excessive pathogen gathering and retention in the stomach cavity and indicates excess patterns. If the stomach cavity is pǐ but more with distension or stuffiness, is soft when pressed and is without pain; this is mostly due to deficiency and weakness of the stomach and indicates deficiency patterns.
    b. Chest accumulation pattern: chest or thoracic accumulation is due to excess pathogens blocking and stagnating the movement of qi.
        ① Minor chest accumulation pattern:
            The patient experiences distension and oppression in the stomach cavity, and the area is painful when pressed.
        ② Major chest accumulation pattern:
            The chest, stomach, and abdomen are all hard, full, painful and dislike being pressed.
    c. The stomach cavity is distended and painful when being pressed, on palpation it sounds like water is being pushed, this is due to water in the stomach.

B. Abdominal area:
Examination of this area can be used for detecting disorders of the small intestine, large intestine, bladder, uterus and appendix.
    a. A cold sensation of the skin when pressed with preference for warmth, indicates cold patterns.
    b. A feverish sensation of the skin when pressed with a preference for cold, indicates heat patterns.
    c. Abdominal pain with a preference for pressure indicates deficiency patterns.
    d. Abdominal pain with an aversion to pressure indicates excess patterns.
    e. Abdominal fullness:
        ① Fullness which is felt on palpation as having elasticity and where there is tenderness, indicates excess patterns.
        ② Softness which is felt by palpation and lacks elasticity or tenderness, indicates deficiency patterns.
    f. Abdominal distension: the abdomen is distended rounded and large, just like a

drum.
> ① The abdomen has fluctuations like a bag of water when tapped and indentations made by pressure remain when pressure is removed, this is called water drum distension.
> ② The abdomen does not fluctuate when tapped and immediately returns to normal once any pressure is relieved, is called qi drum distension.

g. Accumulation and gathering: Lumps in the abdomen, either swelling or pain.
> ① Immobile abdominal lumps with fixed pain, are called concretions or accumulations, and indicate blood disease.
> ② Mobile abdominal lumps with migratory pain, or no sensation on palpating, are called conglomerations or gatherings, and indicate qi disease.

h. Rope-like matter, which is found in the left lesser abdomen, is mostly due to hard stool stuck in the intestines.

i. Pain in the right lesser abdomen, with a mass when pressed, is mostly seen with an intestinal abscess.

j. A fluctuating abdominal mass when pressed, which has no definite place or peristaltic movements like an earthworm, is mostly due to worm accumulation.

3. Palpating the skin (cubit skin)

Palpating the skin means touching the skin at various locations. By examining some aspects, such as if it is cold or hot, moist or dry, slippery or rough, feelings of pain, swellings, and/or ulcers, the physician can identify the cold or heat, and deficient or excessive nature of the disease, as well as exuberance or debilitation of yin and yang.

The normal skin is warm, moist, lustrous, resilient and without rashes, swellings, distension, pain, ulcers or nodes, etc.

(1) Palpating to discern the coldness or heat of the skin

A. If the skin is cold and the general temperature of the body is low, this indicates deficiency of yang.

B. Cold of the skin due to reverse flow of qi and blood (when limbs become progressively colder from the extremities inwards, also called reversal cold), profuse sweating, white face and weak pulse, is a sign of yang collapse.

C. If the skin is scorching hot and the body temperature is high, this is due to exuberance of yang and indicates excessive heat patterns.

D. Warm skin accompanied by greasy sweating and a racing and weak pulse, is a sign of yin collapse.

E. A hot body and cold limbs indicates true heat with false cold.

F. An externally contracted disease, sweating, feverishness, and cold body, indicates an exterior pathogen.

G. An externally contracted disease, no sweat, and hot skin, is due to extreme heat.

H. If fever is severe to the initial touch but gets milder when touched for longer; this indicates heat in the exterior.

I. A hot sensation, which becomes even more severe when touched for longer, indicates heat in the interior.

(2) Investigating moistness or dryness, slipperiness or roughness of the skin

A. Investigating whether moist or dry:

Palpating can be used to detect for the presence of sweating as well as exuberance or debilitation of body fluids.

    a. Dry skin indicates no sweat or insufficiency of fluids.
    b. Dry and shriveled skin indicates deficiency of body fluids.
    c. Moist skin suggests sweating.

B. Investigating whether slippery or rough:

Palpating can be used to differentiate the increase or decrease of the qi and blood.

    a. Lubricated skin indicates prosperity of qi and blood.
    b. Dry and rough skin means shortage of qi and blood.
    c. Scaly skin suggests blood deficiency or blood stasis.

(3) Investigating the pain

A. If pain is soft and if any pain is decreased by palpating, this indicates deficiency patterns.

B. If pain is hard, full and extremely painful after palpating, this indicates excess patterns.

C. Pain felt with mild pressure indicates the location of the disease is superficial.

D. Pain felt with heavy pressure indicates the location of the disease is deep.

(4) Palpating the swelling

Swelling due to water (oedema) or swelling due to qi disorder can be differentiated by heavy palpating. If a depression appears after palpation and the skin does not return to normal (pitting oedema), it is swelling due to water; while if the depression in the skin rapidly returns to normal (non-pitting oedema), it is swelling due to qi disorder.

(5) Palpating sores and ulcers

A. Swelling, hardness, with no heat sensation, indicates cold patterns.

B. Swelling, heat, a burning sensation and pain with pressure, indicates heat patterns.

C. Diffuse and flat swelling indicates yin patterns.

D. Constricted swelling with prominence indicates yang patterns.

E. If the affected area is hard; this indicates there is no pus inside.

F. If the top of the swelling is soft and the sides are hard; this indicates there must be pus inside.

(6) Palpation of the forearm skin

According to the conditions of chronic and acute, slippery and rough, cold and heat of the forearm skin, the practitioner can often judge the nature of disease.

A. Extreme heat of the forearm skin and with a surging, slippery rapid pulse indicates warm-heat diseases.

B. Cold forearm skin with a thready and small pulse can be seen in diarrhoea and weak breathing.

C. Rough forearm skin just like dry scales of a fish, suggests insufficient essence-blood or blood stasis or phlegm-rheum.

4. Palpating the hands and feet

The purpose of feeling the hands and feet is to identify cold or heat patterns, deficiency or excess states, and internal or external conditions, as well as favourable or unfavourable prognosis.

The normal hands and feet are usually warm and moist.

A. Palpating the dorsal surfaces, palms and soles of the hands and feet:
   a. The dorsal surfaces of the hands and feet are more feverish than the palms and soles, indicating externally contracted fever (exogenous factors).
   b. The palms and soles are more feverish than the dorsal aspects of the hands and feet, indicating internal damage fever.
   c. The forehead is more feverish than the palms, indicating exterior heat patterns.
   d. The palms are more feverish than the forehead, which indicating interior heat patterns.
B. Palpating the hands and feet of the child:
   a. Coldness of the finger-tips may indicate convulsions.
   b. Only the middle finger is hot, indicates an exterior wind-cold pattern.
   c. Only the tip of the middle finger is cold, is a sign of the onset of measles.
C. Investigating the existence or depletion of yang:
   a. Yang deficiency with four limbs still warm, means yang is still preserved.
   b. Yang deficiency with coldness of the four limbs due to reverse flow of qi indicates a bad prognosis.
   c. Coldness of both hands and feet, indicates cold patterns.
   d. Heat of both hands and feet, indicates heat patterns.

5. Palpating the transport points (*shū* points)

The qi of the meridians, when converging on the body surface, will infuse into certain transport points (*shū* points), where some pathological changes inside the body will often be reflected; so this is a method in which special *shū* points on the body are palpated and pressed, to identify the changes and reactions of the points in order to identify some disorders of the *zang-fu* organs.

In palpating acupuncture points, one should pay particular attention to the changes in the acupuncture points or *shū* points, which include the appearance of nodules or cord-like substances, and abnormal reactions such as tenderness, red reactions or sensitivity to touch.

The frequently used transport points in diagnosis are:

(1) LU 1 (*zhōng fǔ*), BL 13 (*fèi shù*), LU 9 (*tài yuān*) can be used for diagnosing lung diseases.

(2) RN 14 (*jù quē*), RN 17 (*dàn zhōng*), PC 7 (*dà líng*) can be used for diagnosing heart diseases.

(3) LV 14, (*qī mén*), LU 1 (*gān shù*), LV 3 (*tài chōng*) can be used for diagnosing liver diseases.

(4) LV 13 (*zhāng mén*), SP 3 (*tài bái*), BL 20 (*pí shù*) can be used for diagnosing spleen diseases.

(5) RN 6 (*qì hǎi*), K 3 (*tài xī*) can be used for diagnosing kidney diseases.

(6) ST 25 (*tiān shū*), BL 25 (*dà cháng shù*) can be used for diagnosing large intestine diseases.

(7) RN 4 (*guān yuán*) can be used for diagnosing small intestine diseases.

(8) GB 24 (*rì yuè*), BL 19 (*dǎn shù*) can be used for diagnosing gallbladder diseases.

(9) BL 20 (*wèi shù*), ST 36 (*zú sān lǐ*) can be used for diagnosing stomach diseases.

(10) RN 3 (*zhōng jí*) can be used for diagnosing bladder diseases.

CHAPTER 8
Pattern Differentiation According to the Eight Principles

The eight principles are: interior-exterior; hot-cold; excess-deficiency; yin-yang. They are used as the foundation for all the other methods of pattern identification. It is the basic groundwork of pattern identification in Chinese medicine, allowing the practitioner to identify the location and nature of the disharmony, as well as to establish the principles of treatment.

SECTION 1
CONCEPT OF PATTERN DIFFERENTIATION ACCORDING TO THE EIGHT PRINCIPLES

The eight principles refer to the eight categories of pattern identification, namely, yin, yang, exterior, interior, heat, cold, excess and deficiency. These are the basic methods and principles of Chinese medicine pattern identification. Therefore, based on clinical experiences, the eight principles can assist in understanding the depth of the disease, the nature of the disease, the exuberance and weakness of the *xié* (pathogenic factors) and *zhèng* (healthy qi) and disharmony between yin and yang.

The method of pattern identification according to the eight principles differs from all the others in so far as it is the theoretical basis for all of them and is applicable in every case. It allows us to distinguish exterior from interior, hot from cold, and excess from deficiency.

SECTION 2
THE BASIC PATTERNS OF THE EIGHT PRINCIPLES

Exterior and Interior

The categories of exterior and interior are a pair of principles that determine the severity and depth of the disease and its location.

Exterior and interior are relative concepts. But generally, they have a concrete location (Table 8-1).

Table 8-1 Concepts of exterior and interior clinical manifestations

Key concepts on exterior and interior		Exterior	Interior	Clinical manifestations
Relative property of exterior and interior	Superficial portion of the body and *zang-fu* organs	Superficial portion of the body	*Zang-fu* organs	Transmission of pathogens from exterior to interior (aggravation) Transmission of pathogens from interior to exterior (alleviation)
	Zang organs and *fu* organs	*Fu* organs	*Zang* organs	
	Channels and networks and *zang-fu* organs	Channels and networks	*Zang-fu* organs	
	Three yang channels and three yin channels	Three yang channels	Three yin channels	
	Skin, bones and muscles	Skin	Bones and muscles	
In general		Skin, body hair, striated muscles, channels	*Zang-fu* organs, marrow	Exterior pattern: relatively mild Interior pattern: relatively severe

1. Exterior pattern

Concept: The exterior pattern refers to the slight and superficial symptoms caused by the invasion of the six exogenous pathogenic factors via the skin, hair, mouth and nose. It is mainly seen in the early stage of diseases caused by exogenous pathogenic factors.

Causes: Invasion of exterior pathogenic factors.

Clinical manifestations:
- General symptoms: Fever, aversion to cold (or wind), headache and body pain, thin and white tongue coating, floating pulse.
- Respiratory symptoms: Stuffy nose, runny nose, sneezing, sore throat, cough, sweating or no sweating.

Characteristics:
- Simultaneous onset of fever and aversion to cold, floating pulse, no marked symptoms from *zang-fu* organs.
- Sudden onset, superficial and mild, short course.
- Mainly seen in the early stage of diseases caused by exogenous pathogenic factors.

Analysis: See Fig. 8-1.

Types: Signs and symptoms of exterior patterns are very complicated. The reasons for this complexity is due to the various constitutions that people have and the variety of pathogens there are. This exterior pattern is usually divided into three types (Table 8-2).

Diagnostics in Chinese Medicine

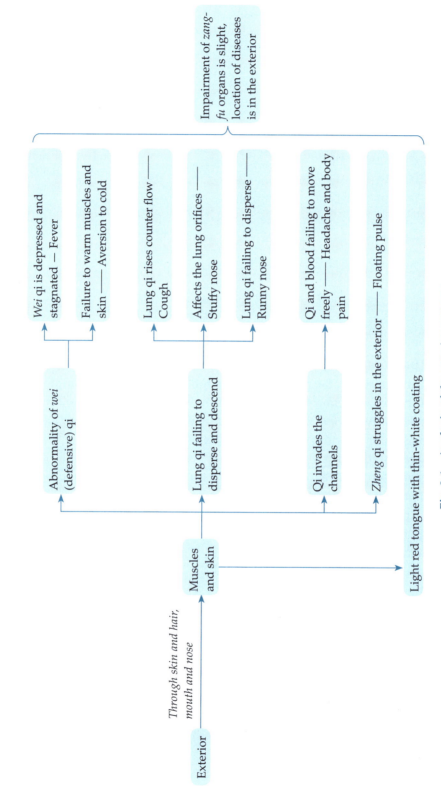

Fig. 8-1 Analysis of the exterior patterns

Table 8-2 Clinical manifestation of the three types of exterior patterns

Types	Causes	Clinical manifestation
Attack of cold	Cold pathogen	Severe aversion to cold with slight fever, no sweating, headache and body pain, thin white and moist coating, floating and tense pulse
Attack of wind	Wind pathogen	Aversion to wind with slight fever, sweating, floating pulse
Attack of wind-heat	Wind-heat pathogen	Severe fever and slight aversion to cold, thirst, sore throat, normal tongue body or slightly red in the tip and sides, thin-white and dry coating or thin and slightly yellow coating, floating and rapid pulse

2. Interior patterns

Concept: Generally refers to the pattern that has its location in the interior. Pathogens invade the *zang-fu* organs, qi-blood and marrow. Anything that is not an exterior pattern is ascribed to an interior pattern.

Causes:
- The exterior pattern is not resolved and enters the interior to invade the *zang-fu* organs.
- Direct invasion of pathogens on the *zang-fu* organs.
- Functional disturbance of the *zang-fu* organs by emotional factors, improper diet or overstrain.

Clinical manifestations: These are difficult to summarise.

Characteristics:
- Cold or heat symptoms, marked symptoms from *zang-fu* organs.
- Acute or chronic onset, severe conditions, long course.
- Mainly seen in the middle or late stage of diseases caused by exogenous pathogenic factors.

Signs and symptoms of an interior pattern vary. Pattern identification of cold-heat and deficiency-excess in this chapter and also pattern identification of qi-blood and body fluids, *zang-fu* organs, channels and networks in the following chapters, all are related to the interior patterns.

3. Distinguishing Exterior and Interior Patterns (Table 8-3)

Table 8-3 Comparison of exterior and interior patterns

Items Types	Course	Cold or heat patterns	Symptoms of internal organs	Tongue	Pulse
Exterior pattern	Short	Aversion to cold and fever	Are not obvious, but mainly seen with body pain and headache, stuffy nose or sneezing	Mostly unchanged	Floating pulse
Interior pattern	Long	Fever without aversion to cold or aversion to cold without fever	Are obvious and mainly seen with cough, panting, palpitations, abdominal pain, vomiting or diarrhoea	Mostly with changes	Deep pulse

Cold and Heat

Cold and heat are the principles used to differentiate the nature of the disease. Cold patterns and heat patterns reflect the relative exuberance and debility of the yin and yang of the body. For instance, the manifestation of yin excess or yang deficiency indicates a cold pattern, and the manifestation of yang excess or yin deficiency indicates a heat pattern.

1. Cold pattern

Concept: A cold pattern is a pattern that manifests in diminished function and movement of the body mechanism owing to yang deficiency, yin excess or an invasion of a cold pathogen.

Clinical manifestations: Signs and symptoms vary with different types of cold patterns. The common ones are aversion to cold or aversion to cold with a preference for warmth, cold limbs and curling up in bed, a pale complexion, absence of taste in the mouth, lack of thirst, clear sputum, saliva and nasal discharge, clear and profuse urine, loose stool, pale tongue with white moist and slippery coating, and a slow or tense pulse.

Analysis: See Fig. 8-2.

2. Heat pattern

Concept: A heat pattern is a pattern that manifests in hyperactivity of the body mechanisms owing to yang excess, yin deficiency or invasion of a heat pathogen.

Clinical manifestations: Signs and symptoms vary with different types of patterns. The common symptoms are fever, aversion to heat with preference for cold, red complexion and eyes, thirst with a desire for cold drinks, restlessness, insomnia, thick-yellowish sputum and nasal discharge, haematemesis (vomiting of blood), epistaxis (nose bleeding), scanty deep-yellow urine, constipation, red tongue with dry yellowish coating and rapid pulse, etc.

Analysis: See Fig. 8-3.

3. Distinguishing cold and heat patterns (Table 8-4)

Cold and heat patterns are the reflection of excess and deficiency of yin and yang and are the main nature of the diseases. So, we should observe the general manifestation of diseases, paying special attention to preference or aversion to cold and heat, thirst or lack of thirst, red or pale complexion, and also pay attention to urine, stool, tongue, pulse and etc.

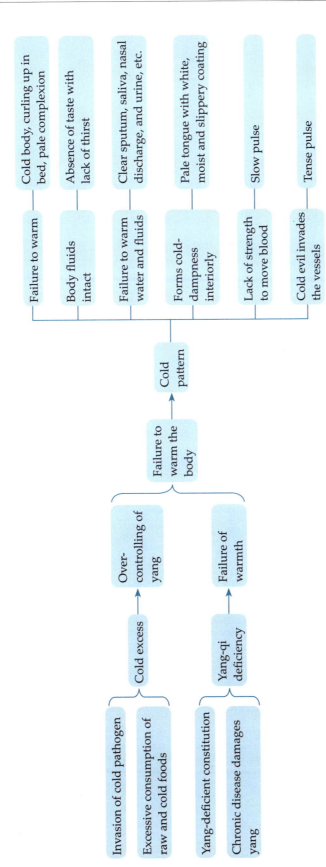

Fig. 8-2 **Analysis of cold patterns**

Diagnostics in Chinese Medicine

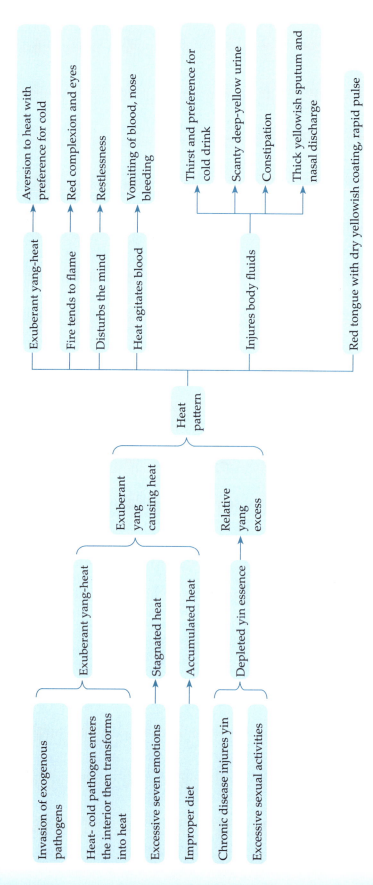

Fig. 8-3 Analysis of heat patterns

Table 8-4 Distinguishing cold and heat patterns

Items \ Types	Preference for cold or heat	Thirst	Complexion	Limbs	Behaviour	Sputum and nasal discharge	Urine and stool	Tongue	Pulse
Cold pattern	Aversion to cold and preference for warmth	No	Pale	Cold	Curling up in bed with little movement	Clear and white	Loose stool, profuse clear urine	Pale tongue with moist slippery and white coating	Slow or tense
Heat pattern	Aversion to heat and preference for cold	Thirst with a desire for cold drinks	Red	Hot	Restlessness	Thick and yellow	Dry stool, scanty deep-yellow urine	Red tongue with yellow and dry coating	Rapid

Excess and Deficiency

Excess and deficiency are the two principles that differentiate the strength and weakness of the body's *zheng* qi and the exuberance and debility of the pathogenic qi.

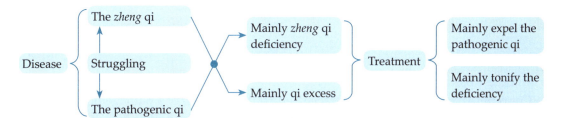

Fig. 8-4 A schematic diagram of the pathogenesis and therapeutic principles of excess and deficiency patterns

1. Deficiency pattern

Concept: A deficiency pattern includes all kinds of symptoms due to the weakness or deficiency of the *zheng* qi. The deficiency patterns suggest weak and insufficient *zheng* qi and absence of pathogenic qi.

We can distinguish four types of deficiency:
- qi deficiency, see chapter 10 (P.165);
- blood deficiency, see chapter 10 (P.170);
- yin deficiency see chapter 8 (P.140);
- yang deficiency, see chapter 8 (P.138);

Analysis: See Fig. 8-5.

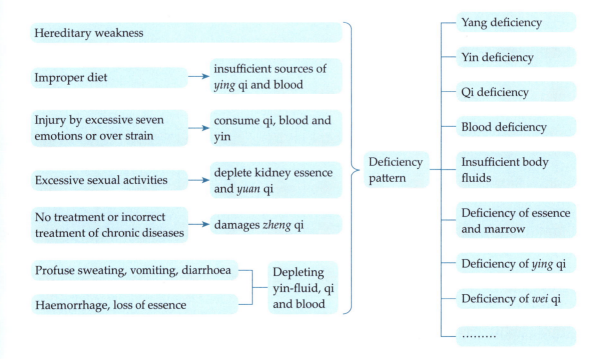

Fig. 8-5 Analysis of deficiency patterns

2. Excess pattern

Concept: An excess pattern is characterised by the presence of a pathogenic factor (which may be interior or exterior) of any kind, and by the fact that the body's qi is relatively intact, so qi fights against the pathogenic factor and this results in the occurrence of the signs and symptoms.

The formation of an excess pattern has two aspects:
- An external pathogen attacks the body.
- Dysfunction of the internal organs leading to the formation and retention of secondary pathological products such as phlegm, fluids and blood stasis.

Clinical manifestations: The signs and symptoms vary with different types of excess pattern. The common signs and symptoms are: fever, abdominal distending pain that the patient is reluctant to have pressed, restlessness, fullness in the chest, coma and delirium, coarse breathing, profuse sputum and saliva, dry stool, or dysentery, tenesmus, dribbling or inhibited urination, or difficult and painful urination, tough tongue with thick and greasy coating, and a forceful pulse.

Analysis: See Fig. 8-6.

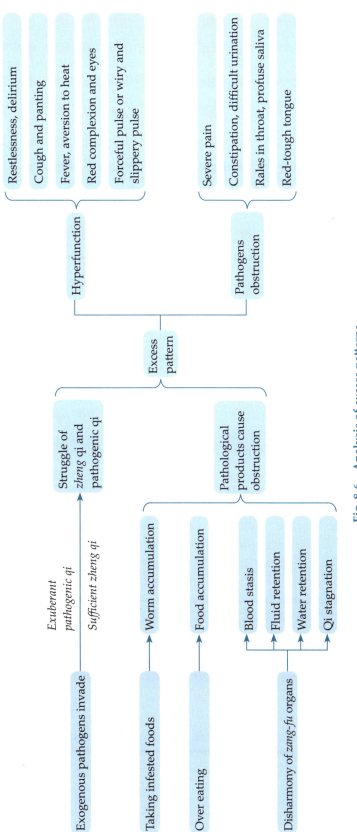

Fig. 8-6 Analysis of excess patterns

Yin and Yang

- **Yin and yang are the keys to the application of the eight principles**

Yin and yang represent two contradictory, yet complementary opposites. Yin and yang represent the general principle of the nature of the disease. CM uses the theory of yin and yang to explain the relationship of opposition and unity within human physiology and pathology. In addition, yin and yang are a summary of the other six principles in a general sense (see Table 8-5).

Table 8-5 Distinguishing yin and yang patterns

Types	Characteristic	Symptoms	Characteristics of the disease
Yang pattern	Exterior, heat, excess: active, restless, hyperfunction, bright, etc.	Outward, upward, and easily observed	Caused by yang pathogen, the state of the disease changes relatively quick
Yin pattern	Interior, cold, deficiency: quiet, restrained, hypofunction, dull, etc.	Inward, downward, and difficult to observe	Caused by yin pathogens, the disease changes relatively slow

- **Yin-yang has actual patterns**

In CM, yin-yang is not only a philosophical concept but also has many specific patterns. These patterns include:
  ○ yin deficiency and yang deficiency,
  ○ yin excess and yang excess,
  ○ collapse of yin and collapse of yang.

1. Yang deficiency pattern

Concept: This is due to yang qi deficiency and consequent hypofunction; lack of warmth; lack of movement and lack of qi transformation.

Causes: Chronic disease damaging yang qi, further development of qi deficiency, kidney deficiency with old age, living in a cold environment, taking too much bitter or cold medicines will all lead to hypofunction of the *zang-fu* organs, yang qi deficiency and failure of warmth.

Clinical manifestations: Aversion to cold, cold limbs, lack of thirst or thirst with a desire for hot drinks, spontaneous sweating, profuse clear urine or scanty urine, general oedema, loose stool, pale complexion, enlarged pale tongue with moist and slippery whitish coating, and a deep, slow and weak pulse, along with qi deficiency symptoms such as fatigue and shortness of breath. Yang deficiency is mainly seen in chronic diseases and has a chronic onset.

Analysis: See Fig. 8-7.

> **Key points for differentiation:** Manifests in chronic diseases or in those with weak constitutions. Symptoms are mainly aversion to cold, cold limbs, low spirits, fatigue, pale complexion, and a light/pale tongue.

NOTE:
① Yang deficiency often combines with qi deficiency, which is known as a yang qi

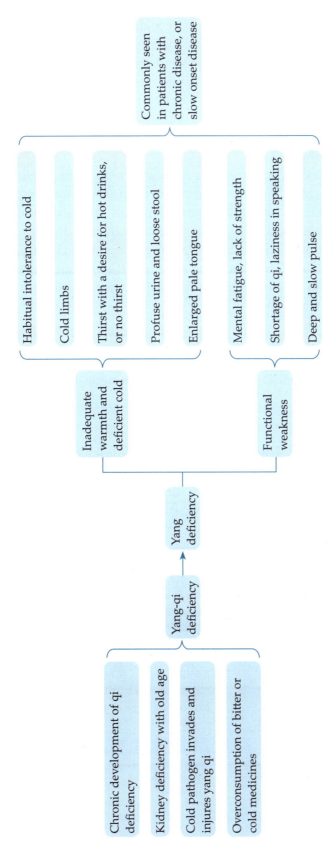

Fig. 8-7 Analysis of yang deficiency patterns

deficiency pattern. Yang deficiency will lead to cold, so there must be cold manifestations and the person will be easily susceptible to a cold pathogen. Yang deficiency can lead to yin deficiency (both yin and yang deficiency) and yang depletion. Yang deficiency can also bring about qi stagnation, blood stasis, water retention or phlegmatic fluid.

② Yang deficiency often involves multiple *zang* and *fu* organs such as the heart, spleen, kidney, stomach and uterus.

2. Yin deficiency pattern

Concept: A yin deficiency pattern refers to yin deficiency failing to control yang.

Causes: Injury of yin at the late stage of warm diseases, consumption of yin fluids due to emotional problems, excessive sexual activities, taking too much warm and dry medicines, etc. Yin deficiency fails to control yang and generates interior heat.

Clinical manifestations: Slim body, dry mouth and throat, tidal fever, red cheeks (malar flush), feverishness in the chest, palms and soles, night sweating, scanty urine, dry stool, red and dry tongue with little coating, thready and rapid pulse, etc. Yin deficiency usually has a long course with slow onset.

Analysis: See Fig. 8-8.

> **Key points for differentiation:** Manifests in a weak constitution due to chronic disease; characterised by emaciation, red cheeks and tongue, tidal fever, dry mouth, and a rapid pulse.

NOTE:

① Yin deficiency could coexist with or be a reciprocal causation with other patterns such as qi deficiency, blood deficiency, yang deficiency, yang hyperactivity, fluid deficiency, dryness (external or internal). Yin deficiency can also develop into yang deficiency and yin exhaustion. Yin deficiency could lead to wind stirring, qi stagnation, blood stasis and water retention, etc.

② Yin deficiency is always related to the heart, liver, lung, kidney and stomach.

For identification of yin deficiency and yang deficiency, see Table 8-6.

Table 8-6 Distinguishing yang deficiency and yin deficiency patterns

Types	Cold or heat	Complexion	Thirst	Urine and faeces	Pulse	Tongue
Yang deficiency	Aversion to cold and cold limbs	Pale	A bland taste, no thirst, or thirst and preference for warm drinks	Clear urine, loose stool	A slow and powerless pulse	A light and enlarged tongue, a white and moist coating
Yin deficiency	Feverish sensation in the five centres or steaming bones and tidal fever	Flushed cheeks	Dry mouth and throat	Brownish urine, dry stool	A thready and rapid pulse	A red tongue with scant coating and fluid

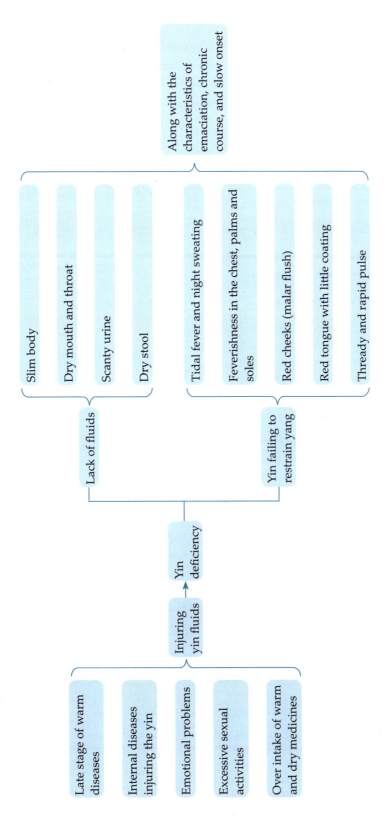

Fig. 8-8 Analysis of yin deficiency patterns

3. Yin excess pattern (excess-cold pattern)

Causes: Invasion of cold pathogen.

Clinical manifestations: Aversion to cold, preference for warmth, pale complexion, cold limbs, abdominal pain which dislikes pressure, borborygmus and diarrhoea, wheezing, phlegm, cough, panting, tastelessness, profuse saliva, profuse clear urine, thick whitish and greasy coating on the tongue and a slow or tense pulse.

Analysis: See Fig. 8-9.

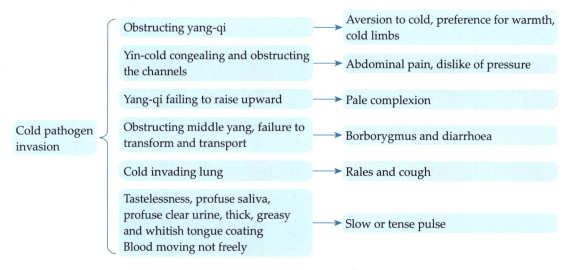

Fig. 8-9 Analysis of a yin excess pattern

4. Yang excess pattern (excess-heat pattern)

Causes: Yang-heat pathogen invades the body from the exterior to the interior leading to an excess-heat pattern.

Clinical manifestations: High fever, preference for cold, thirst with a desire for cold drinks, flushed face and red eyes, restlessness and delirium, abdominal distending pain, refusal of pressure, constipation, scanty dark urine, red tongue with dry-yellow coating, bounding, rapid, and forceful pulse.

Analysis: See Fig. 8-10.

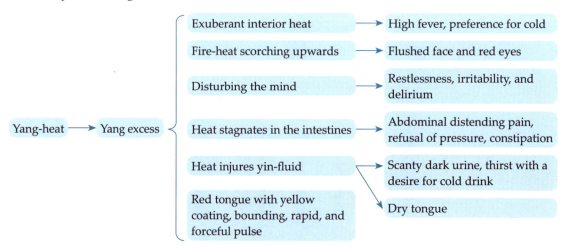

Fig. 8-10 Analysis of yang excess patterns

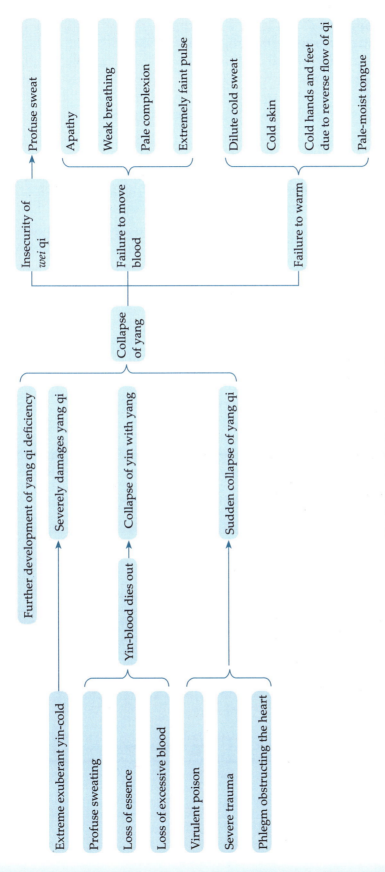

Fig. 8-11 Analysis of a yang collapse

5. Collapse of yang

Concepts: An extremely severe state of yang deficiency.

Clinical manifestations: Profuse cold and dilute sweating, apathy, cold limbs and cold skin, cold of the hands and feet due to reverse flow of qi, weak breathing, pale complexion, pale and moist tongue, faint pulse, etc.

Analysis: See Fig. 8-11.

> **Key points for differentiation:** A long disease history of yang deficiency or factors that lead to sudden collapse of yang qi; manifesting as cold sweat, coldness of limbs due to reverse flow of qi, a pale complexion, weak breathing and a faint pulse.

Yang collapse pattern generally refers to yang qi collapse of the heart and kidney. According to the theory of interdependence of yin and yang, yang collapse will lead to yin fluid exhaustion.

6. Collapse of yin

Concept: An extremely severe state of yin deficiency, which manifests as signs of extreme exhaustion of yin fluid.

Clinical manifestations: Profuse, warm, sticky or oily sweating, hot skin, hot limbs, restlessness, aversion to heat, thirst with a desire for drink, withered skin, scanty urine, red complexion, dry lips and tongue, thready, rapid and forceless pulse, etc.

Analysis: See Fig. 8-12.

> **Key points for differentiation:** Pathological basis for severe yin fluid consumption. Manifests as sticky sweating, hot limbs and body, vexation, thirst, dry lips, flushing, and a thready and rapid pulse.

Yin collapse commonly involves the heart, liver and kidney. If yin collapse is not treated at the appropriate times and properly, yang qi will inevitably be consumed.

For a comparison of yang collapse with yin collapse, see Table 8-7.

Table 8-7 Distinguishing between yang collapse and yin collapse

Types	Sweating	Four limbs	Breathing	Complexion	Behaviour	Tongue	Pulse
Yang collapse	Dilute, cold and bland sweat	Cold due to reverse flow of qi	Faint	Pale	Fatigued	Pale and moist	Faint and thready
Yin collapse	Sticky, hot and salty sweat	Warm	Coarse	Flushed cheeks	Restless	Red and dry	Thready, rapid and powerless

Chapter 8   Pattern Differentiation According to the Eight Principles   Section 2

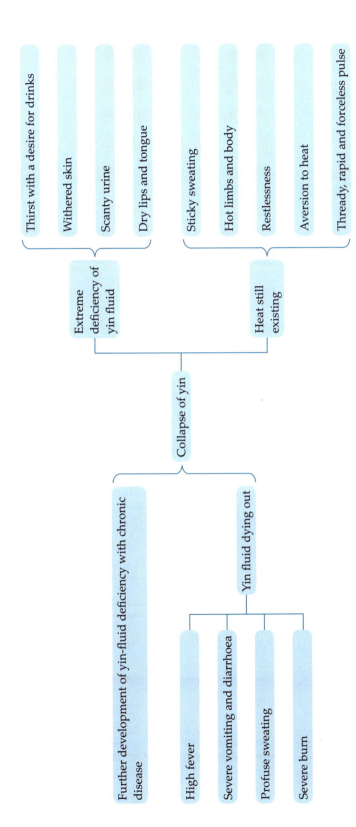

Fig. 8-12   Analysis of yin collapse

Section 3
The Relationship Among the Eight Principles Patterns

The relationship among the eight principles patterns can mainly be divided into three aspects: combination, transformation, false and true.

Combined Patterns

This is where two patterns of the eight principles mix together. They include a simultaneous exterior and interior pattern, hot and cold pattern, and excess and deficiency pattern (Table 8-8).

Table 8-8 Simultaneous exterior and interior pattern

Type	Cause of disease	Signs and symptoms
Internal-external cold	• Cold in the interior along with the exterior cold • Invasion of exterior cold along with internal damage by cold food and drink	Headache, body pain, aversion to cold, cold limbs, abdominal pain, vomiting, diarrhoea, slow pulse, etc.
Internal-external heat	Innate interior heat along with invasion of wind-heat	Fever, panting, sweating, dry pharynx with a desire for cold drink, restlessness, delirium, constipation, scanty urine, red tongue with dry and yellow coating or prickly coating, rapid pulse, etc.
Cold on the exterior-heat in the interior	• Exterior cold has not resolved with the interior heat • Interior heat with invasion of cold pathogen	Aversion to cold, fever, headache, body pain, thirst with a desire for drink, and heart vexation.
Heat on the exterior-cold in the interior	• Innate yang deficiency or damage by cold and raw foods • *Shaoyin* pattern with fever at the beginning and deep pulse • Exterior heat pattern is not resolved with excess intake of cold natured medicinals causing spleen and stomach qi deficiency	Fever, sweating, difficult digestion, loose stool, enlarged tongue, slight yellow coating, etc.
Internal-external excess	Exterior cold pathogen is not resolved with stagnated phlegm and food accumulating inside	Aversion to cold, fever, no sweating, body pain and headache, abdominal distension, forceful pulse, etc.
Internal-external deficiency	Deficiency of both qi and blood and deficiency of yin and yang	Spontaneous sweating, aversion to wind, dizziness, palpitations, poor appetite, loose stool, forceless pulse, etc.
External deficiency and internal excess	Stagnated phlegm and food accumulating internally, but insecurity of *wei* qi externally	Spontaneous sweating, aversion to wind, abdominal distension, refusal of pressure, constipation, thick tongue coating, etc.
External excess and internal deficiency	Congenital weakness and invasion of exterior pathogen	Aversion to cold, fever, no sweating, general aching and headache, abdominal pain at times, poor appetite or vomiting, etc.

1. Simultaneous exterior and interior pattern (Fig. 8-13)

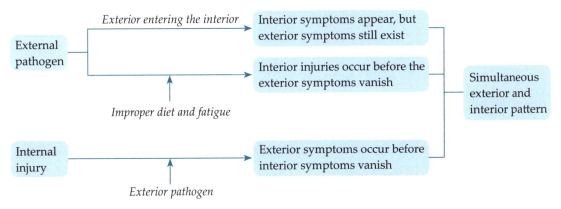

Fig. 8-13 Analysis of simultaneous exterior and interior pattern

2. Mixed cold and heat pattern

This can be divided into two parts:

(1) Exterior and interior: A pattern of exterior cold and interior heat and a pattern of exterior heat and interior cold. Details of this were discussed in **Simultaneous exterior and interior patterns**.

(2) Upper and lower: A pattern of upper heat and lower cold (Fig. 8-14) and a pattern of upper cold and lower heat (Fig. 8-15).

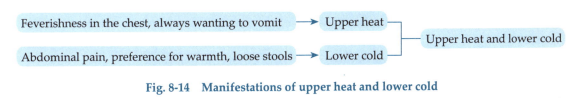

Fig. 8-14 Manifestations of upper heat and lower cold

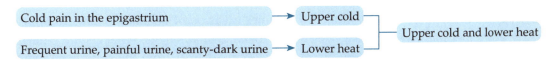

Fig. 8-15 Manifestations of upper cold and lower heat

3. Mixed excess and deficiency pattern

There are three patterns as follows: An excessive pattern accompanied by a deficient pattern, a deficient pattern accompanied by an excess pattern and both severe deficiency and severe excess (Fig. 8-16).

Transformation of Patterns

This refers to the contradictory patterns of the eight principles' patterns, which under some conditions can transform into each other. Pattern transformation mainly refers to transformation of one pattern into its contradictory pattern, completely changing the nature of the pattern.

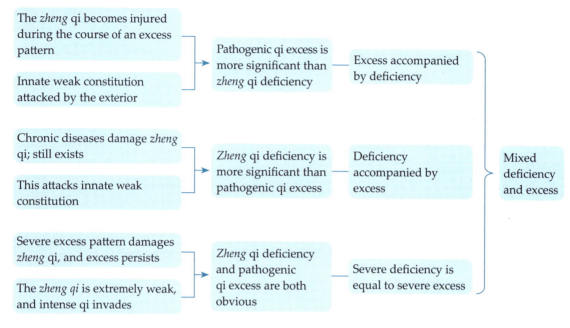

Fig. 8-16 The mechanism of mixed deficiency and excess pattern

1. The exterior and interior and moving out or entering in of the pattern

During the development of a disease, the exterior pattern, which has not been relieved through the struggle between *zheng* qi and the pathogen, can move into the interior and then forms an interior pattern, which is called an inner invasion of an exterior pattern. Alternatively, some pathogens leading to interior patterns can reach to the exterior from the interior. This is called an interior pathogen moving out to the exterior.

Inner invasion of an exterior pattern: This refers to the phenomenon when there is an exterior pattern at first, and then the interior pattern is appearing while the exterior is disappearing. That is to say, the pathogenesis of an inner invasion of an exterior pattern is the invasion of an exogenous pathogen. The inner invasion of an exterior pattern appears mostly at the beginning of disease caused by exogenous pathogens, which is the reflection of the pathological condition of the disease developing deeper from the superficial regions (Fig. 8-17).

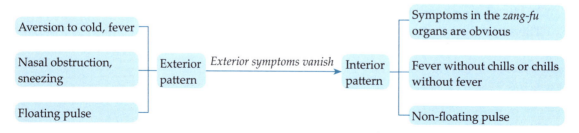

Fig. 8-17 Forming process of an inner invasion of an exterior pattern

Interior pathogen moving out to the exterior: This refers to the phenomenon when an interior pathogen has the tendency to move outwards. When an interior pathogen moves outwards this is generally a good sign because the pathogen has found a way to move out of the body and this usually suggests a good prognosis for the course of a disease.

For example in measles: when measles cannot come out fever, dyspnoea, cough and restlessness appear. Once the pathogen that causes measles has moved out, then the measles resolves and the restlessness, dyspnoea and cough disappear. During an exterior warm-heat disease, interior heat such as high fever can be dispersed by sweating. If pathogenic-heat invades yin-blood, general fever and restlessness will be relieved when maculae appear. However, this is not the transformation of an interior pattern into an exterior pattern (Fig. 8-18).

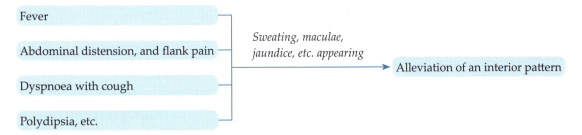

Fig. 8-18 Interior pathogen moving out to the exterior

2. Transformation between cold and heat

There are essential differences between a cold pattern and heat pattern. However, in some conditions a cold pattern can transform into a heat pattern and vice versa a heat pattern can transform into a cold pattern.

A cold pattern transforming into a heat pattern refers to the condition, which originally is a cold pattern and then the cold pattern disappears with the appearance of a heat pattern. For instance, if bronchial wheezing is due to cold, manifesting in a white coating and thin-whitish sputum, then after a prolonged course, the appearances change to a red tongue with a yellowish coating and thick-yellowish sputum this is transformation of a cold pattern into a heat pattern. Alternatively, symptoms of blockage by a cold pattern are a heavy cold feeling and numbness, and then owing to unsuitable treatment or delayed treatment, they are converted into redness, swelling and burning pain of the involved area, this is another example of the conversion of a cold pattern into a heat pattern (Fig. 8-19).

A heat pattern transforming into a cold pattern refers to the pattern, which is originally a heat pattern, but where the heat pattern disappears with the appearance of the cold pattern. An example of the transformation of a heat pattern into a cold pattern is a patient with a high fever, where, due to continuous sweating, the heat drains through the sweat; or, if there is excessive vomiting and diarrhoea, the yang follows the loss of fluids. These manifest as a sudden drop in temperature, cold limbs, pale complexion and a deep and thin pulse or an extremely faint pulse. This is caused by the original heat pattern transforming into a cold pattern (Fig. 8-20).

The key point in transformation of heat and cold patterns is whether yang qi is sufficient or not. If yang qi is sufficient, the cold pattern is prone to transform into a heat pattern; if

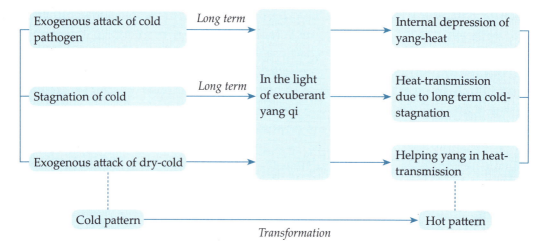

Fig. 8-19 Analysis of a cold pattern transforming into a heat pattern

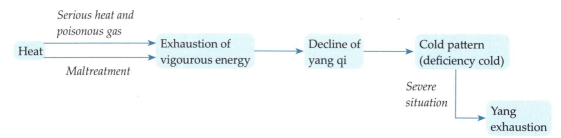

Fig. 8-20 Analysis of a heat pattern transforming into a cold pattern

yang qi is insufficient, the heat pattern is prone to transform into a cold pattern.

3. Transformation between deficiency and excess

In the course of a disease, an excess pattern can transform into a deficient pattern and a deficient pattern can transform into an excess pattern because of changes in the *zheng* qi and pathogenic qi. Although an excess pattern transforming into a deficiency one is common in clinic and generally happens in the course of a disease, a deficiency pattern transforming into an excess one is rare in clinic.

An excess pattern transforming into a deficiency pattern: This conversion can happen in clinic due to lack of treatment or inappropriate treatment, the course of the disease is lingering, then the pathogenic qi is gradually expelled, but the *zheng* qi is also damaged, consequently it gradually becomes a deficiency pattern (Fig. 8-21).

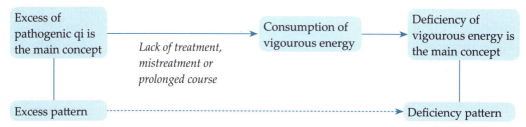

Fig. 8-21 An excess pattern transforming into a deficiency pattern

A deficiency pattern transforming into an excess pattern: This conversion usually happens in clinic due to insufficiency of *zheng* qi, leading to an inability to transport and transform, causing the accumulation and retention of an excess pathogen such as qi stagnation or phlegm production, etc. It should be regarded as a mixed excess and deficiency pattern (Fig. 8-22).

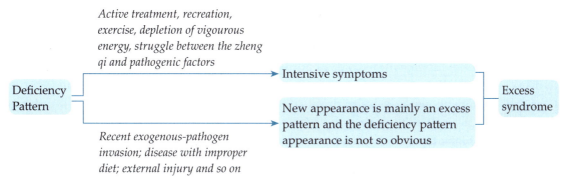

Fig. 8-22   Deficiency pattern transforming into excess

True and False Pattern

Some diseases have some false manifestations, which are contrary to the nature of the disease. We should precisely distinguish the nature of a pattern; subsequently we can make a precise diagnosis.

1. True or false & cold or heat patterns

Some false manifestations, which are contrary to the nature of the disease appear when the disease develops into extremes of cold or heat. For instance "the pattern of extreme cold appearing with heat signs" is real cold with pseudo-heat manifestations and "the pattern of extreme heat appearing with cold signs" is real heat with "pseudo-cold manifestations" (Table 8-9).

Table 8-9   Comparison between a pseudo-heat pattern and pseudo-cold pattern

Category	Synonym	Mechanism	Signs and symptoms
False heat pattern	Up floating of yang or excessive yin rejecting yang	Deficient and weak yang-qi, internal excess of yin cold, yang deficiency floating upward	• "True" cold: watery diarrhoea with undigested food in the stool, clear and profuse urine, pale tongue with white coating, etc. • "False" heat: reddish complexion, general fever, thirst, rapid pulse
False cold pattern	Excessive yang keeping yin externally or excessive heat causing cold	Internal excess of a heat pathogen, internal loading of yang qi will not reach outside	• "True" heat: thirst and desire for drinking, dry pharynx and halitosis, coma and delirium in the serious condition, dark-yellow urine and dry stool or heat dysentery and prolapsed sensation, red tongue with dry-yellow coating, rapid and powerful pulse • "False" cold: Peripheral coldness, deep and tense pulse

(1) Real cold with a pseudo-heat pattern or a false-heat pattern is the internal true cold with an external pseudo-heat manifestation.

(2) Real heat with a pseudo-cold pattern or a false-cold pattern is the internal true heat with an external pseudo-cold manifestation.

Caution: Complexion in a false-heat pattern is reddish, but the colour only appears on the cheeks, and it has an intermittent course and also it is different from the flushed complexion in a true-heat pattern. Although in a false-heat pattern the body is hot, the patient desires to be covered with clothes and quilt. Alternatively, the patient has a feverish dysphoria (ill at ease restlessness) but there will not be burning heat in the chest and abdomen, and the limbs will be cold. In addition, if the patient is thirsty but has no desire to drink, or drinks little, or prefers to drink warm liquids, then this is different from the true heat-pattern patients who desire to drink cool liquids. A floating, rapid and weak pulse is different from a surging, bounding and powerful pulse of the true-heat pattern.

The limbs in the false-cold pattern are cold, but the patient has aversion to heat and will have burning heat in the chest and abdomen. In this case although the pulse is deep, it is rapid and powerful. Therefore, we can conclude that cold limbs, rapid and powerful pulse are all signs of a false-cold pattern.

(3) Key points for distinguishing between true or false, and cold or heat patterns (see Table 8-10)

Table 8-10 Key points for true or false & cold and heat pattern differentiation

Key points for differentiating	False symptoms	True symptoms
Course of the disease	Often appears in the various stages of the disease	Usually runs through the whole course of the disease
Organs	Often manifests in the limbs, skin and face	Qi, blood, body fluid, tongue, pulse, etc.
Signs and symptoms	The appearance in pseudo-heat is the reddish colour, which only appears on the cheeks, but the complexion is pale. It has an intermittent course	The red colour covers the whole face in the true heat pattern
Signs and symptoms	The appearance in a pseudo-cold pattern usually is peripheral coldness, but there is burning heat in the chest and abdomen. Or the whole body is cold, but there is no desire to be covered with clothes and quilt	The patient likes to lie down and curls up, and there is a desire to be covered with clothes and quilt
Drinking test	In pseudo-heat, there is no desire for drinking. Sometimes vomiting after drinking	Thirst with desire for cool drinks
Drinking test	The pseudo-cold patient has a preference for drinking	Patient has no thirst and no desire for drinking

2. True or false & deficiency or excess patterns

Similarities between true and false patterns appear when the disease progresses to the serious and complicated stage.

(1) A deficiency pattern with a pseudo-excess pattern

This is a severe deficiency pattern with manifestations of an excess pattern.

(2) An excess pattern with a pseudo-deficiency pattern

This is a severe excess pattern with manifestations of a deficiency pattern.

Table 8-11 Distinguishing of true or false & deficiency or excess patterns

Deficiency-excess & true-false	Synonym	Mechanism	Signs and symptoms
Deficiency pattern with pseudo-excess pattern	Extreme deficiency with signs of excess	Disturbance in qi movements is caused by extraordinary deficiency of energy	• "True" deficiency: pain alleviated by pressure, shortness of breath, pale tongue and physically weak body and weak pulse due to chronic course of disease • "False" excess: abdominal distension and fullness, sonorous voice and coarse breathing, blockage in urination or defaecation
Excess pattern with pseudo-deficiency pattern	Extreme excess with signs of deficiency	Internal resistance of an excess pathogen, extraordinary accumulation, blockage of meridians, disturbance of qi-blood, failure to warm periphery and brain	• "True" excess: loud voice and coarse breathing, fullness in the chest, abdominal distension and pain which is aggravated by pressure, powerful pulse, etc. • "False" deficiency: quiet appearance, lassitude and no desire to speak, emaciation, thready and feeble pulse, etc.

Caution: Abdominal distension of a deficiency pattern with pseudo-excess is different from abdominal distension of an excess pattern. In the abdominal distension of an excess pattern the patient is reluctant to be pressed; while the abdominal distension of a deficiency pattern with pseudo-excess is intermittent and the patient is not reluctant to be pressed, or the pain is alleviated by pressure, or the feeling of pressure is soft. The voice in an excess pattern with pseudo-deficiency should be loud, though the person usually has a quiet appearance, but it would be different from a pure deficiency pattern, which has a low voice, shortage of qi and no desire to speak. An excess pattern with a pseudo-deficiency patient should be powerful, though the patient is reluctant to move while the symptoms can be alleviated after the movement, but the symptoms of a pure deficiency pattern are aggravated after the movement. In an excess pattern with pseudo-deficiency the patient feels comfortable after defaecation, though the stool is loose, while in a pure deficiency pattern the patient feels more tired after defaecation. The other signs and symptoms of an excess pattern with pseudo-deficiency are powerful pulse, rigid tongue, and thick and greasy coating.

(3) Key points for true or false & deficiency or excess

The key points are pulse taking and tongue inspection. Yang Cheng-liu, an ancient CM doctor, pointed out that here we should pay particular attention to the tongue inspection. All in all we should focus on the following points:

A. Pulse: forceful or forceless pulse, floating or deep pulse. Pay more attention to the pulse when palpated at a deep posistion.

B. Tongue: rigid tongue (excess pattern) or flaccid tongue (deficiency pattern); and coating: thick, greasy coating or thin or no coating.

C. Voice: loud voice or low voice.

D. Constitution of patient, the cause of the disease, long (chronic) disease or short (acute) disease, as well as the course of the treatment.

In addition, we should pay attention to suspicious and complex symptoms.

CHAPTER 9
Differentiation of Patterns According to Pathogenic Factors

This pattern identification requires analysis of the signs and symptoms, as well as any real life experiences, in order to grasp the cause or aetiology of the disease. It is always important to determine the cause, or aetiology, in Chinese medicine.

In addition, the identification of patterns according to pathogenic factors involves analysing the clinical manifestations of the patient in the light of the characteristics of the pathogenic factors.

Pathogenic factors are usually divided into "external", "internal" and "others" according to the classification of Chen Yan, a doctor in the *Song* Dynasty. The external causes reflect the six kinds of normal manifestations of changes in weather, which are called the six exogenous pathogenic factors and this category also includes epidemic pestilence. The seven emotional factors are usually considered as internal causes; whilst others, may include improper diet; overstrain; infestation or injury by parasites, insects, snakes and other animals; and trauma etc.

SECTION 1
PATTERN IDENTIFICATION OF THE SIX EXOGENOUS PATHOGENIC FACTORS

The six exogenous pathogenic factors include wind, cold, summer-heat, dampness, dryness and fire. The sources of these are the six qi, which are six kinds of normal manifestations of changes in weather. The reasons the six qi can create disease is either weakness of the body due to insufficiency of *zheng* qi, or alternatively if there are abnormal changes in the weather at inappropriate times, for any particular weather condition. When any of these six qi cause disease they are called the six pathogens. In addition, epidemic pestilence such as infectious damp-heat is also considered an exterior pathogen.

Characteristics of the six exogenous pathogenic factors:

① Disease caused by the six pathogens has a relationship to seasonal weather. Generally, as one might imagine, in the winter cold disease predominates whereas summer-heat disease commonly occurs in summer.

② The six pathogens can cause disease alone, or the six qi can combine, leading to more complex disease patterns, for example, wind-cold or wind-damp-heat, etc.

③ Initially, the six pathogens enter through the skin, mouth, and nose leading to the emergence of exterior patterns; after further development they may cause interior patterns.

Wind Pattern (Table 9-1)

Wind is yang in nature and tends to injure blood and yin. Wind is often the vehicle through which other climatic factors invade the body. The clinical manifestations due to wind mimic the characteristics of wind; for instance it arises quickly and changes rapidly, it moves swiftly, blows intermittently and moves upwards to sway the tops of the trees. Wind is divided into interior and exterior wind. Interior wind can cause paralysis of the limbs while exterior wind can cause facial paralysis or simple stiffness of the neck. Interior wind will be discussed later in Chapter 11 - Differentiation of Syndromes According to the *Zang-fu* Organs (p.186).

Disorders caused by pathogenic wind are characterised by:
- Sudden onset.
- Rapid changes in symptoms such as stiffness, paralysis, tremors, and convulsions.
- It affects the top part of the body.
- It affects the lung first.
- It affects the skin.
- It causes itching.

Table 9-1 Analysis of wind patterns

Types		Pathogenesis	Clinical manifestations
Attack of wind	Wind pathogen invading the exterior	Leads to insecurity of *wei qi* and opens the pores	Fever with aversion to wind, sweating
		Affects the top of the body and attacks superficial channels	Headache
		Lung fails to disperse causing disturbances of the lung system	Cough, stuffy nose, runny nose
		Wind interferes with the circulation of *wei* qi	Thin-white coating, floating and moderate pulse
Wind *bì* (migratory arthralgia)		Invasion of wind combined with cold and dampness in the joints and channels	Wandering pain in the joints and limbs
Wind-water		Wind invading the lung causes failure of the lung to regulate water passages	Fever, aversion to wind, facial oedema, puffy face and eyes, scanty urine
Urticaria		Wind interferes with the circulation of qi and blood under the skin	Wandering itchy skin, skin rashes which are of sudden onset and migratory
Wind-stroke in the networks		Wind pathogen invading the channels and networks and obstructing the channels	Facial paralysis: sudden facial numbness, deviation of the mouth and eyes
Tetanus			Neck rigidity, lockjaw, convulsions, spasm, opisthotonus

Key symptoms: Aversion to wind, mild fever, sweating, floating and moderate pulse, or sudden onset of wheals, itchy skin, numbness, wandering pain in joints and limbs.

Cold Pattern (Table 9-2)

Cold is a yin pathogenic factor and has a tendency to injure yang. The nature of cold is congealing and stagnating. Cold contracts the tissues and it hinders the circulation of yang qi. These effects of cold can lead to pain, which typically can be eased with warmth.

Disease patterns caused by cold pathogens can be divided into attack of cold and cold strike. The former is due to cold pathogen settling in the exterior of the flesh; the latter is caused by cold pathogens directly invading certain organs. Yang deficiency patterns can also generate internal cold, but this does not belong to the six pathogenic qi. Internal cold and cold pathogens may interact with each other, that is to say, patients with yang deficient constitutions are more easily invaded by pathogenic cold and pathogenic cold more easily invades a body already damaged by yang qi deficiency. When these two pathogens interact the internally generated cold is more severe and more difficult to resolve.

Table 9-2 Analysis of cold patterns

Types	Pathogenesis		Clinical manifestation
Cold attack	Cold pathogen congealing under the skin	Cold constrains *wei* qi and the pores are tightly closed	Fever, aversion to cold, no sweating
		Cold invades channels	Headache, painful body
		Lung fails to disperse and descend	Cough, panting, stuffiness in the chest, stuffy nose
		Cold invading the exterior	Thin-white coating, floating and tight pulse
Cold strike	Cold damages the spleen and stomach yang leading to spleen failure to rise and stomach failure to descend, and abnormal transportation and transformation		Clear vomit, intestinal rumbling, diarrhoea, sudden severe cold pain in the epigastrium and abdomen which is aggravated by cold, thick-white coating, deep and tight or taut pulse
Cold *bì*	Cold invades muscles, channels and joints leading to qi and blood stagnation		Pain of the joints and limbs, spasm, disturbance in joint movements, all of which are aggravated by cold

Summer-Heat Pattern (Table 9-3)

Summer-heat is a yang pathogenic factor and reflects the oppressive heat of summer. This summer-heat tends to consume qi and injure yin, it is often accompanied by damp. In severe cases, summer-heat can invade the pericardium and cause clouding of the mind which is often referred to as heat-stroke; this is not to be confused with wind-stroke which is very different.

Table 9-3 Analysis of summer-heat patterns

Types	Pathogenesis		Clinical manifestations
Attack of summer-heat	Acute warm disease, rapid transformation, tendency for injury to fluids and damage to qi, qi blocking pattern and liver wind pattern	Summer-heat steams fluids	Fever, profuse sweating, thirst with a desire to drink, dark urine, red tongue
		Copious sweating, loss of qi with sweating	Fatigue, lack of strength, deficient rapid pulse
		Combination of summer-heat and dampness invades the upper *jiao*	Poor appetite, nausea, vomiting, stuffiness in the epigastrium and abdomen, loose stool
Summer-heat stroke	Taxing work or other activities for a relatively long time when summer-heat is strong	Summer-heat disturbs the mind	Sudden faint
		Summer-heat damages qi and injures fluids	Sudden fever, copious sweating, thirst, hasty panting
		Damage to fluids and qi, agitation of liver wind, yang qi not reaching the extremities	May even lead to coma or convulsions
		Exuberant summer-heat injures *ying* qi	Dry crimson tongue, rapid or large and deficient pulse
Summer-heat-damp	Summer-heat combined with dampness leading to copious sweating which damages qi and fluids	Summer-heat injures fluids and damages qi	Sudden onset, high fever, profuse sweating, thirst, scanty urine, red tongue with yellow coating, surging and rapid pulse
		Summer-heat invades the pericardium and agitates liver wind	May even lead to coma or convulsions

Dampness Pattern (Table 9-4)

Dampness is the governing qi of late summer (the sixth month of the traditional Chinese (lunar) calendar). Dampness can result not only from damp weather or humidity, but also from damp living or working conditions.

The main characteristics of dampness are: dampness is a yin pathogenic factor and tends to injure yang, it easily disturbs the normal flow of qi as it is turbid and sticky. Diseases due to pathogenic damp tend to be prolonged and intractable. Damp is characterised by viscosity and stagnation, it is heavy and in the body produces feelings of sluggishness, it tends to go downward, and it causes repeated attacks.

The spleen likes dryness and dislikes dampness so dampness is liable to impair spleen yang. Damp fills up the whole body and tends to accompany other pathogens, leading to summer-heat-dampness, damp-heat, damp-cold etc.

Table 9-4 Analysis of dampness patterns

Types	Pathogenesis	Clinical manifestations
Attack of dampness	Invades the exterior and encumbers *wei* qi	Aversion to cold, fever, distending headache
	Blocks the qi activity and encumbers spleen yang	Chest stuffiness, poor appetite, epigastric fullness, nausea, no thirst
	Blocks the qi dynamic and encumbers clear yang	Heaviness of the body, fatigue, lack of strength
	Invades the upper and blocks the qi dynamic	Thin-pale coating, soggy or soft and moderate pulse
Dampness *bì*	Dampness is heavy and turbid and causes stagnation in the limbs and joints	Pain and heavy sensation of the joints and limbs, disturbance in joint movements
Warm-dampness	Retention of heat due to dampness encumbering	Mild fever, which is relieved in the morning and aggravated in the evening, sweating with no resolution of the fever, epigastric stuffiness, poor appetite, loose stool with a sensation of incomplete defaecation, fatigue of limbs and body, etc.
Eczema	Dampness spreads under the skin	See observation of skin in Chapter 2

Dryness Pattern (Table 9-5)

Dryness is the governing qi of the autumn and dryness syndrome arises mostly in this season. Dryness is a yang pathogenic factor and it tends to injure blood and fluids and usually attacks the lung via the mouth and nose.

Table 9-5 Analysis of dryness patterns

Types	Pathogenesis	Clinical manifestations
Cool dryness	Deeper into autumn, when the weather turns cool, cool-dryness invades the lung	Slight headache, aversion to cold, absence of sweating, cough, dry throat and lips, stuffy nose, dry and pale tongue, floating pulse
Warm dryness	A surplus of summer qi at the beginning of autumn. Warm-dryness invades the lung and injures fluids	Fever, sweating, thirst, dry throat, dry cough, chest pain if the cough is serious, blood-tinged sputum, dry nose, dry tongue with yellow coating, floating and rapid pulse

Fire Pattern (Table 9-6)

The nature of fire and heat are the same and fire is an extreme form of heat. Fire patterns can derive from direct invasion of a warm heat pathogen or it can also transform from the five qi of wind, cold, summer-heat, damp and dryness. Here, there follows a discussion on the externally generated fire pattern.

Fire is a yang pathogenic factor. Fire tends to move upward and dry out and damage the blood vessels; it can even generate wind to affect the mind. The clinical manifestations include high fever, thirst, sweating, coma, delirium, mania and convulsions, vomiting of blood or other kinds of bleeding.

Table 9-6 Analysis of fire patterns

Types	Pathogenesis	Clinical manifestations
Excess fire	In the qi level	Flushed face, red eyes, high fever, sweating, thirst with a desire for cold drinks, heart vexation, constipation, dark-yellow urine, yellow tongue coating, bounding and rapid pulse
	In the *ying* level	Severe fever at night, thirst with a desire to drink in small sips, heart vexation and sleeplessness, crimson tongue, rapid pulse
	In the blood level	Dark purple maculopapular eruptions, vomiting of blood, or other kinds of bleeding
	Disturbs the mind	Coma and delirium
	Generates wind	Convulsions
Fire toxin	Fire is depressed and stagnated to form a fire toxin, obstructing in the flesh to form corrupted flesh and blood	Skin ulcers, red swelling of the surrounding skin, accompanying pus and blood, high fever, dry mouth and tongue, coma, delirium, mania, red tongue, powerful and rapid pulse, etc.

SECTION 2
PATTERN IDENTIFICATION OF THE SEVEN EMOTIONS

The seven emotions are: joy, anger, anxiety, thought, sorrow (grief), fear and fright. Different emotions have different effects upon the internal organs. The normal expression of the seven emotions is healthy and cannot lead to disease. Disease is caused by an external stimulus, which leads to hyperactive or hypoactive emotional reactions, which can damage the internal organs. Each of the emotions has a particular influence on qi and affects a certain organ, which is seen in the Table 9-7.

Table 9-7 Analysis of the seven emotions

Syndromes	Pathogenesis	Clinical manifestations
Joy damage	Excessive joy impairs qi activity and disturbs the heart	Restlessness, incoherent speech, erratic behaviour
Anger damage	Anger damages the liver driving the qi upwards, and blood follows the qi upwards	Red face and red eyes, staring of the eyes, bursts of anger, vomiting of blood, even unconsciousness, sudden syncope
Anxiety damage	Anxiety damages the lung and spleen and causes the qi activity to become blocked and inhibited	Depression, lassitude, mental fatigue, poor appetite

Syndromes	Pathogenesis	Clinical manifestations
Thought damage	Thought damages the heart and spleen leading to failure of transportation and transformation	Poor appetite, fatigue, forgetfulness, palpitations, insomnia, thin body, withered yellow facial colour
Sorrow damage	Sorrow damages the lung and results in qi dispersal	Pale complexion and miserable expression, shortage of qi, laziness in speaking
Fear damage	Fear results in qi descending and affects the kidney	Apprehensiveness and lack of peace, often closing the door as if someone were coming to seize or arrest the person, urinary incontinence
Fright damage	Fright scatters qi and affects the kidney and heart	Palpitations, worry, panic, chaotic mind, uncontrollable talking nonsense, erratic behaviour

Section 3
Pattern Differentiation of Diseases due to Improper Diet, Overstrain or Lack of Exercise (Table 9-8)

Table 9-8 Analysis of pattern differentiation of diseases due to improper diet and activity, and excessive sexual activity

Types		Pathogenesis		Clinical manifestations
Improper diet		Excessive consumption of fatty and sweet foods, irregular dietary habits, abnormal transportation and transformation	It damages the stomach	Stomachache, intolerance of food smells, poor appetite, fullness and distension in the epigastrium and chest, rotten belching, acid regurgitation, thick and sticky tongue coating, powerful and smooth pulse
			It damages the spleen and intestines	Abdominal pain, diarrhoea
			Intake of poison by mistake	Nausea, vomiting, or alternating vomiting and diarrhoea, abdominal colicky pain
Improper activity	Overstrain and stress	May consume *yuan* (original) qi		Lassitude, preference for lying down, lack of strength, drowsiness, laziness in speaking, poor appetite, large and moderate pulse, or floating or thready pulse
	Lack of physical exercise	May lead to stagnation of qi and blood, and deficiency of qi		Obesity, difficulty in walking, shortness of breath on exertion, palpitations, weakness of the limbs

Continued

Types	Pathogenesis		Clinical manifestations
Excessive sexual activity	Depletes essence	May lead to yin deficiency and yang hyperactivity	Cough, haemoptysis, tidal fever, palpitations, night sweating
		May lead to yang deficiency and failure of warmth	Impotence, premature ejaculation, cold limbs, back and knee pain, nocturnal emissions

Section 4
External Injury or Trauma (Table 9-9)

External injury includes falls, incisions, knife wounds, gunshots, contusions, fractures, burns, frostbite, insect and animal bites, etc.

Table 9-9   Analysis of trauma

Types	Pathogenesis		Clinical manifestations
Knife wounds	Leading to injury or rupture of the channels and networks in the related area		Injury to some regions or organs, excessive bleeding, severe pain; generally excessive loss of blood, pale complexion, dizziness, etc.
	Tetanus		Fever, aversion to cold, tension and spasm, a tightly closed jaw, bitter smile on the face, muscular spasms and clonic convulsions, opisthotonus, profuse sputum, etc.
Insect and animal bites	Insect bites		Slight: redness, swelling and pain of the area, numbness, or papulae Severe: severe pain or numbness of the limbs, dizziness, chest stuffiness
	Rabies (dog bite)		Excitement, fearfulness, agitation, fear of water, fear of light, sweating
Falls, contusions	Falls and contusions cause qi and blood stagnation, collapse of blood, brain damage		Swelling, pain, bleeding, fractures in an injured area In severe cases or falls from a high place: vomiting of blood, or other kinds of bleeding In brain damage: dizziness, aphasia, syncope, coma

CHAPTER 10
Pattern Differentiation According to Qi, Blood and Body Fluids

Identification of patterns according to the theory of qi, blood, and body fluids is used to analyse and identify different patterns by applying the theory of qi, blood, and body fluids on the basis of their physiological and pathological characteristics.

There are some overlaps between these patterns and identification of patterns according to the eight principles and *zang-fu* organs. For instance, the pattern of qi deficiency is essentially similar to qi deficiency according to the eight principles. Qi, blood and body fluids pattern identification are important, since they complete the clinical picture emerging from the eight principles and internal *zang-fu* organs patterns.

Section 1
Patterns of Qi

Symptoms of qi diseases are various. *Plain Questions: Pain* (*Sù Wèn: Jǔ Tòng Lùn*, 素问·举痛论) says: "Various diseases arise from qi disorders". This text points out the extensiveness of qi diseases but these patterns of qi can be classified into:

- qi deficiency
- qi sinking
- collapse of qi
- qi stagnation
- qi counterflow
- qi blocking pattern

(Fig. 10-1)

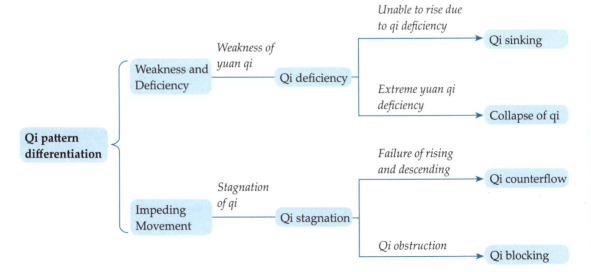

Fig. 10-1 Analysis of qi patterns

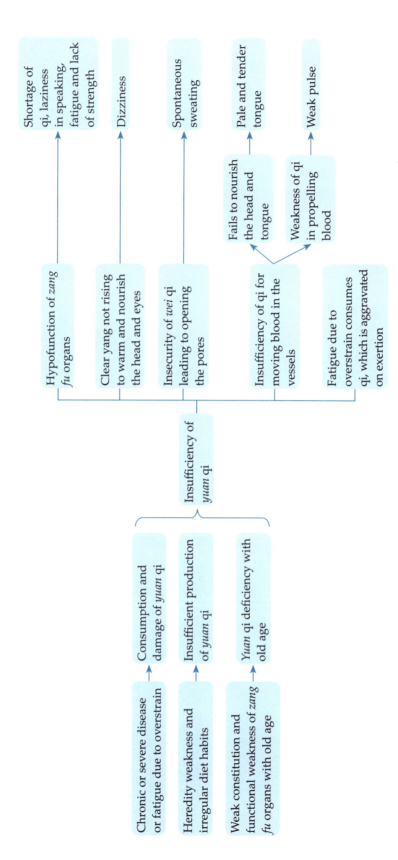

Fig. 10-2 Analysis of qi deficiency

Qi Deficiency Pattern

Concept: A qi deficiency pattern refers to *yuan* (original, primordial or primary) qi deficiency and weakness of the qi function. The normal qi functions such as its dynamic activities, warming, holding, defense and transformation are reduced and this can lead to hypofunction of the *zang-fu* organs.

Clinical manifestations: Shortage of qi can result in laziness in speaking, mental fatigue, lack of strength, dizziness, spontaneous sweating, all of which are aggravated on exertion. The complexion will be pale, the tongue may be pale and tender, whilst the pulse will be weak and deficient.

Analysis: Insufficiency of *yuan* qi and hypofunction of the *zang fu* organs result in shortage of qi, lack of strength, and fatigue, all of which are aggravated on exertion (Fig. 10-2).

> **Key symptoms:** Shortage of qi, lack of strength, fatigue, all of which are aggravated on exertion, deficient and forceless pulse.

Impairment of *yuan* qi usually results in functional weakness of the *zang-fu* organs; consequently there are various patterns such as heart qi deficiency, lung qi deficiency, stomach qi deficiency, spleen qi deficiency, liver and gallbladder qi deficiency, and kidney qi deficiency patterns. Furthermore some of these can happen at the same time.

Pathological changes of qi deficiency: Qi deficiency arises due to many reasons, and it can result in many kinds of pathological changes (Fig. 10-3).

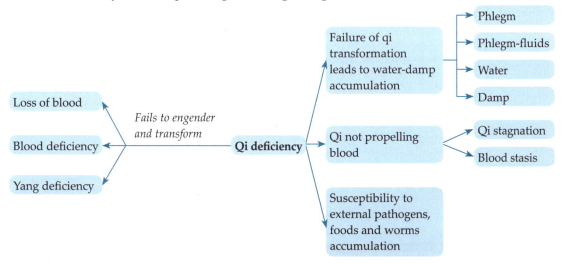

Fig. 10-3 Analysis of pathological changes of qi deficiency

Identification: Both qi deficiency patterns and yang deficiency patterns include shortage of qi, mental fatigue, lack of strength, spontaneous sweating, a pale and tender tongue, a weak and deficient pulse and other symptoms of functional weakness. However, a yang deficiency pattern is the further development of a qi deficiency pattern. In addition to the symptoms of qi deficiency, the yang deficiency pattern includes cold manifestations such as aversion to cold; cold limbs; pale, enlarged, and slippery tongue and a deep, slow and weak pulse.

Qi Sinking Pattern

Concept: This is due to further development of qi deficiency and is characterised by weakness in holding the internal organs, and their subsequent prolapses. In addition qi deficiency can prevent the clear yang qi from rising, and cause it to fall. It is also called spleen deficiency along with qi sinking.

Clinical manifestations: Dizziness, shortage of qi, tiredness, chronic diarrhoea, the abdominal area has a sagging and distending sensation, prolapse of the rectum, the uterus or another internal organ, and a pale tongue, with a weak pulse.

Analysis: The internal organs of the human body have a fixed location. They are inseparably correlated with flourishing of the *zheng* (healthy) qi. If *zheng* qi is deficient, or qi is weak, it often results in prolapse of an internal organ. Hence qi sinking generally has qi deficiency accompanied by a bearing down sensation of the abdomen or in serious cases, there is prolapse of the internal organs (Fig. 10-4).

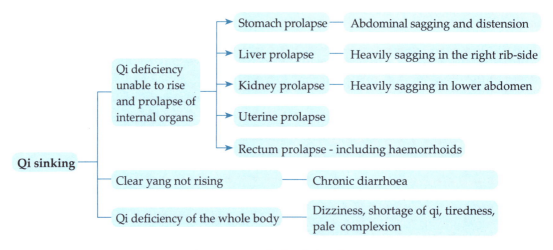

Fig. 10-4 Analysis of qi sinking

Key symptoms: Qi deficiency accompanied by visceroptosis.

Qi Collapse Pattern

Concept: This refers to critical manifestations of extreme qi deficiency and functional exhaustion of the *zang-fu* organs.

Clinical manifestations: Sudden fainting, pale complexion, weak breathing, profuse sweating, mouth opening and eyes closing, cold limbs due to reverse flow of qi, urinary and bowel incontinence, pale tongue, floating and large pulse without root or faint pulse.

Analysis: Generally, collapse of qi is the further development of qi deficiency. If it is caused by copious loss of blood, it is called collapse of qi with collapse of blood. Collapse of qi and yang usually appear simultaneously. Their symptoms are almost the same, except that the numbness of the limbs and cold body and cold limbs are the primary characteristics of the collapse of yang, but weak breathing is the primary feature of the collapse of qi. Therefore, it is usually called collapse of yang qi (Fig. 10-5).

Chapter 10 Pattern Differentiation According to Qi, Blood and Body Fluids **Section 1**

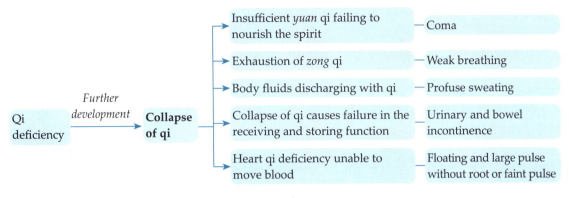

Fig. 10-5 Analysis of qi collapse

Key symptoms: Qi deficiency accompanied by spontaneous sweating; urinary, bowel, menstrual or essence incontinence.

Qi Stagnation Pattern

Concept: Qi stagnation happens in a particular portion of the body or in a *zang fu* organ where qi is impeded and obstructed.

Clinical manifestations: This pattern is described by stuffiness, distension and distending pain, wandering pain in the chest, epigastrium, hypochondrium and abdomen. Distension and pain wax and wane and are relieved after belching or flatus, and are often related to emotional changes. There is a taut pulse, and normal tongue.

Analysis: The key symptoms are: Stuffiness, distension and pain in a certain portion of the body (Fig. 10-6).

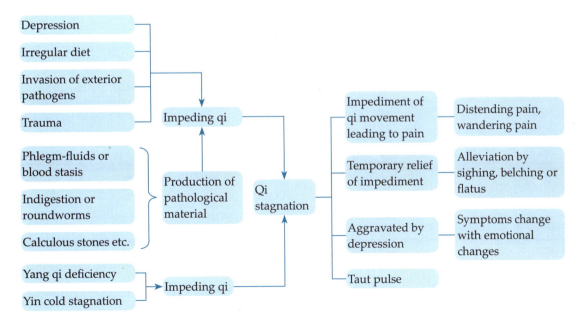

Fig. 10-6 Analysis of qi stagnation

Diagnostics in Chinese Medicine

> **Key symptoms:** Local distension, oppression and pain.

The causes of qi stagnation vary, and the locations are different, the symptoms have respective features. There are various patterns such as liver qi stagnation, stomach and intestine qi stagnation, liver and stomach qi stagnation.

Pathological changes of qi stagnation: If qi stagnation is prolonged, various patterns may appear (Fig. 10-7).

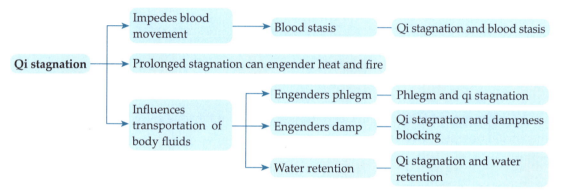

Fig. 10-7 Analysis of pathological changes of qi stagnation

Qi Counterflow (Perversion) Pattern

Concept: This is due to abnormal function of qi when rising and descending, which leads to upward disturbance of qi. This syndrome is mainly seen in the lung, stomach, and liver.

Clinical manifestations: When lung qi moves upward, this will result in cough and laboured breathing. When stomach qi counterflows upwards, this will result in nausea, vomiting, belching, hiccoughs and regurgitation, and liver qi rebellion results in headache, dizziness, syncope, coma or haematemesis (vomiting of blood).

Analysis: See Fig. 10-8.

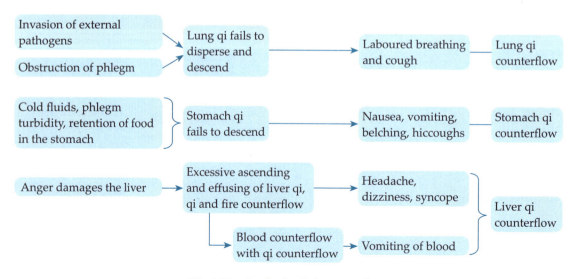

Fig. 10-8 Analysis of qi counterflow

Qi Blocking Pattern

Concept: This is due to an exuberant wind pathogen, phlegm, fire, or static blood causing rebellion and disorder of the qi dynamic, disharmony of yin and yang, and blocking of the qi dynamic.

Clinical manifestations: Sudden fainting, clouded spirits, loud breathing with phlegm gurgling in the throat, locked jaw, both hands grasping firmly, constipation and stranguria, slippery and rapid pulse or powerful wiry and rapid pulse or hidden pulse.

Analysis: See Fig. 10-9.

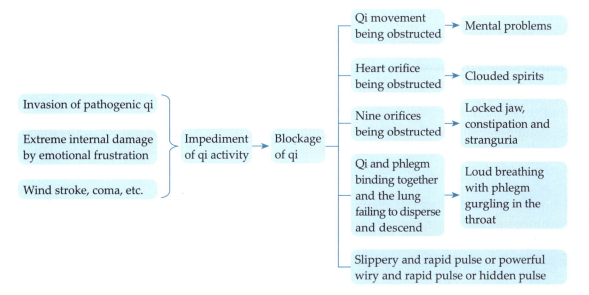

Fig. 10-9 Analysis of the qi blocking pattern

Key symptoms: Sudden syncope or colic pain, enuresis, defaecation, coarse breathing, excess pulse.

Identification: Qi blocking pattern and qi collapse pattern (Table 10-1).

Table 10-1 Comparison of the qi blocking pattern and collapse of qi

Patterns	Nature	Similarity		Distinction
		Features	Symptoms	
Qi blocking pattern	Excess	Sudden onset, changes quickly	Cloudy spirit or coma	Nine orifices being obstructed, locked jaw, hands are clasped firmly, constipation and stranguria, loud breathing, scanty or no sweat, powerful pulse
Collapse of qi pattern	Deficiency			Weak breathing, profuse sweating, mouth opening and eyes closing, cold limbs due to reverse flow of qi, incontinent urination and defaecation, pale tongue, floating and large pulse without root or faint and expiring pulse

Section 2
Patterns of Blood

Blood moves in the vessels, inwards to the *zang-fu* organs, and outwards to the superficial portion of the body. If an external pathogen invades the body, subsequently *zang-fu* organs will be disturbed, which can cause abnormal function of the blood. There are four patterns for blood disturbances:
- blood deficiency
- blood stasis
- blood heat (heat in the blood)
- blood cold (cold in the blood)

Blood Deficiency Pattern

Concept: This pattern is due to blood deficiency failing to nourish the *zang-fu* organs and vessels and manifests as weak symptoms.

Clinical manifestations: Pallor or sallow complexion, pale lips and nails, dizziness, cardiac palpitations, insomnia, numbness of the limbs, hypomenorrhoea, delayed menstruation or amenorrhoea, a pale tongue with a white coating, a thready and weak pulse.

Key symptoms: Pale complexion, lips, nails, tongue, mucous membrane and the skin, accompanied by failure of nourishment of the *zang-fu* organs (mainly heart and liver).

Analysis: See Fig. 10-10.

> **Key Symptoms:** Pale face, lips, nails and tongue, general weakness.

Blood Stasis Pattern

Concept: Blood stasis refers to blockage of blood in the meridians or vessels or in the *zang-fu* organs. Such blood turns into condensed clots, which have no ability to carry out normal physiological functions, therefore, a blood stasis pattern is caused by static blood blocking.

Clinical manifestations: Stabbing pain in a fixed location usually aggravates at night. Glomus lumps, which are blue-purplish colour when they are on the surface of the body. The repeated bleeding cause dark purple blood mixed with blood clots to result in ecchymosis; the stool is dark like the colour of asphalt; a dark and dusky complexion; blue purplish lips and nails; purple maculae under the skin; scaly dry skin; telangiectasia (coarse or fine red capillaries or a discoloured point with radiating lines under the skin); distending pain in the legs; amenorrhoea or metrorrhagia. In addition there will be a dark purple tongue, which sometimes has petechiae (purple spots), congested varicose veins under the tongue or blue-purple veins in the sides of the tongue, a thready and choppy pulse, or knotted and intermittent pulse, or sometimes no evident pulse.

Analysis: See Fig. 10-11.

> **Key symptoms:** Stabbing pain, glomus lumps, bleeding, dark purple colour in the mucous membranes or under the skin and a choppy pulse.

Chapter 10 Pattern Differentiation According to Qi, Blood and Body Fluids   Section 2

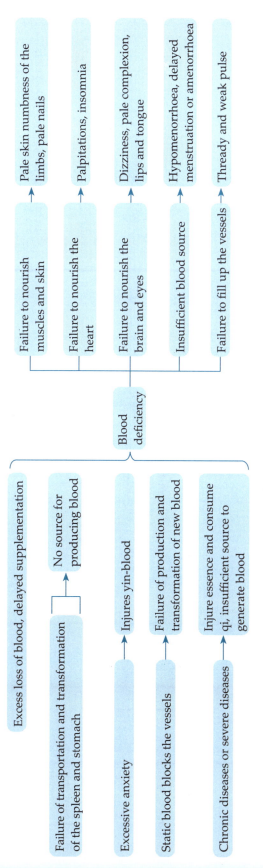

Fig. 10-10 Analysis of blood deficiency

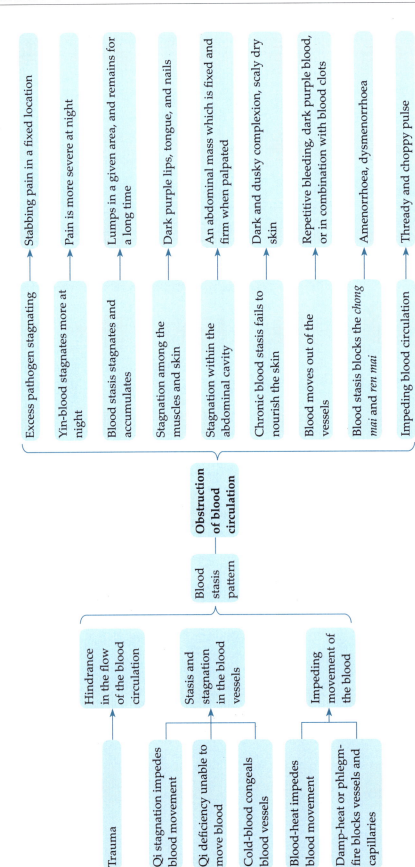

Fig. 10-11 Analysis of blood stasis

The domain of pathological changes of blood stasis or blood stagnation is extensive. For example:
- Stagnation and impediment in the heart vessels can result in chest stuffiness and pain
- Stagnation and impediment in the brain networks can result in coma, mania and headache
- Stagnation and impediment in the liver and gallbladder can result in jaundice
- Stagnation and impediment in the lung can result in chronic coughing and laboured breathing
- If blood stasis happens in the channels, it can result in pain, paralysis or numbness
- If blood stasis occurs in the five senses and nine orifices, it may cause functional abnormalities of the ears and eyes, dysphasia, and constipation, etc.

Blood Heat Pattern

Concept: This pattern is due to exuberant heat and fire in the internal organs agitating the blood.

Clinical manifestations: Haemoptysis, haematemesis (vomiting of blood), haematuria and haemafaecia (blood in the urine and stools), early menstruation, bright red and thick menses, accompanied by fever, thirst, red-crimson tongue, powerful and rapid pulse.

Analysis: Generally this is caused by depressed emotions leading to qi depression, which transforms into fire, or by excessive indulging in alcohol, or by excessive consumption of acrid and spicy foods, or by excessive sexual activity resulting in yin deficiency and fire flourishing that assail the blood (Fig. 10-12).

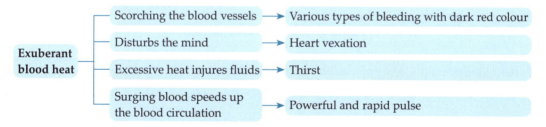

Fig. 10-12 Analysis of blood heat

Key symptoms: All kinds of haemorrhage, and symptoms of a heat pattern.

Identification: Blood-heat pattern and blood level pattern (Table 10-2).

Table 10-2 Differentiation between a blood-heat pattern and blood level pattern in warm heat (*wen bing*) diseases

Patterns	Similarity		Distinction	
	Causes	Symptoms	Features	Symptoms
Blood heat	Heat	Haemorrhage accompanied by a heat pattern	Slow onset, long course	Generally no high fever
Blood level pattern in warm heat diseases			Critical stage of warm heat disease, tendency to infection, sudden onset and short course	Usually accompanied by high fever, mania and delirium

Blood Cold Pattern

Concept: Cold in the blood is caused by retention of cold in the blood, which stagnates qi and impedes the blood circulation. Usually it arises from invasion of a cold pathogen.

Clinical manifestations: Cold pain mostly occurring in the limbs which can be relieved by warmth, pain in the lower abdomen, cold body and limbs, dark purple and cold skin, delayed menstruation with purple menstrual blood accompanied by blood clots, a purple tongue, a white tongue coating, and deep, slow and choppy pulse.

Analysis: See Fig. 10-13.

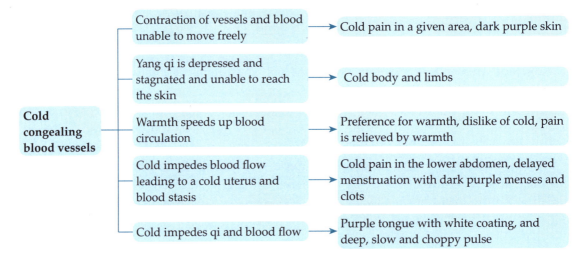

Fig. 10-13 Analysis of blood cold

Key symptoms: Cold pain in the limbs or lower abdomen, dark purple skin and complexion.

Section 3
Simultaneous Qi and Blood Disease Pattern Identification

Qi and blood depend upon each other for their existence. Qi is yang and blood is yin. Qi propels blood and blood contains qi. Qi is the commander of blood while blood is the mother of qi. When there are pathological changes, they may influence each other. So qi and blood diseases can occur at the same period, namely, simultaneous qi and blood disease.

The commonly seen patterns of both qi and blood include:
- deficiency of both qi and blood
- loss of blood due to deficiency of qi
- collapse of qi resulting from excessive haemorrhage
- stagnation of blood due to deficiency of qi
- blood stasis due to stagnation of qi

(Fig. 10-14).

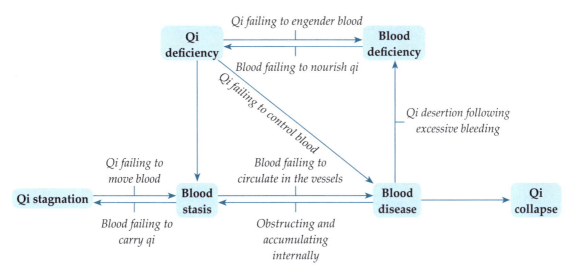

Fig. 10-14 Mutual relationship of qi and blood disease

Qi Stagnation and Blood Stasis

Concept: This refers to the pattern of depression and stagnation of qi resulting in obstruction and stasis of blood movement.

Clinical manifestations: Distension, fullness and wandering pain in the chest and hypochondria, irritability, abdominal masses, stabbing pain. Dysmenorrhoea, a dark purple menstruation mingled with blood clots. A purple tongue or sometimes tongue with ecchymosis and a choppy pulse.

Analysis: The liver dominates the free flow of qi. Emotional depression causes failure of the liver in organising the free flow of qi and blood, thus leading to irritability, distension and wandering pain in the chest and hypochondria, consequently stagnation of qi gives rise to blood stasis, thus causing abdominal masses (Fig. 10-15).

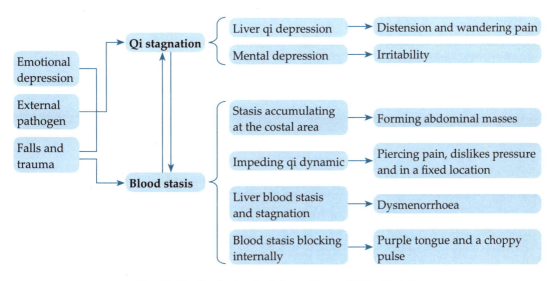

Fig. 10-15 Analysis of qi stagnation and blood stasis

Qi Deficiency and Blood Stasis

Concept: This pattern is caused by failing to propel the blood due to qi deficiency, which leads to stasis and stagnation of blood circulation.

Clinical manifestations: A pale complexion, tiredness and lack of strength, shortness of breath and laziness in speaking, stabbing pain which the patient is reluctant to have pressed, and commonly occurring in the chest area, a purple tongue or sometimes a tongue with ecchymosis, and a deep and choppy pulse.

Analysis: See Fig. 10-16.

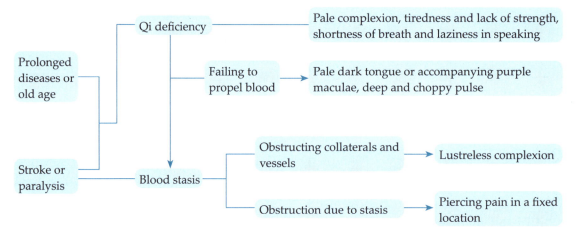

Fig. 10-16 Analysis of qi deficiency and blood stasis

Key symptoms: Qi deficiency and blood stasis occur simultaneously, and clinically the location of the pain is usually in the chest area.

Deficiency of Both Qi and Blood

Concept: This refers to the simultaneous symptoms of qi deficiency and blood deficiency.

Clinical manifestations: Dizziness, shortness of breath and laziness in speaking, lack of strength, spontaneous sweating, pallor or sallow complexion, heart palpitations and insomnia, a pale and tender tongue and a fine and weak pulse.

Analysis: See Fig. 10-17.

Key symptoms: Pale or sallow complexion, palpitations, insomnia, dizziness and debility.

Loss of Blood due to Deficiency of Qi (Qi Failing to Control Blood)

Concept: This pattern refers to haemorrhage or extravasations of blood due to qi deficiency.

Clinical manifestation Vomiting of blood, blood in the stool, subcutaneous ecchymosis, copious menstruation, shortness of breath, tiredness and lack of strength, pale complexion, pale tongue and a thready weak pulse.

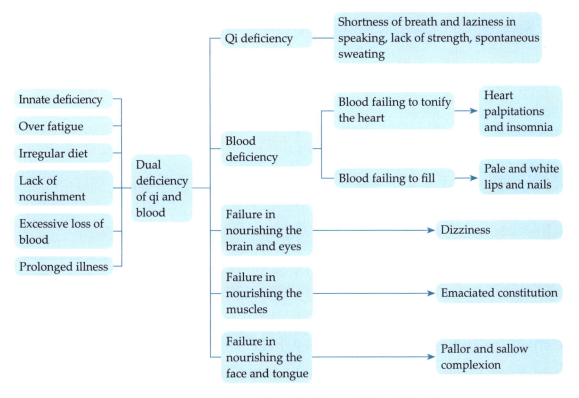

Fig. 10-17 Analysis of dual deficiency of qi and blood

Analysis: This is usually due to chronic disease, which damages qi, or chronic blood loss, which exhausts qi and consequently causes qi failing to hold blood (Fig. 10-18).

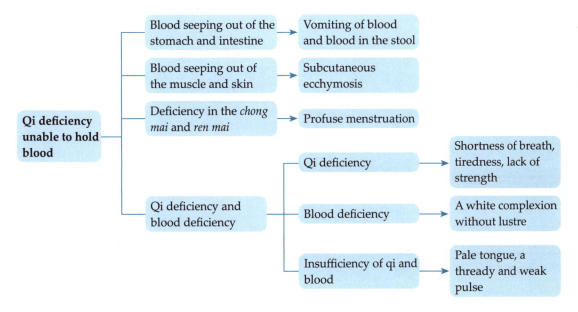

Fig. 10-18 Analysis of qi not holding blood

Key symptoms: Qi deficiency and haemorrhage occurring simultaneously.

Identification: Loss of blood due to deficiency of qi, and a blood heat pattern (Table 10-3).

Table 10-3   Differentiation between loss of blood due to deficiency of qi, and a blood heat pattern

Patterns	Course of disease	Nature	Colour and quality of blood	Symptoms	Tongue and pulse
Qi failing to hold blood	Usually chronic, transforming slowly	Deficiency pattern	Pale and thin	Shortness of breath, laziness in speaking, tiredness, lack of strength	A pale tongue, a thready and weak pulse
Bleeding due to blood heat	Usually acute, transforming quickly	Excess pattern	Bright red and dense	General fever, heart vexation, thirst	A purple-red tongue, a string-like and rapid pulse

Collapse of Qi Resulting from Haemorrhage

Concept: This is caused by qi collapse due to excessive haemorrhage.

Clinical manifestations: Excessive bleeding, pallor, cold limbs and profuse cold sweating, dizziness, an extreme weak pulse or fading or faint pulse.

Analysis: This pattern is often caused by trauma with profuse bleeding, excessive functional uterine bleeding, and excessive postpartum haemorrhage (Fig. 10-19).

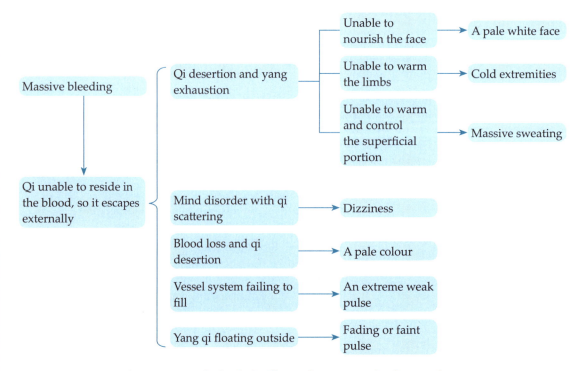

Fig. 10-19   Analysis of qi collapse due to excessive haemorrhage

Key symptoms: Excessive haemorrhage and collapse of qi.

Identification: Collapse of qi resulting from haemorrhage and qi failing to hold blood (Table 10-4).

Table 10-4 Differentiation between collapse of qi resulting from haemorrhage, and qi failing to hold blood

Patterns	Similarity	Difference	
		Cause and pathogenesis	Progress
Collapse of qi resulting from haemorrhage	Bleeding and qi deficiency	Massive bleeding first, then qi collapse due to no blood to support it	Abrupt and quick bleeding accompanied by critical symptoms of qi collapse and yang exhaustion
Qi failing to hold blood		Qi deficiency and inability to hold blood inside the vessels	Slow onset with bleeding in a small amount

SECTION 4
PATTERNS OF BODY FLUIDS

Body fluid is the general name of normal fluids in the human body. It has the functions of nourishing the *zang-fu* organs, lubricating the joints, nourishing the muscle and skin etc. Production and transportation of body fluids mainly have a close relationship with the transportation and transformation action of the spleen, the harmonisation action of the lung and steaming function of the kidney. Generally, the pathological changes of the body fluids includes two aspects:
- insufficiency of body fluids
- stagnation and accumulation of fluid

Insufficiency of Body Fluids Pattern

Insufficiency of body fluids refers to the pattern resulting from lack of nourishment and moistening of the whole body or some organs such as *zang-fu* organs due to body fluid deficiency. This pattern is also called an internal dryness pattern.

Clinical manifestations: These include a dry throat and lips, dry or splitting lips, depressed eyeballs, dry skin or even dehydration and emaciation, thirst, scanty urine, dry stools, a red tongue with little fluid, a fine and rapid pulse.

Analysis: See Fig. 10-20.

Key symptoms: Dryness of lips, tongue, throat and skin, and scanty urine and dry stool.

Clinically, according to different reflections of internal organs, an insufficiency of body fluids pattern can be divided into insufficiency of body fluids due to lung dryness, stomach dryness, or intestinal dryness.

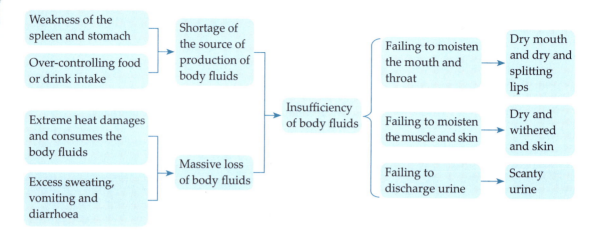

Fig. 10-20 Analysis of insufficiency of body fluids

Retention of Body Fluids Pattern

Six exogenous pathogenic factors and internal damage by seven emotions will influence the transportation and distribution function of the *zang-fu* organs, channels, vessels, and *sanjiao*, all of which impede the distribution and excretion of body fluids and create retention of fluids in a local area or in the whole body. Though pathological changes of this pattern vary, oedema and phlegm-fluids are clinically the most commonly found of retained fluids.

1. Oedema

Water retention in the body overflowing into the skin leading to puffiness of the head and face, limbs, chest, abdomen, and even all over the body, is called oedema. Clinically, it is divided into yang oedema and yin oedema; and it is appropriate to be able to distinguish between yang oedema and yin oedema in clinic.

A. Yang oedema:

This oedema is excess in nature. It is usually caused by a wind pathogen invasion, or invasion of water-damp in the interior, or failure of the spleen in transporting and transforming. The following two patterns are frequently seen in clinic.

a. Wind-water fighting the lung pattern

Concept: This includes a wind pathogen impairing the lung's function of dispersing and descending, leading to disturbances in regulating the water passage and so causes water overflowing in the skin and muscles.

Clinical manifestations: Oedema starting at the eyelid and face, then rapidly spreading all over the body; oliguria (scanty urine) occurs abruptly; the skin is thin and bright, accompanied by aversion to cold (wind-cold), no sweat, a thin and white tongue coating and superficial and tight pulse; or there may be swelling of the throat, a red tongue and a superficial and rapid pulse (wind-heat).

Analysis: See Fig. 10-21.

Key symptoms: Abrupt swelling of the eyelid, head and face.

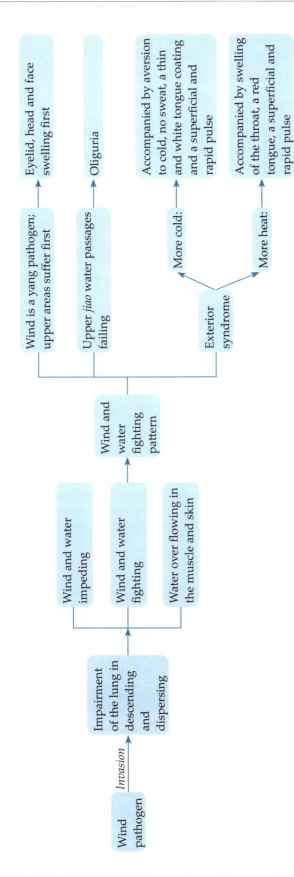

Fig. 10-21 Analysis of wind and water fighting

b. Water-damp obstructing the spleen

Concept: Water-dampness impairs the function of the spleen leading to failure of the spleen in transforming and transporting, subsequently accumulated water overflows in to the subcutaneous tissue causing oedema. The onset of this type of oedema develops slowly.

Clinical manifestations: General oedema, which occurs slowly, the practioners fingers become submerged on palpation, heavy limbs and drowsiness, oliguria (scanty urine), and fullness in the epigastrium, anorexia, nausea and a white and greasy tongue coating, and deep pulse. If this pattern transforms into a heat pattern, urine will be yellow and scanty; there will be a red tongue with yellow and greasy coating, and a deep rapid pulse or a soft rapid pulse.

Analysis: See Fig. 10-22.

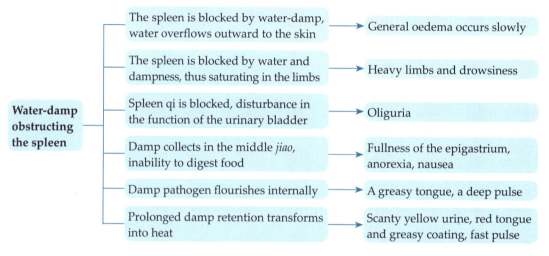

Fig. 10-22 Analysis of damp pathogen obstructing the spleen

B. Yin oedema:

Concept: This oedema is deficient in nature. It is usually caused by deficiency of the *zheng* (healthy) qi after prolonged illness, fatigue or internal damage, and/or incorrect treatment of yang oedema.

Clinical manifestations: Oedema which is more serious below the lumbar region, pitting oedema (indentation remains after pressure), oliguria, epigastric fullness and abdominal distension, anorexia and loose stool, pallor or sallow complexion, tiredness and heavy limbs, pale tongue with slippery coating and a deep pulse. If oedema aggravates increasingly, there will be difficulty in micturition (urination), cold limbs, chilly feeling, fatigue, white and grey complexion, pale and plump tongue, white and slippery tongue coating and a deep, slow, and forceless pulse.

Analysis: See Fig. 10-23.

Key symptoms: This oedema forms slowly and starts from below the lumbar region and shows indentation on pressure, subsequently oedema occurs firstly in the feet and then in severe cases below the waist.

Identification: Yin oedema and yang oedema (Table 10-5).

Chapter 10 Pattern Differentiation According to Qi, Blood and Body Fluids Section 4

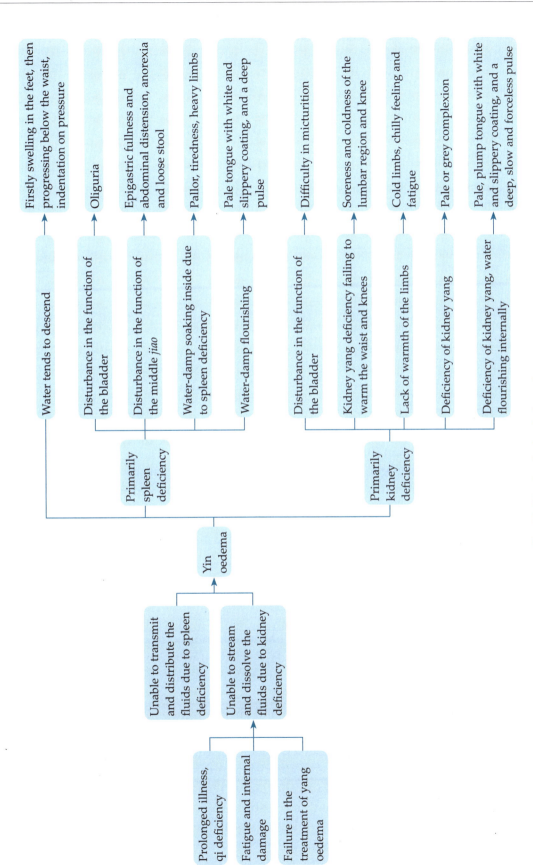

Fig. 10-23 Analysis of yin oedema

Table 10-5 Differentiation between yang oedema and yin oedema

Pattern	Causes	Nature	Onset	Features of oedema	Symptoms	Tongue	Pulse
Yang oedema	Wind pathogen, water-damp soaking, damp heat collecting internally	Excess, heat	Acute	At first in the eyelids, head and face and is more serious in the upper body	Exterior pattern, or tiredness, heavy limbs, fullness of epigastrium	White, greasy or thin, white coating	Superficial or deep, forceful pulse
Yin oedema	Prolonged illness and deficiency of the *zheng* qi, fatigue and internal damage, failure in treatment of yang oedema	Deficiency, cold	Chronic	Usually the feet suffer at first, below the waist is more serious	Cold and tired limbs and tired mind, cold pain in the waist and knees	Pale, plump, tender, with white and slippery coating	Deep, slow and forceless pulse

2. Phlegm-fluid retention (turbidity)

Both phlegm and pathogenic fluid (turbidity) are pathological products of the body fluid, which result from disturbance of water-fluid metabolism. Phlegm is dense, while turbidity is thin. In clinic, their manifestations are different though they are in the same category.

A. Phlegm pattern:

Concept: Phlegm is caused by fluid condensation, which can block every part of the body.

Clinical manifestations: Cough and panting (asthma), chest distress, rattle sound of phlegm in the throat, expectoration. Fullness in the chest, abdominal masses, anorexia, nausea, dizziness and vertigo, coma, uncontrolled and excited behaviour (mania), numbness of the limbs, hemiplegia, scrofula, goitre, tumour, subcutaneous nodules, nodules of the breast and foreign body sensation in throat, a white greasy or yellow greasy tongue coating, and a slippery pulse (Fig. 10-24).

Analysis: The symptoms of phlegm vary and change frequently. Phlegm has various manifestations in different organs such as obstruction in the chest and diaphragm, accumulation in the intestine and stomach, or blockage in the meridians, limbs, and tissues. It flows everywhere by means of the rising and falling of qi, so the symptoms are innumerable. Mostly, strange and extraordinary signs and symptoms are caused by phlegm. Ancient doctors believed that "most strange diseases arise from phlegm". In general, phlegm can be divided into two kinds, visible (narrowly defined) phlegm and invisible (broadly defined) phlegm. Visible phlegm is easy to identify, such as sputum after expectoration, vomiting of phlegm, rattle sound of phlegm in the throat, subcutaneous

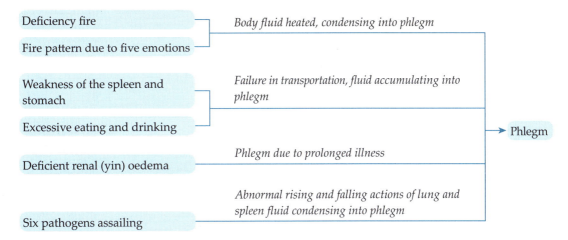

Fig. 10-24　Pathogenesis of phlegm

nodules etc.. Invisible phlegm is hard to make a definite diagnosis, such as insomnia, uncontrolled and excited behaviour (mania), dizziness, obstructed feeling in the throat (Globus Hystericus), and chest distress, shortness of breath, paralysis and numbness of the limbs. In clinic, diagnosis can be made according to signs of greasy or sticky tongue coating, and slippery or smooth pulse (Fig. 10-25).

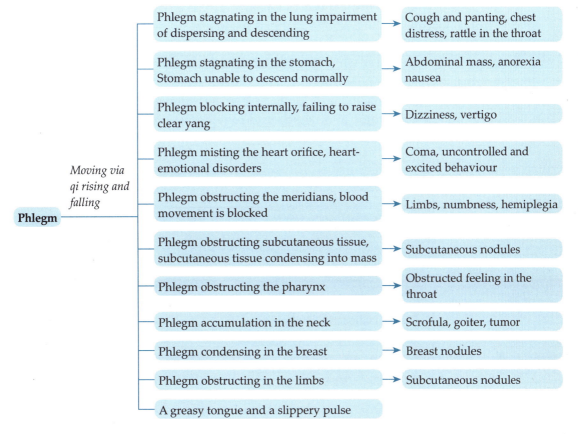

Fig. 10-25　Analysis of the phlegm pattern

B. Fluid retention pattern:

This pattern is caused by retention of thin fluid between the stomach, intestines, heart, lung, chest and hypochondria.

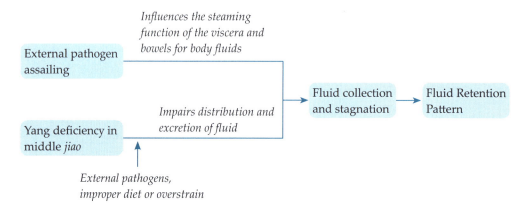

Fig. 10-26 Analysis of the fluid retention pattern

a. Fluid-retention stagnating in the stomach and intestines

Concept: This refers to the pattern resulting from cold fluid-retention collecting in the stomach and intestines. It is the "narrow" meaning of phlegm turbidity in the book of *Essentials from the Golden Cabinet*.

Clinical manifestations: Abdominal distension and fullness, splashing sounds in the stomach and intestines, vomiting of clear fluid, a lack of the sense of taste, a lack of thirst, dizziness, white greasy tongue coating and a deep, slippery pulse.

Analysis: This is usually due to uncontrolled eating and drinking, overstrain causing internal damage, injury to the spleen and stomach, failure of the central yang (middle *jiao* yang), all of which lead to retention and stagnation of fluid in the stomach and intestines (Fig. 10-27).

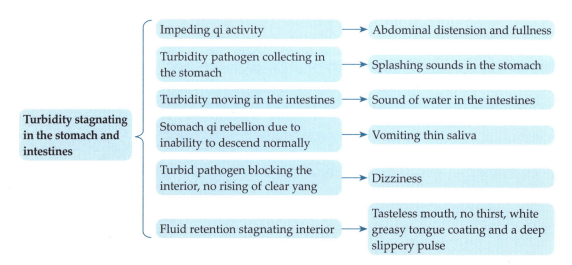

Fig. 10-27 Analysis of turbidity stagnating in stomach and intestines

Key symptoms: Splashing sounds in the stomach and intestines, abdominal distension and fullness.

b. Fluid-retention stagnating in the lung
   Concept: This is caused by cold fluid-retention obstructing the lung and impairment in the ascending and descending function of the lung. In the book *Essentials from the Golden Cabinet*, it is called retention of fluid in the diaphragm and hypochondrium, which is under the category of internal medicine lung distension diseases.
   Clinical manifestations: Cough with panting (asthma), chest distress or dyspnoea and fullness of the chest, which makes it difficult to lie supine (flat on the back), shortness of breath, rattling sound of phlegm in the throat, in serious cases there may be heart palpitations and puffiness, a white and greasy tongue coating, and string-like and taut pulse.
   Analysis: Retention of fluid in the lung is usually due to yang deficiency of the spleen and kidney leading to recurrent fluid-retention in the lung, this disease occurs when the patient is exposed to cold places and it is difficult to manage (Fig. 10-28).

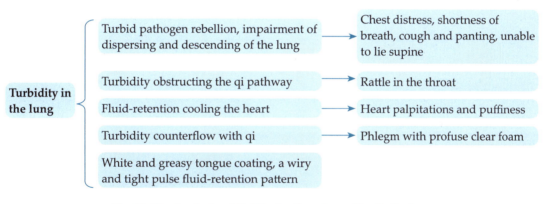

Fig. 10-28 Analysis of fluid-retention stagnating in the lung

Key symptoms: Cough with panting and dyspnoea and expectoration of thin and foamy sputum.

c. Fluid-retention in the chest and hypochondrium
   Concept: The primary mechanism of this pattern is retention of fluid in the chest and hypochondrium, subsequently qi activity is blocked leading to symptoms such as fullness in the chest and hypochondrium, cough, expectoration, and pain during breathing. In Western medicine it is called pleural effusion.
   Clinical manifestations: Distension, fullness and pain in the chest and hypochondrium, pain is more serious when expectorating and coughing, fullness between the ribs, short and quick breathing, dizziness, pain occurring in the chest and hypochondrium during respiration or turning the body laterally.
   Analysis: This disease is usually due to yang deficiency failing to transform

Diagnostics in Chinese Medicine

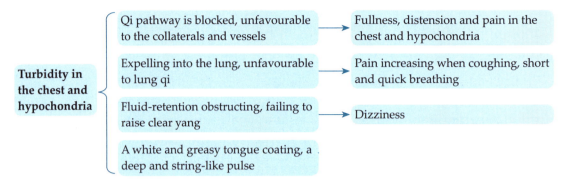

Fig. 10-29 Analysis of turbidity in the chest and hypochondria

and transport body fluids leading to fluid retention and stagnation, or due to invasion of exterior pathogenic factors causing failure in the function of the lung, consequently leading to collection and stagnation of fluid which then flows into the pleural cavity (the space between lung and ribs) (Fig. 10-29).

Key symptoms: Fullness, distension and pain in the chest and hypochondria, pain when coughing, expectorating or breathing.

Chapter 11
Differentiation of Patterns According to the *Zang-Fu* Organs

The differentiation of patterns according to the theory of the *zang-fu* organs is based on the clinical manifestation of the internal organs when the harmony between qi and blood is out of balance.

This method of pattern identification is mostly used for interior and chronic diseases. However, it may also apply for a few exterior and acute patterns.

The eight principles pattern identification classifies the patterns according to the disharmony, which may happen in the body. For example, according to the eight-principle method the signs and symptoms of qi deficiency (*xū*) include shortness of breath, feeble voice, pale complexion, lassitude and lack of appetite. Although the eight principles consist of one single method, which is a chief one among all the differentiation methods used to identify the common features of patterns, this method cannot precisely identify patterns concerning which organs are involved. Consequently, according to the theory of the *zang-fu* organs, for instance, the above symptoms can be further classified as lung qi deficiency (*xū*) in respect of shortness of breath and feeble voice, or spleen qi deficiency in respect of lassitude and lack of appetite. This method may be more applicable and significant in clinical application, because this method is a differentiation method, which gives concrete indications in order to locate the diseased organ. The differentiation of patterns according to the theory of the *zang-fu* organs is very useful, particularly for identification of internal chronic diseases (Table 11-1).

The characteristics of pattern differentiation according to the theory of the *zang-fu* organs:

In this section the patterns relating to each organ will be discussed in detail. It is important to know that, in reality, not all the symptoms and signs described need necessarily appear at the same time. These patterns often actually describe the advanced cases of disharmony in a particular organ. In some cases, even only two symptoms will be sufficient to identify a specific internal organ pattern. In fact, the real art of diagnosis in Chinese medicine is to detect a certain disharmony in the body and not to find some specific clinical manifestation.

(1) Moreover, Chinese medicine will help to develop a deeper understanding of the aetiology and pathology of a given disharmony. The goal of this method, therefore, is not to classify signs and symptoms according to organ patterns, but to understand how the signs and symptoms arise and how they interact with each other, in order to identify the current organ disharmony.

(2) The organ patterns are not like the diseases in biomedicine as they are not just a collection of signs and symptoms, but rather an expression of existing disharmony in a patient. Signs and symptoms are used to identify the characteristics and nature of a disharmony, which can give an indication for the method and strategy to carry out treatment.

Table 11-1 The main content of *zang-fu* pattern differentiation

No.	Heart and small intestine patterns	Lung and large intestine patterns	Spleen and stomach patterns	Liver and gallbladder patterns	Kidney and bladder patterns	Combined patterns
1	Heart-qi deficiency	Wind-cold invading the lung	Spleen qi deficiency	Liver blood deficiency	Kidney yang deficiency	Disharmony between the heart and kidney
2	Heart yang deficiency	Wind-heat invading the lung	Spleen qi deficiency and sinking	Liver yin deficiency	Kidney deficiency and water flooding	Heart and kidney yang deficiency
3	Sudden desertion of heart yang	Lung-dryness	Spleen yang deficiency	Liver yin deficiency	Kidney yin deficiency	Heart and lung qi deficiency
4	Heart blood deficiency	Cold-pathogen congesting the lung	Spleen failing to control blood	Liver constraint and qi stagnation	Kidney essence deficiency	Dual deficiency of the heart and spleen
5	Heart yin deficiency	Phlegm-damp obstructing the lung	Cold-dampness encumbering the spleen	Intense liver fire	Kidney qi insecurity	Heart and liver blood deficiency
6	Intense heart fire	Intense lung heat	Damp-heat accumulating in the spleen	Ascendant hyperactivity of liver yang	Kidney failing to grasp qi	Spleen and lung qi deficiency
7	Heart vessel obstruction	Phlegm-heat obstructing the lung	Stomach-cold	Liver wind agitating within	Bladder damp-heat	Kidney and lung yin deficiency
8	Phlegm misting the heart spirit	Lung qi deficiency	Stomach-heat	Damp-heat in the liver and gallbladder		Liver fire insulting the lung
9	Phlegm-fire harassing the heart	Lung yin deficiency	Stomach yin deficiency	Cold stagnation in the liver channel		Liver-stomach disharmony
10	Blood stasis obstructing the brain networks	Intestinal damp-heat	Retention of food in the stomach	Depressed gallbladder with phlegm harassing		Liver constraint and spleen deficiency
11	Small intestine excess-heat	Intestinal heat and bowel excess	Blood stasis in the stomach			Liver and kidney yin deficiency
12		Intestinal dryness and liquid depletion				Kidney and spleen yang deficiency
13		Worm accumulation in intestine				
14		Large intestine deficient-cold				

(3) The clinical manifestations, which belong to each pattern usually describes the whole manifestations of a certain pattern; but it is important to know that *zang-fu* patterns appear in different degrees of severity. For instance, kidney yin deficiency (*xū*) is defined by tinnitus; dizziness; soreness and weakness of the lumbar region; feverish sensation in the chest, palms and soles; night sweating; afternoon fever; malar flush and thready and rapid pulse. In fact, this constellation of signs and symptoms generally describe an advanced case of kidney yin deficiency. However, if kidney yin deficiency is just developing, a patient might only suffer from backache, slight night sweating and a slightly rootless coating. Significantly, these manifestations would be enough to warrant a diagnosis of kidney yin deficiency.

(4) Clinically, several patterns may occur at the same time, the combination of these patterns can be as below:

A. Two or more patterns from one yin organ (e.g. heart qi deficiency and heart-yang deficiency)

B. Two or more patterns from different yin organs (e.g. heart and kidney yang deficiency)

C. One or more patterns from a yin organ with one or more patterns from a yang organ (e.g. spleen qi deficiency and bladder damp-heat)

D. An interior pattern, accompanied by an exterior pattern (e.g. retention of damp-phlegm in the lungs and an exterior attack of damp-cold on the lungs)

E. The interior organ pattern and a channel pattern (e.g. lung-qi deficiency and painful obstruction pattern of the large intestine channel)

(5) There is no correspondence between the *zang-fu* organ patterns of Chinese medicine and organ diseases of biomedicine. For example, according to Chinese medicine a patient can suffer from kidney yin deficiency, yet without any recognisable clinical manifestations defined for kidney disease in biomedicine; conversely, a patient may suffer from kidney disease from the viewpoint of biomedicine but the clinical manifestations do not correspond to characteristics of a kidney pattern in Chinese medicine.

(6) In identification of patterns according to the theory of the *zang-fu* organs the following topics will be discussed:
- a brief summary of the functions of the organ,
- the clinical manifestations of internal organ patterns,
- the pathology (the structural and functional changes that result from disease processes), and
- the aetiology (the cause or origin of a disease or disorder as determined by diagnosis).

SECTION 1
HEART AND SMALL INTESTINE PATTERN DIFFERENTIATION

The heart is located within the upper *jiao* and protected externally by the pericardium. The heart channel of the hand *shaoyin* runs along the posterior border of the medial aspect of the arms, then goes down to connect with the small intestine; the heart and small intestine have an exterior-interior relationship through their channels. The heart opens into the tongue and governs the pulse; the state of the heart can be reflected in the complexion. One of the main physiological functions of the heart is to govern blood and vessels, to promote the continuous blood circulation in the vessels. On the other hand, the function of the heart is to house the mind; consequently, mental activity, consciousness, spirit, and thinking reside in the heart of a human being.

The pathological changes of the heart mainly manifest as disturbances of the heart and also disturbances in controlling the blood, vessels and mind. Therefore, the common symptoms of heart diseases include: palpitations, chest pain, insomnia, dreaming, forgetfulness, coma, mental confusion, knotted, intermittent and rapid pulse, etc. In addition, some pathological changes of the tongue are associated with the heart diseases, such as pain of the tongue and ulceration of the tongue (Table 11-2).

Table 11-2 The main functions of the heart and small intestine and their pathological changes

Physiological Functions	Pathology	Common Symptoms
Controlling the blood and vessels	Obstruction of qi-blood circulation	Palpitations, suffocating feeling in the chest, shortness of breath, chest pain, knotted and intermittent pulse
	Abnormal circulation of blood	Haematemesis (vomiting blood), non-traumatic haemorrhage, haematuria (blood in the urine), bruises, pyodermal diseases (ulcers and pus), etc.
	Unsupported heart due to blood deficiency	Palpitations, dizziness
Controlling the mind	Unsupported mind due to blood deficiency	Insomnia, dream-disturbed sleep, poor memory
	Heat in the heart disturbing the mind	Mild: mental restlessness and sadness Severe: aggressive and violent behaviour, mania, coma
The heart opens into the tongue	Hyperactivity of heart fire	Red tongue, prickly tongue, tongue ulcers
	Blood stasis	Purple tongue, sometimes with purples spots
	The tongue out of control due to obstruction by pathogenic factors	Curled-up tongue, stiff tongue, waggling tongue, difficulty in speaking
The heart manifesting in the complexion	Deficiency of qi or blood or yang	Pale or light pale face
	Blood stasis	Dim and purple face
Heart links with the small intestine	The heart transmits heat to the small intestine	Oliguria (low levels of urinary output), haematuria (blood in the urine), urgency, burning pain in the urethra

Heart patterns include excess and deficiency patterns (see Table 11-3, Fig. 11-1)

Table 11-3 The classification of common heart diseases

	Pathogenesis	Common patterns
Deficiency pattern	Inherent deficiency, weakness of the qi of the five zang organs, heart injury due to chronic illness	Deficiency of heart blood, deficiency of heart yin, deficiency of heart qi, deficiency of heart yang, sudden collapse of heart yang
Excess pattern	Stagnation of phlegm, fire disturbance, cold coagulation, stagnated qi, blood stasis, etc.	Hyperactivity of heart fire, obstruction of the heart vessel, mental confusion due to phlegm and phlegm-fire disturbing the mind

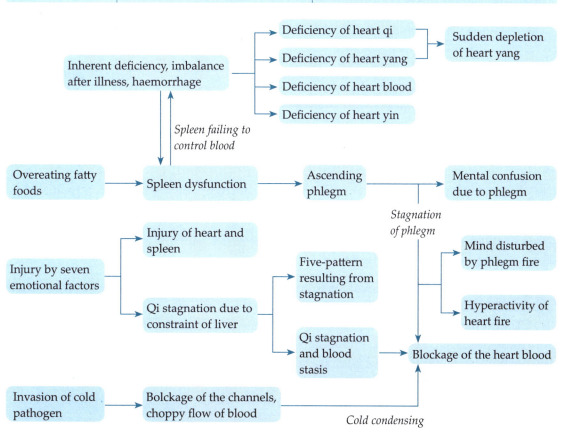

Fig. 11-1 Description of the pathogenesis and pathology of heart diseases

The brain (heart-included) is the mind of the heart, thus the pattern of stagnation in the brain collaterals is associated with heart disease.

Heart Qi Deficiency Pattern

The heart qi deficiency pattern results from weakness of heart qi in pushing blood flow, i.e. circulating blood.

Clinical manifestations: Palpitations, shortness of breath and chest distress, lassitude, symptoms worsening with physical exertion, pale complexion, spontaneous sweating, and pale tongue body with white tongue coating, weak pulse or rapid weak pulse, knotted or intermittent pulse.

Analysis: The pattern is mainly caused by prolonged weakness of the body, or qi deficiency of the five zang organs, etc. (Fig. 11-2).

Diagnostics in Chinese Medicine

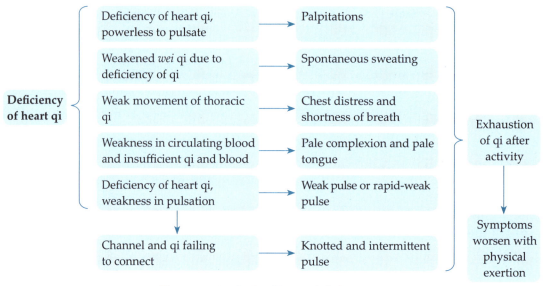

Fig. 11-2 Analysis of heart qi deficiency

Key symptoms: Palpitations, chest distress, shortness of breath, and symptoms of qi deficiency.

Heart Yang Deficiency Pattern

Deficiency of heart yang develops from the deficiency of heart qi, and the appearance of a deficient-cold pattern.

Clinical manifestations: Palpitations, chest distress or chest pain, chilly with cold limbs, shortness of breath, lassitude, spontaneous sweating, pale complexion, a pale and moist tongue body with white tongue coating, faint, knotted and intermittent pulse, or deep weak and slow pulse.

Analysis: Symptoms are always secondary to the deficiency of heart qi (Fig. 11-3).

Key symptoms: Palpitations, chest distress or chest pain, and general symptoms of yang deficiency.

Sudden Collapse of the Heart Yang Pattern

Sudden loss of heart yang is a critical condition due to extreme exhaustion of heart yang and sudden loss of yang qi.

Clinical manifestations: Apart from the symptoms of heart yang deficiency, some other symptoms will appear, such as sudden profuse cold sweating, cold limbs, weak breath, pale complexion, or sharp heart pain, cyanotic (blue) lips, indistinct pulse, or even unconsciousness and coma.

Analysis: This pattern is the further development of heart yang deficiency. It may be caused by severe impairment of heart yang by pathogenic cold or obstruction of the heart by phlegm (Fig. 11-4).

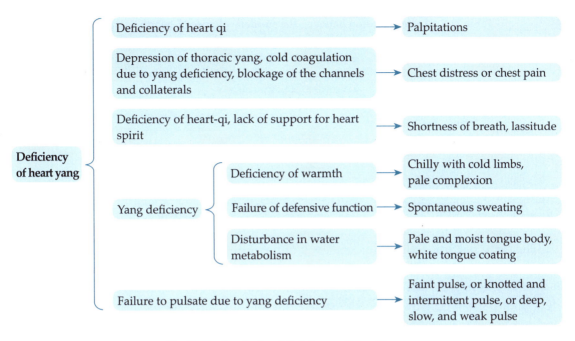

Fig. 11-3　Analysis of deficiency of heart yang

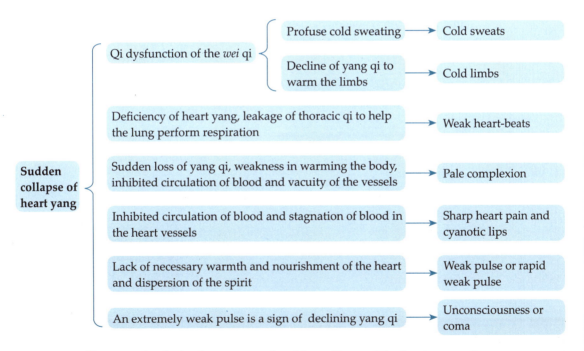

Fig. 11-4　Analysis of symptoms of sudden collapse of the heart yang pattern

Key symptoms: Manifestations of heart yang deficiency and declination of yang qi.

Identification: Sudden collapse of heart yang pattern and collapse of yang pattern (Table 11-4), heart qi deficiency pattern, heart yang deficiency pattern and sudden collapse of heart yang pattern (Table 11-4).

Table 11-4 Differentiation between the sudden collapse of heart yang pattern and collapse of yang pattern

Pattern	Common	Difference	
		Cause and pathogenesis	Key points for differentiation
Sudden collapse of heart yang	Both are critical conditions due to sudden depletion of yang qi, of which clinical manifestations are basically the same	Disease is located in the heart and occurs on the basis of heart yang deficiency	Symptoms of obstruction of the heart vessels including palpitations, chest oppression and pain as well as dull purplish complexion, lips, and nails can usually be seen
Collapse of yang		Depletion of yang qi due to various factors	Some symptoms of primary yang deficiency appear before onset

The three patterns which are deficiency of heart qi and heart yang and sudden collapse of heart yang relate to three progressively worsening phases of the heart function; from lack of function, to further loss of function to acute and serious loss of function. The heart qi deficiency pattern is characterised by such symptoms as palpitations, and chest oppression, and is accompanied by a qi deficiency pattern. The heart yang qi deficiency pattern forms on the basis of yang deficiency and is therefore characterised by a deficient cold pattern, which includes chest pains, aversion to cold and cold limbs (Table 11-5).

Table 11-5 Differentiation between a heart qi deficiency pattern and heart yang deficiency pattern and sudden collapse of heart yang pattern

Syndrome	Cause	Pathogenesis	Symptoms	
			Common symptoms	Different symptoms
Deficiency of heart qi	Usual weakness of the body, lack of effective treatment and care for protracted disease, weakness in old age	No power to push the blood due to heart qi deficiency	Palpitations and fearful throbbing, oppression in the chest, shortness of breath, aggravated by exertion, spontaneous sweating	Accompanying qi deficiency symptoms: pale or pallid complexion, pale tongue, white coating, weak pulse
Deficiency of heart yang	Further development of deficiency of heart qi	Weakness to propel and internal production of deficiency cold due to deficiency of heart yang		Accompanying deficiency cold symptoms: aversion to cold, and cold body, central chest pains, pallid or gloomy complexion, pale and enlarged tongue, white and slippery coating, thready pulse
Sudden collapse of heart yang	Further development of heart yang deficiency. It may be caused by severe impairment of heart yang by pathogenic cold or obstruction of the heart by phlegm	Sudden collapse of heart yang due to extreme exhaustion of heart yang		Accompanying deficiency of yang qi symptoms: sudden profuse cold sweating, cold limbs due to reverse flow of qi, weak breath, pale complexion, cyanotic lips, unconsciousness or coma (red or dark tongue, indistinct pulse)

Heart Blood Deficiency Pattern

Concept: Pattern caused by deficiency of heart blood failing to nourish the heart.

Clinical manifestations: Palpitations, insomnia and dream-disturbed sleep, dizziness, poor memory, withered-yellowish or pale complexion, pale lips and nails, pale tongue, a thready and weak pulse.

Analysis: This pattern is usually caused by spleen deficiency failing to produce blood, or severe haemorrhage, or chronic diseases impairing blood, or prolonged anxiety and worry consuming the blood (Fig. 11-5).

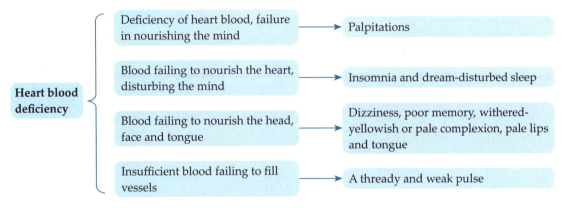

Fig. 11-5 Analysis of heart blood deficiency

Key symptoms: Palpitations, insomnia, accompanied by symptoms of blood deficiency.

Heart Yin Deficiency Pattern

Deficiency of heart yin generates internal deficient-heat, which then leads on to the internal disturbances.

Clinical manifestations: Palpitations, insomnia and dream-disturbed sleep, vexing heat in the chest, palms and soles, tidal fever in the afternoon, night sweating, red cheeks, red tongue with diminished fluids, a thready and rapid pulse.

Analysis: This pattern is mainly caused by excessive and prolonged apprehension and anxiety, which gradually injures heart yin. It may be caused by yang pathogenic factors such as summer-heat, dryness, and fire which may damage body fluids thus causing deficiency of heart yin directly, or kidney and liver yin deficiency which may lead to deficiency of heart yin. This pattern can also be caused at the late stage of warm diseases due to consumption of yin fluids (Fig. 11-6).

Key symptoms: Palpitations, insomnia, accompanied by symptoms of yin deficiency.

Identification: Heart blood deficiency and heart yin deficiency (Table 11-6).

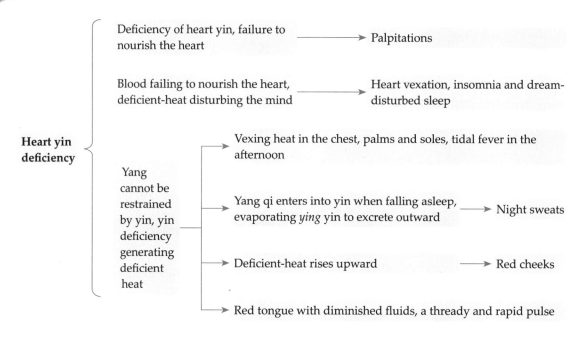

Fig. 11-6 Analysis of heart yin deficiency

Table 11-6 Differentiation of heart blood deficiency and heart yin deficiency

Pattern	Aetiology	Pathogenesis	Symptom Common	Symptom Different
Heart blood deficiency	Usually caused by spleen deficiency failing to produce blood, or severe haemorrhage, chronic diseases impairing blood, or prolonged anxiety and worry consuming the blood	Deficiency of heart blood fails to nourish the heart	Palpitations, dream-disturbed sleep	Accompanied by symptoms of blood deficiency such as: dizziness, pale complexion, pale lips and nails, pale tongue, a thready and weak pulse
Heart yin deficiency	Usually caused by excessive and prolonged anxiety and apprehension gradually injuring heart yin, or kidney and liver yin deficiency causing deficiency of heart yin, or consumption of yin fluids at the late stage of warm diseases	Deficiency of heart yin generates internal deficient heat, which then leads on to internal disturbances		Accompanied by symptoms of yin deficiency with internal deficient heat such as: tidal fever, vexing heat in the chest, palms and soles, night sweating, red cheeks, red tongue with diminished fluids, a thready and rapid pulse

Heart Fire Hyperactivity Pattern

Concept: Manifestations of heart fire flaming upward.

Clinical manifestations: Ill at ease and restlessness with a hot sensation in the chest, insomnia, red complexion, thirst, yellow urine and dry stool, red tongue with red-crimson tip of the tongue or ulceration and pain of the tongue, a powerful and rapid pulse, or mania and delirium, haematemesis (blood vomiting), epistaxis (nose bleeding), pyodermic diseases such as skin ulceration, pus and swelling e.g. acne or dermal burning pain.

Analysis: This pattern is usually caused by long-term depression of the seven emotions causing qi stagnation which turns into fire; or by invasion of the exogenous fire pathogen, or by indulgence in fatty food or alcoholic drinks, which can accumulate and turn into fire over a long time (Fig. 11-7).

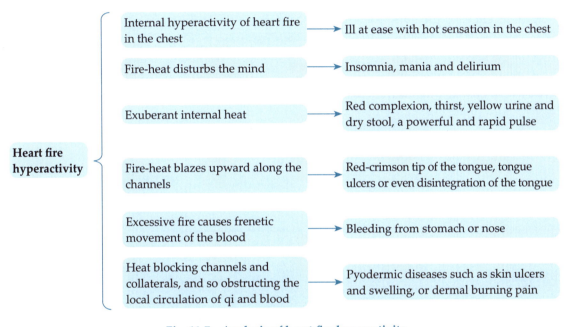

Fig. 11-7 Analysis of heart fire hyperactivity

Key symptoms: Feeling ill at ease and restless with a hot sensation in the chest; insomnia; heart vexation; mania and delirium; red tongue with red-crimson tip of the tongue or tongue ulcers; accompanied by symptoms of a full-heat pattern.

Caution: Both heart fire hyperactivity and heart yin deficiency clinically manifest as common symptoms of the heart and heat patterns, but the former is an excess pattern, while the latter is a deficiency pattern.

Obstruction of the Heart Vessel Pattern

This disease is mostly due to blood stasis, retention of phlegm, cold coagulation, or stagnation of qi, all of which block the heart vessel.

Clinical manifestations: Palpitations, a suffocating feeling and pain in the chest radiating to the shoulder, back, and the inner aspect of the arm; the pain is sometimes present and sometimes not.

In cases with stabbing pain, dark tongue with blue and purple spots, and a thready and choppy pulse, knotted or intermittent pulse, this pertains to blood stasis in the heart vessel.

In cases of obesity with excessive phlegm, heaviness of the body, suffocating pain, white greasy coating, and deep and slippery or deep and choppy pulse, this refers to the retention of phlegm in the heart vessel.

In cases with sudden attacks of severe pain, which can be relieved by warmth, cold limbs, a pale tongue with a white coating, and a deep and slow or deep and tense pulse, this indicates stagnation of cold or cold coagulation obstructing the heart vessel.

In cases with distending pain, rib-side distension, frequent sighing, with the attacks being often related to emotional factors, a pale red tongue, a thin and white tongue coating, and a wiry (bow-string) pulse, this refers to qi stagnation in the heart vessel.

Analysis: This disease may be derived from the other heart patterns, particularly heart yang deficiency, so the symptoms vary according to the different pathogenic factors. The pathogenesis of this disease is divided into four patterns:

- blood stasis,
- retention of phlegm,
- cold coagulation, and
- stagnation of qi,

all of which obstruct the heart vessel (Fig. 11-8).

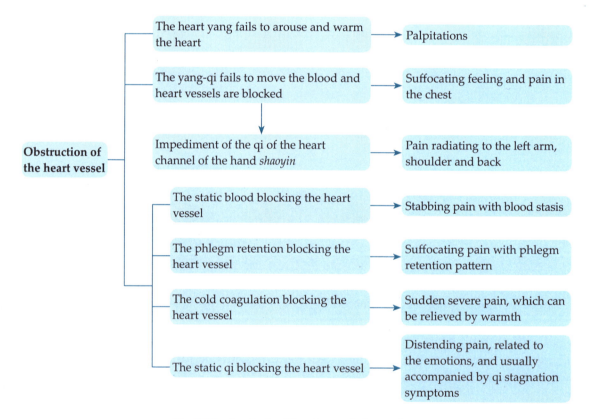

Fig. 11-8 Analysis of heart vessel obstruction

Key symptoms: Palpitations, a suffocating feeling and pain in the chest radiating to the shoulder, back, and the inner aspect of the arm, accompanied by symptoms of other heart patterns which can obstruct the heart vessel (Table 11-7).

This pattern may be simply caused by blood stasis or a pathogenic cold pathogen. However, pathogenic factors mostly exist in combination, such as qi stagnation combines with blood stasis, qi stagnation with phlegm retention, and qi stagnation with blood stasis and phlegm retention, cold obstruction combines with qi stagnation and blood stasis, etc. Phlegm retention is usually accompanied by blood stasis. Therefore, only when the main symptoms of different patterns are precisely differentiated, then an accurate diagnosis will be made.

Table 11-7 Differentiation of various pathological factors in the obstruction of the heart vessel

Disease	Symptoms	Patterns	Characteristics of symptoms
Obstruction of the heart vessel	Palpitations, a suffocating feeling and pain in the chest radiating to the shoulder, back, and the inner aspect of the arm; the pain comes and goes	Blood stasis	Dark tongue with blue and purple spots, and a thready and choppy pulse
		Phlegm retention	Excessive phlegm, heaviness of the body, suffocating pain, white greasy coating, a deep and slippery pulse
		Cold obstruction	Sudden attacks of severe pain which can be relieved by warmth, cold limbs, pale tongue with a white coating, and deep and slow or deep and tense pulse
		Qi stagnation	Distending pain, which is related to emotional factors, pale red tongue and a wiry pulse

Phlegm Misting the Heart Orifices Pattern

Concept: In this pattern the heart is misted by the phlegm, leading to disturbances of the mind.

Clinical manifestations: Various mental derangements, such as depressive-psychosis, epilepsy or syncope (sudden unconsciousness) disorders.

A. Depressive-psychosis: depression, apathy, dementia, soliloquy, abnormal behaviour, with a greasy tongue coating, and slippery pulse.

B. Epilepsy: sudden fainting, loss of consciousness, drooling, a gurgling sound in the throat, convulsions, upward staring of the eyes, shouting which sounds like a pig or a sheep, then returning quickly to a normal condition after awaking, with a greasy tongue coating, and slippery pulse.

C. Phlegm syncope: sallow complexion, fullness in the epigastrium and chest oppression, nausea, vomiting, cloudy consciousness (mental confusion), glossolalia (non-meaningful speech), a rattling sound in the throat, and even loss of consciousness and fainting, with a white and greasy coating, and a slippery pulse.

Analysis: This pattern is mainly caused by transformation of pathogenic dampness into phlegm; or by stagnation of qi activity due to emotional depression, which causes retention of body fluids, resulting in phlegm collection; then the heart becomes misted by the phlegm, leading to derangement of the mind. This pattern can also result from flaring up of liver wind, which causes rising of hidden phlegm (in the heart channel) and misting of the mind, so the phlegm is sent by the wind to agitate the mind (Fig. 11-9).

Key symptoms: Mental disorders, accompanied by phlegm patterns, such as a gurgling sound in the throat, drooling, greasy tongue coating, slippery pulse, etc.

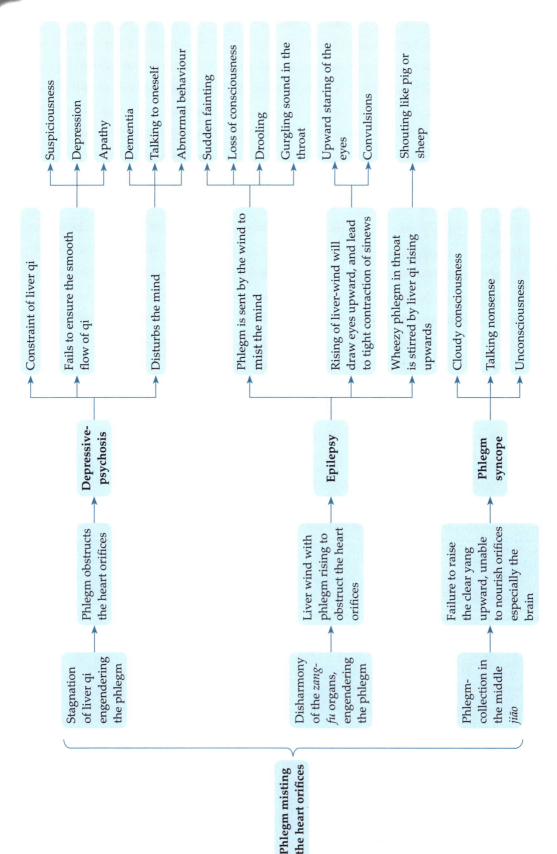

Fig. 11-9 Analysis of the heart vessel phlegm misting the heart orifices

Phlegm Fire Harassing the Heart Pattern

Concept: This pattern is due to a combination of phlegm and fire obstructing the heart orifices and harassing the mind, resulting in mental disorders.

Clinical manifestations: Fever, mental restlessness, reddish complexion, red eyes, thirst, coarse breathing, constipation and yellow urine, yellow and sticky sputum or a rattling sound in the throat, insomnia, a suffocating feeling in the chest, heart vexation, even mania or delirium, violent and aggressive behaviour, such as a tendency to hit or scold people and destroy objects, incoherent speech, uncontrolled weeping and laughing without obvious reason, a red tongue, yellow and greasy coating, a slippery and rapid pulse.

Analysis: This pattern is mainly caused by severe emotional irritation, leading to stasis of qi which turns into fire, and fire scorching and changing the fluids into phlegm; or by exterior pathogenic damp-heat which accumulates inside the body, resulting in phlegm fire, or by invasion of exterior pathogenic heat which burns the fluids into phlegm, and phlegm-fire harassing the heart (Fig. 11-10).

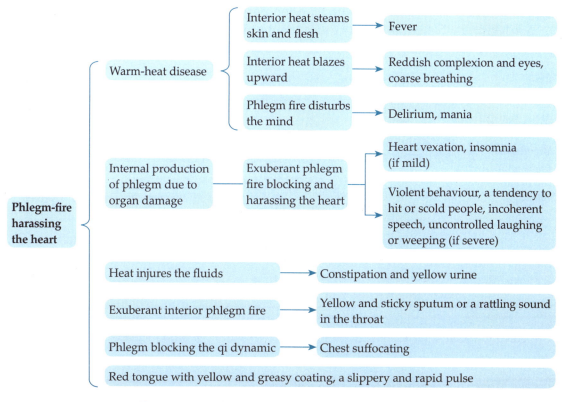

Fig. 11-10 Analysis of phlegm fire harassing the heart

Key symptoms: Mental disorders and manifestations of interior phlegm fire such as yellow and sticky sputum, a red tongue, yellow and greasy coating, a slippery and rapid pulse, etc.

Identification: Phlegm misting the heart orifices and phlegm fire harassing the heart (Table 11-8).

Table 11-8 Differentiation of phlegm misting the heart orifices and phlegm fire harassing the heart

Pattern	Nature	Similar symptoms	Different Symptoms
Phlegm misting the heart orifices	Yin pattern	Mental disorders, accompanied by a phlegm pattern	Clouding of consciousness, apathy, depression, dementia, etc. without a heat pattern
Phlegm-fire harassing the heart	Yang pattern		Mania, delirium, violent behaviour, reddish complexion, fever, etc. with an obvious dry-heat pattern

Blood Stasis Obstructing the Brain Collaterals Pattern

Concept: This pattern is ascribed to blood stasis affecting the brain and blocking its networks (collaterals), and manifests as headache, dizziness, etc.

Clinical manifestations: Headache, chronic dizziness, stabbing pain fixed in one place, poor memory, insomnia, palpitations, or coma after head trauma, dark and dusky complexion, dark-purple tongue, with blue and purple spots, a thready and choppy pulse.

Analysis: The pattern is mainly caused by head trauma, or chronic disease eventually affecting networks leading to blood stasis, which obstructs brain collaterals (Fig. 11-11).

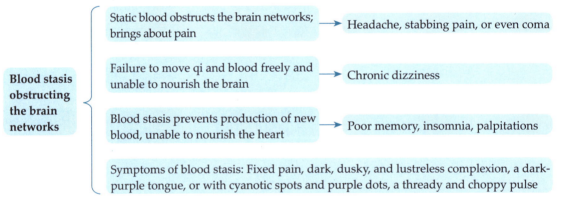

Fig. 11-11 Analysis of blood stasis obstructing the brain networks

Key symptoms: Headache, dizziness with symptoms of blood stasis.

Excess Heat in the Small Intestine Pattern

Concept: This pattern results from exuberant heat in the small intestine.

Clinical manifestations: Heart vexation (irritability), insomnia, thirst with desire for cold drinks, tongue and mouth ulcers, dark and scanty urine, burning pain on urination, haematuria (blood in the urine), red tongue with a yellow coating, and a rapid pulse.

Analysis: This pattern is caused by heat in the heart shifting to the small intestine (Fig. 11-12).

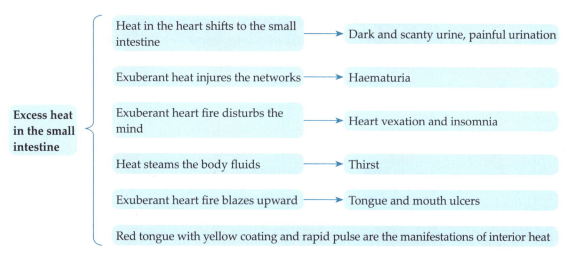

Fig. 11-12 Analysis of excess heat in the small intestine

Key symptoms: Symptoms of exuberant heart fire, accompanied by dark and scanty urine, and burning pain on urination.

SECTION 2
LUNG AND LARGE INTESTINE PATTERN DIFFERENTIATION

The lung, located in the upper *jiao*, connects with the windpipe (trachea) and throat, and opens into the nose orifice. It dominates dispersing, descending and depurating and is related externally to the skin and manifests on the body hair. Its channel originates from the middle *jiao* and runs down to connect with the large intestine; the lung and large intestine are internally-externally connected. The main function of the lung is to govern qi and respiration; it inhales clear air and stores it in the chest to help produce *zōng* (gathering) qi which assists the heart to push blood to the extremities. There are two sayings in the *Yellow Emperor's Inner Classic*, the first supports this function as it states that *"The lung is the master of qi"*. However, the lung also governs the regulating of water passages; this function ensures dispersal of qi and fluids to warm and moisten the skin and body hair and to regulate water passages. This is why there is a second saying that states *"The lung is the upper source of water"*. The function of the large intestine is to govern transmission and discharge of waste material.

The pathological changes in the lung are mainly reflected in the functional weakness of the lung system such as the hypofunction of respiration, disturbances in regulating the water passages and lack of distribution of *wei* qi, etc. (Table 11-9).

The lung patterns can be classified into two types: deficiency and excess. The former is caused by deficiency of qi or deficiency of yin, which occurs in chronic diseases or chronic cough or in *zang-fu* impairments, whilst the latter results from invasion of wind cold, dryness heat or retention of fluid in the lung (Fig. 11-13).

Table 11-9 The physiological function, pathological changes and primary symptoms of the lung and large intestine patterns

Physiological function	Pathological changes	Primary symptoms
Governs qi and respiration dominates dispersing and descending	Hypofunctional activity	Shortage of qi, feeble voice
	Fails to govern dispersing and descending	Cough, asthma Shortness of breath, chest pain
Regulates the water passage	Fails to disperse fluids	Fluid retention oedema
Controls the skin and body hair	Insecurity of *wei* (defensive) qi	Spontaneous sweating, aversion to wind, tendency to catch cold
	Fails to nourish the skin and body hair	Dry hair and lustreless skin
Opens into the nose orifice	Nasal functional weakness	Stuffy nose, runny nose, sneezing
Takes the throat as a window	Affects the throat	Itchy throat, sore throat, hoarseness, loss of voice
The large intestine governs transmitting and discharging of waste material	Unable to transmit	Constipation, diarrhoea

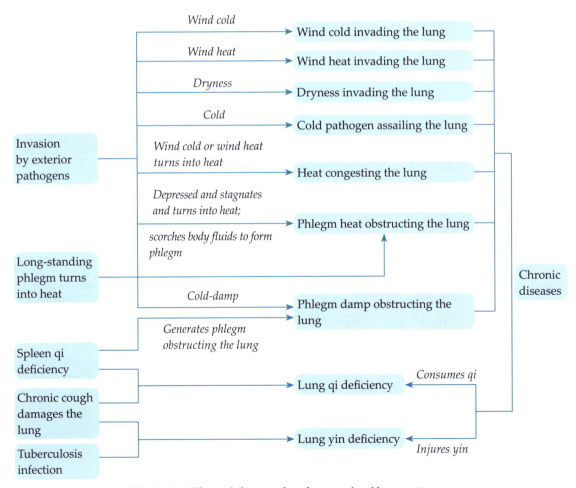

Fig. 11-13 The aetiology and pathogenesis of lung patterns

Wind-Cold Invading the Lung Pattern

Concept: Wind-cold pathogen invading the *wei* qi level of the lung system and impairing the lung dispersing function.

Clinical manifestations: Cough, clear watery sputum, aversion to cold with slight fever, stuffy nose with clear watery mucus, absence of sweating, head and body pain, thin-white coating, a floating and tight pulse.

Analysis: This pattern is mainly caused by the exterior wind-cold pathogen invading the *wei* qi level of the lung system and impairing the lung's dispersing function (Fig. 11-14).

> **Key symptoms:** Cough, clear watery sputum, along with symptoms of an exterior wind-cold pattern.

Identification: Wind cold invading the lung pattern and an exterior wind-cold pattern (Table 11-10).

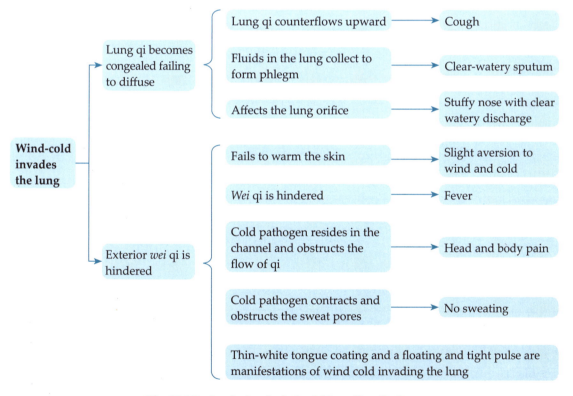

Fig. 11-14 Analysis of wind cold invading the lung

Table 11-10 Comparison of wind cold invading the lung pattern and an exterior wind cold pattern

Type	Classification in the eight principles	Primary symptoms	Secondary symptoms
Wind cold invading the lung	Exterior and interior	Cough	Slight symptoms of an exterior wind-cold pattern
Exterior wind cold	Exterior	Aversion to cold, fever	Occasional slight cough

Wind-Heat Invading the Lung Pattern

Concept: Wind-heat pathogen invading the *wei* qi level of the lung system.

Clinical manifestations: Cough with sticky yellow sputum, stuffy nose with thick yellow nasal discharge, fever with slight aversion to wind-cold, slight thirst, or sore throat, the front of the tongue is red with a thin-yellow coating, and a floating and rapid pulse.

Analysis: This pattern is mainly caused by the exterior wind heat pathogen, which invades the *wei* qi level of the lung system (Fig. 11-15).

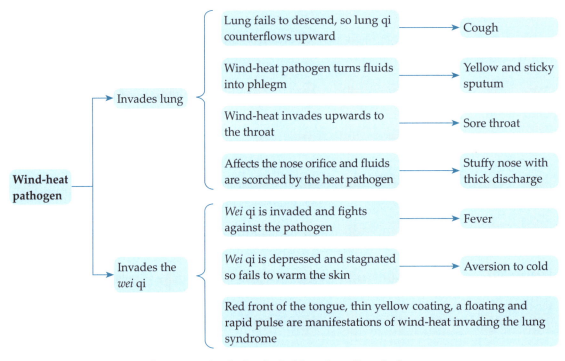

Fig. 11-15 Analysis of wind-heat invading the lung

Key symptoms: Cough and symptoms of exterior wind-heat patterns (Fig. 11-15).

Identification: Wind-heat invading the lung pattern and exterior wind-heat pattern (Table 11-11).

Table 11-11 Comparison of wind-heat invading the lung pattern and the exterior wind-heat pattern

Type	Classification in eight principles	Primary symptoms	Accompanying symptoms
Wind-heat invading the lung pattern	Interior	Cough	An exterior pattern, such as slight aversion to wind-cold, slight thirst, or sore throat, a red tip of the tongue, a thin-yellow coating, and a floating and rapid pulse
Exterior wind-heat pattern	Exterior	Fever, aversion to cold	Thirst, throat pain, normal tongue with slight red on the sides and tip, thin-white and dry coating or thin yellow coating, a floating and rapid pulse, occasional cough

Lung Dryness Pattern (Invasion of the Lung by Dryness Pattern)

Concept: This is due to an exterior dryness pathogen in autumn, which invades the *wei qi* level and also injures fluids of the lung system. It is also called dryness invading the lung pattern. It is divided into two types: warm-dryness and cool-dryness patterns according to whether the dryness pathogen has a propensity to warm or cool.

Clinical manifestations: Dry cough with scanty sputum, or sticky sputum that is difficult to expectorate, or even chest pain, sputum with blood, dry mouth, lips, nose, and pharynx, or epistaxis (nose bleeding), haemoptysis, dry stool and scanty urine, a thin dry tongue coating with little fluids, fever, slight aversion to wind-cold, no sweating or scanty sweating, a floating and rapid or floating and tight pulse.

Analysis: This pattern is mainly caused by the dryness pathogen invading the lung and injuring lung fluids leading to disharmony of *wei* qi, or by the wind heat pathogen turning into dryness and injuring fluids. Dryness in early autumn has a tendency to warmth; as a result most diseases during this time have a leaning towards warm-dryness, while dryness in the late autumn has a tendency to be cool; and so most diseases then are leaning towards being cool-dryness patterns (Fig. 11-16).

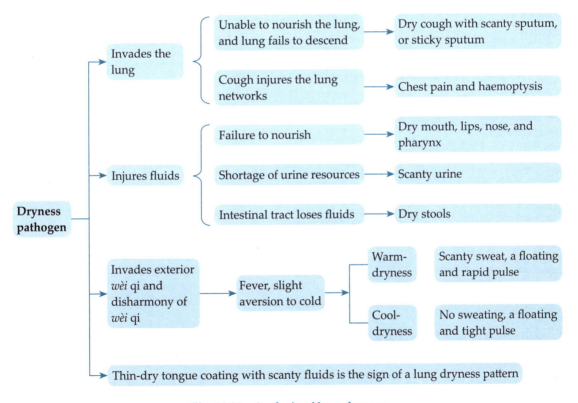

Fig. 11-16 Analysis of lung dryness

Key symptoms: Lung system diseases, along with a dryness and scanty fluids pattern.

Identification: Wind cold and wind heat invading the lung, and a lung dryness pattern (Table 11-12).

Table 11-12 Comparison of wind-cold and wind-heat invading the lung, and a lung dryness pattern

Type	Location	Main symptoms	Accompanied symptoms
Wind cold invading the lung pattern	Lung and the lung system	Cough, clear white and watery sputum	Exterior symptoms of wind cold
Wind heat invading the lung pattern		Cough, yellow thick sputum	Exterior symptoms of wind heat
Lung dryness pattern		Dry cough with scanty sputum that is hard to expectorate, chest pain and haemoptysis (blood in the sputum)	Exterior symptoms of dryness (warm-dryness or cool-dryness)

Cold Pathogen Congesting the Lung Pattern

Concept: This is due to a cold pathogen congesting the lung.

Clinical manifestations: Cough, dyspnoea, white watery sputum, cold body and limbs, pale tongue with white coating, and a slow and moderate pulse.

Analysis: This pattern manifests as a sudden onset of cough and dyspnoea accompanied by a cold pattern as a diagnostic indicator (Fig. 11-17).

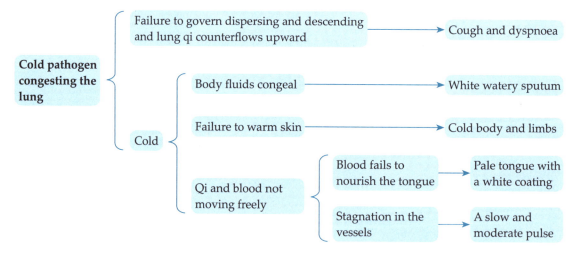

Fig. 11-17 Analysis of a cold pathogen congesting the lung pattern

Key symptoms: Sudden cough and dyspnoea, accompanied by cold signs.

Identification: Cold pathogen congesting the lung pattern and phlegm fluids obstructing the lung pattern have some common symptoms, such as cough, dyspnoea, white watery sputum, etc. however, there are still some differences (Table 11-13).

Table 11-13 Comparison of a cold pathogen congesting the lung, and phlegm-fluids obstructing the lung

Type	Case history	Phlegm		Nature of the pathological change
Cold pathogen congesting the lung pattern	Sudden onset with acute course, usually no past history	White-watery sputum	Scanty sputum	Excess
Phlegm-fluids obstructing the lung	Repeated onset, commonly seen in the autumn and winter, alleviated in the spring and summer, chronic course		Profuse watery frothy sputum	Deficiency in the root and excess in the branch

Phlegm-Damp Obstructing the Lung Pattern

Concept: This is due to spleen qi deficiency or chronic cough damaging the lung or a wind cold-damp pathogen invading the lung, all of which lead the damp phlegm to obstruct and stagnate in the lung.

Clinical manifestations: Cough with profuse white sticky sputum that is easy to expectorate, chest stuffiness, even asthma and wheezing, pale tongue with white greasy coating, and a slippery pulse.

Analysis: This pattern can be seen in both acute and chronic diseases, however mostly seen in chronic diseases (Fig. 11-18).

> **Key symptoms:** Cough with profuse white sticky sputum that is easy to expectorate.

Identification: Wind-cold invading the lung, cold-pathogen congesting the lung, phlegm fluids obstructing the lung, and phlegm-damp obstructing the lung (Table 11-14).

Heat Pathogen Congesting the Lung Pattern

Concept: This is due to a heat pathogen congesting the lung. The invasion of the lung by a heat pathogen impairs the lung's dispersing and descending functions and manifests as excess heat along the lung channel. It is also called a lung heat pattern or lung fire pattern. It belongs to the qi level pattern of the *wei*, qi, *ying*, blood pattern differentiation.

Clinical manifestations: Fever, thirst, cough, dyspnoea, nostrils flaring, chest pain, red, swollen and sore throat, scanty deep-red urine, constipation, red tongue with a yellow coating, a rapid pulse.

Analysis: This pattern is mainly caused by the wind-heat pathogen invading the body, or wind-cold pathogen invading the body then transforming into heat and congesting in the lung (Fig. 11-19).

> **Key symptoms:** Symptoms of lung diseases and symptoms of interior excess heat.

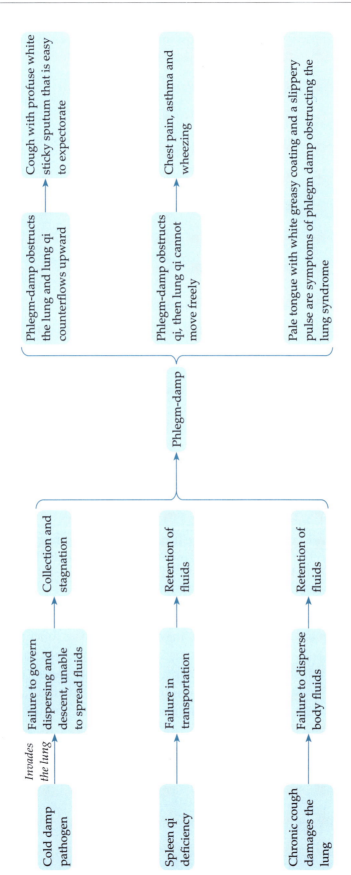

Fig. 11-18 Analysis of phlegm damp obstructing the lung pattern

Table 11-14 Comparison of wind-cold invading the lung, cold-pathogen congesting the lung, phlegm fluids obstructing the lung, and phlegm-damp obstructing the lung

Pattern	Nature	Main symptoms	Secondary symptoms	Coating	Pulse
Wind-cold invading the lung	Excess	Cough, white watery sputum, sneezing, aversion to cold	Stuffy nose with clear-watery discharge, fever, no sweating	Thin-white	Floating
Cold pathogen congesting the lung	Excess	Cough, dyspnoea, white watery sputum	Cold body and limbs without fever	Pale tongue with white coating	Slow and moderate
Phlegm fluids obstructing the lung	Deficiency in the root and excess in the branch	Cough, dyspnoea, profuse white-watery frothy sputum, splashing sounds in the chest, unable to lie down (due to wheezing)	Chest stuffiness, palpitations, oedema in the lower limbs	Pale tongue with white-slippery coating	Fine and slippery, or weak and floating
Phlegm damp obstructing the lung	*Excess pattern*: invasion of an exterior pathogen, sudden-onset. *Deficiency in the root and excess in the branches pattern*: chronic-onset	Cough with plentiful white-sticky phlegm that is easy to expectorate	Chest stuffiness, asthma and wheezing	Pale tongue with thick and greasy coating	Slippery

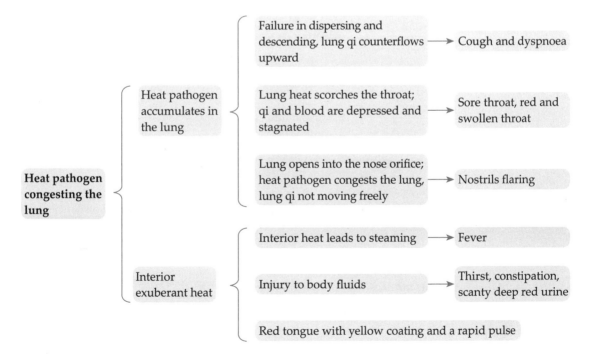

Fig. 11-19 Analysis of a heat pathogen congesting the lung

Phlegm-Heat Obstructing the Lung Pattern

Concept: This is due to phlegm combined with heat obstructing the lung, which leads to impairment in dispersing and descending functions, and consequently manifests as excess heat along the lung channel.

Clinical manifestations: Cough with profuse yellow thick sputum, chest stuffiness, dyspnoea, nostrils flaring, gurgling sound in the throat, vexation and restlessness, fever, thirst, cough and expectoration with foul smelling, pus-like sputum with blood, chest pain, constipation, scanty dark urine, red tongue with yellow-greasy coating, a slippery and rapid pulse.

Analysis: This pattern is mainly caused by pathogens invading the lung, and then stagnating and subsequently turning into heat, which injures lung fluids to form phlegm. Alternatively, it can be caused by long-standing phlegm turning into heat, both of which combine together and obstruct the lung (Fig. 11-20).

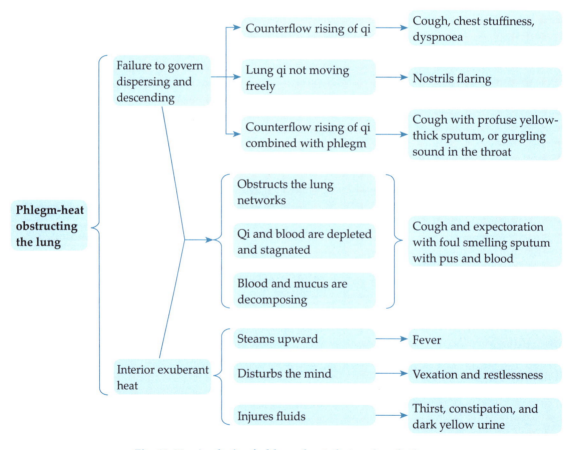

Fig. 11-20 Analysis of phlegm-heat obstructing the lung

Key symptoms: Cough with profuse sputum and symptoms of interior excess heat.

Identification: Wind-heat invading the lung pattern, lung dryness pattern, heat pathogen congesting the lung pattern, and phlegm-heat obstructing the lung pattern (Table 11-15).

Table 11-15 Comparison of wind-heat invading the lung pattern, lung dryness pattern, heat pathogen congesting the lung pattern, and phlegm-heat obstructing the lung pattern

Pattern	Season	Main symptoms	Secondary symptoms	Tongue coating	Pulse
Wind-heat invading the lung pattern	Winter and spring	Cough with yellow sticky sputum	Stuffy nose with yellow thick discharge, fever, aversion to wind, dry mouth, sore throat	Red tip of the tongue with thin yellow coating	Floating and rapid pulse
Lung dryness pattern	Autumn and winter	Dry cough with scanty sticky sputum, dry lips, tongue, pharynx, and nose	Aversion to cold, fever	Red tongue with white or thin yellow coating	Floating and rapid or tense pulse
Heat pathogen congesting the lung pattern	Winter and spring	Cough and dyspnoea with scanty sputum, high fever	Thirst, vexation and restlessness, nostrils flaring, chest pain, sore throat with redness and swelling	Red tongue with yellow coating	Rapid pulse
Phlegm-heat obstructing the lung pattern	Winter and spring	Cough and dyspnoea, with profuse yellow thick sputum, cough and expectoration with foul smelling pus-like sputum with blood, high fever	Thirst, vexation, nostrils flaring, chest pain, chest stuffiness	Red tongue with yellow greasy coating	Slippery and rapid pulse

Lung Qi Deficiency Pattern

Concept: This is due to a declining function of the lung in governing qi and dominating the *wei* (defensive) function.

Clinical manifestations: Weak cough and dyspnoea, shortage of qi, shortness of breath which is worse on exertion, clear-watery sputum, low voice, spontaneous sweating, aversion to wind, a tendency to catch cold, mental fatigue, tiredness, pale complexion, pale tongue with a white coating, and a weak pulse.

Analysis: This pattern is mainly caused by chronic cough damaging the lung qi, or spleen deficiency unable to transform sufficient food into essence qi for nourishing the lung (Fig. 11-21).

> **Key symptoms:** Weak cough, dyspnoea, low voice, and clear watery sputum with other symptoms of qi deficiency.

Diagnostics in Chinese Medicine

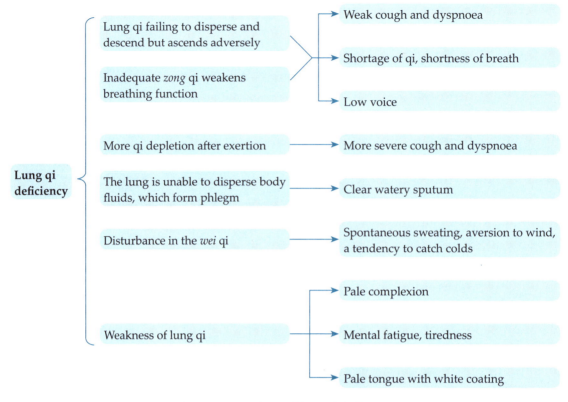

Fig. 11-21 Analysis of lung qi deficiency

Lung Yin Deficiency Pattern

Concept: This is due to lung yin deficiency giving rise to internal heat, which damages the lung and the lung is then unable to dominate descending. If the symptoms of deficient-heat are not obvious, it is called a lung dryness with injured fluids pattern.

Clinical manifestations: Dry cough with scanty sputum or scanty sticky sputum that is difficult to expectorate, a dry mouth and pharynx, emaciation, a feverish sensation in the chest, palms and soles, afternoon fever, night sweating, red cheeks, cough with blood tinged sputum (may be annoying tickly cough at night), hoarseness, red tongue with scanty fluids, a thready and rapid pulse.

Analysis: This pattern is caused by heat-dryness, which injures the lung, or by infection of tuberculosis, or after a febrile disease, or by excessive sweating which depletes the yin fluids, or by enduring cough, which consumes lung yin (Fig. 11-22).

Key symptoms: Dry cough with scanty sticky sputum, and symptoms of deficient-heat, which result from yin deficiency.

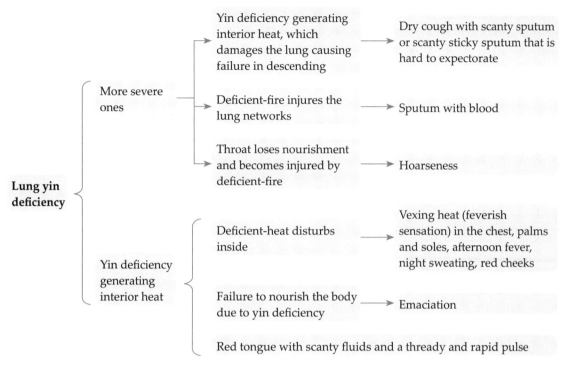

Fig. 11-22 Analysis of lung yin deficiency

Table 11-16 Comparison of lung yin deficiency, and lung dryness patterns

Type	Pathological mechanism	Nature	Common symptoms	Different symptoms
Lung yin deficiency pattern	Heat-dryness injures the lung, or tuberculosis infecting the lung, or excessive sweating depleting the yin fluids, or chronic cough injuring lung yin	Deficiency	Dry cough with scanty sputum, or sticky sputum that is difficult to expectorate, chest pain, haemoptysis (sputum with blood), dry mouth, lips, nose, pharynx, or nose-bleeding, dry stool, scanty urine	Symptoms of yin deficiency: emaciation, vexing heat in the chest, palms and soles, afternoon fever, night sweating, red cheeks, red tongue with scanty fluids, a thready and rapid pulse
Lung dryness pattern	Exterior dryness pathogen in autumn invades the *wei* qi level and injures fluids of the lung system, or a wind-warm pathogen turns into dryness and injures fluids	Excess		Symptoms of disturbance in the *wei* qi: fever, slight aversion to wind-cold, no sweating or scanty sweating, a floating and rapid pulse, or floating and tight pulse

Large Intestine Damp-Heat Pattern

Concept: Damp-heat in the intestinal tract refers to the incapability of the large intestine to transmit caused by damp-heat in the intestinal tract.

Clinical manifestations: Abdominal pain, diarrhoea with blood and mucus, tenesmus (straining with difficulty), spouting diarrhoea with foul smelling stool, a burning sensation of the anus on passing stool, scanty dark urine, fever, thirst with parched mouth but disinclination to drink, red tongue with yellow greasy coating, a slippery and rapid pulse.

Analysis: This pattern is mainly caused by summer-heat dampness assailing the stomach and intestines, or by irregular intake of food, both of which can result in generating damp-heat which brews and becomes binding in the large intestine (Fig. 11-23).

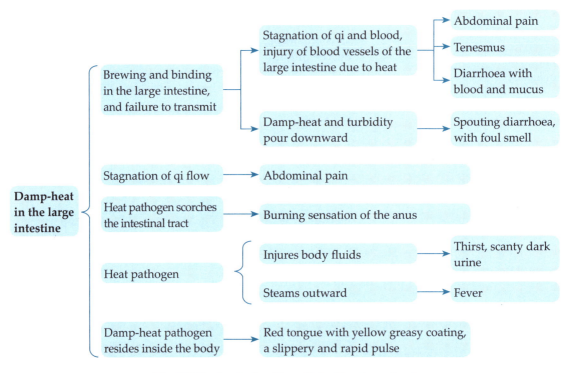

Fig. 11-23   Analysis of large intestine damp-heat

Key symptoms: Dysentery or diarrhoea with a damp-heat pattern.

Heat Obstructing the Large Intestine Pattern

Concept: This is due to when both dry and heat pathogens and the stool combine internally and result in blockage of the large intestine and this pattern manifests as an interior excessive heat pattern. It is classified into: *yangming fu* excess pattern using the six channels (*liù jīng* 六经) pattern differentiation, qi level pattern using the *wèi*, qi, *ying* and blood (*wēn bìng* 温病) pattern differentiation, and the middle *jiao* pattern using the *sanjiao* pattern differentiation.

Clinical manifestations: High fever, or late afternoon fever; distension, fullness, hardness and pain of the abdomen or around the umbilicus which is aggravated by pressure; constipation, or foul smelling stools; sweating; thirst; or mania, coma and delirium; scanty dark urine; red tongue with thick and yellow coating or thorny tongue, and a powerful deep and rapid pulse.

Analysis: This pattern is caused by an exuberant heat pathogen and excessive sweating, or by incorrect treatment with medicinals to induce sweating, all of which leads to an excessive dry-heat pathogen which binds with stool and blocks the intestinal tract.

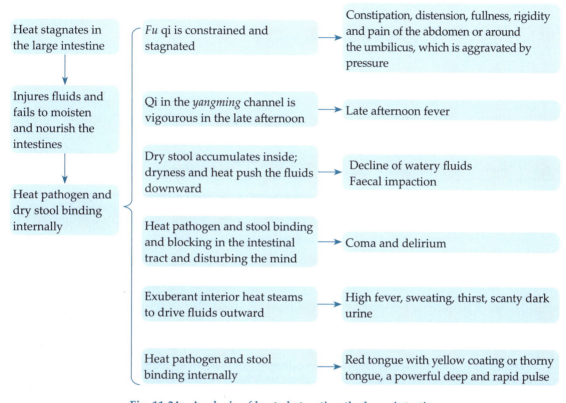

Fig. 11-24 Analysis of heat obstructing the large intestine

Key symptoms: Distension, fullness, rigidity and pain in the abdomen, constipation, with an interior excess heat pattern.

Large Intestine Dryness Pattern

Concept: This is due to deficiency of fluids in the large intestine failing to moisten the intestines, and then this creates dry stool and difficult defaecation.

Clinical manifestations: Dry stool with difficult defaecation, defaecation once every several days, a dry mouth with foul smelling breath, sometimes dizziness, a red tongue with scanty fluids and yellow dry coating, and a thready and choppy pulse.

Analysis: This pattern is caused by innate yin deficiency; or by yin-blood deficiency in old age; or by vomiting and diarrhoea; chronic diseases; the late stage of warm heat disease which consumes and injures yin-fluids; or by blood loss; or from excessive bleeding after delivery; all of which can lead to exhaustion of fluids in the large intestine and thus failure to moisten and nourish the large intestine (Fig. 11-25).

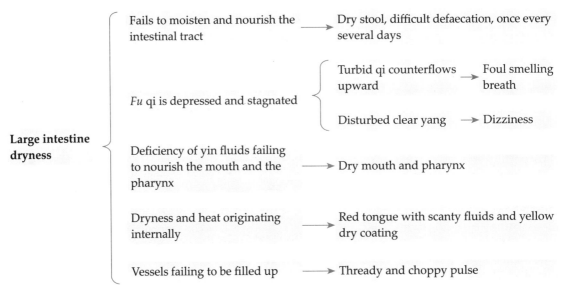

Fig. 11-25 Analysis of large intestine dryness

Key symptoms: Dry stool with difficult defaecation, accompanied by a yin-fluids deficiency pattern.

Identification: Large intestine dryness and heat obstructing the large intestine (Table 11-17).

Table 11-17 Comparison of large intestine dryness, and heat obstructing the large intestine

Pattern	Aetiology	Pathology	Nature of disease	Common symptoms	Different symptoms
Large intestine dryness	Innate yin deficiency, or yin-blood deficiency in old age, or vomiting, diarrhoea, chronic diseases, late stage of warm heat disease leading to consume and injure yin-fluids, or blood loss, excessive bleeding after delivery	Deficiency of fluids in the large intestine and failing to moisten and nourish the large intestine	Deficiency	Dry stools which are difficult to defaecate, defaecation once every several days, a dry mouth, or foul breathing, red tongue with scanty fluids, a yellow dry coating	Dizziness, a thready and choppy pulse, no high fever, abdominal pain with refusal for pressure
Heat obstructing the large intestine	Exuberant heat pathogen and excessive sweating; or depletion of body fluids, accompanied by incorrect usage of medicinals to induce sweating	Dry heat pathogen and faeces binding internally and blocking in the intestinal tract	Excess		High fever or late afternoon fever, rigidity, distension, fullness, and pain of the abdomen which is aggravated by pressure, faecal impaction, sweating, possibly even coma and delirium, mania, a red tongue with a thick and yellow coating, or a thorny tongue, a powerful deep and rapid pulse

Large Intestine Deficient-Cold Pattern

Concept: This is due to yang deficiency of the large intestine.

Clinical manifestations: Rumbling intestines, dull abdominal pain, preference for warmth and pressure, lingering diarrhoea, or faecal incontinence, possibly even tenesmus, rectal or anal prolapse, aversion to cold and preference for warmth, cold body and limbs, fatigue, lack of strength, profuse and clear urine, constipation, a pale tongue with a white-slippery coating, a deep and weak or deep and slow pulse.

Analysis: This pattern is caused by innate yang deficiency, or by over consumption of raw and cold foods, or by chronic diseases or chronic diarrhoea, which damages yang qi.

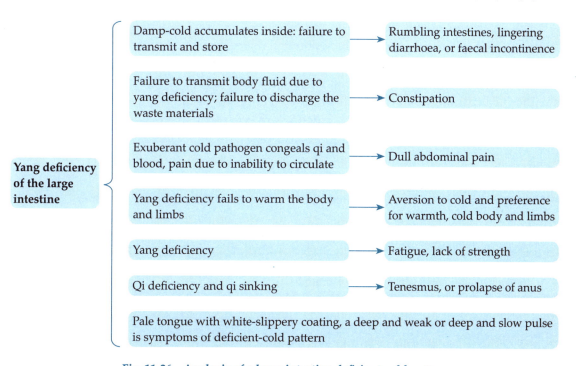

Fig. 11-26 Analysis of a large intestine deficient-cold pattern

Key symptoms: Irregular bowel habits like loose stool or dry stool, with symptoms of a deficient-cold pattern.

Section 3

Spleen and Stomach Pattern Differentiation

The spleen is located in the middle *jiao* and it has an exterior-interior relationship with the stomach. The spleen controls the muscles and the four limbs, it opens into the mouth, and manifests in the lips. The main physiological functions of the spleen are to govern the transportation and transformation (digestion). The spleen transforms the ingested food and drink to extract food-qi or nutritive substances from them and supplies the organs and tissues with adequate nutrition for the maintenance of normal physiological functions; therefore it is a source of qi and blood. Overall, the spleen serves as the source of engendering and transformation of qi and blood and is often called the root of acquired constitution. In addition, the spleen has the function of keeping blood within the blood vessels and preventing extravasation, it helps to send *qing* qi (clear yang qi) upward, it likes dryness and loathes dampness. The stomach also resides in the middle *jiao* and it governs intake and controls the rotting and ripening of food, so it is called the sea of water and food. Contrary to the spleen, the stomach dominates descending of qi and likes dampness and loathes dryness.

The impairment of transportation and transformation of the spleen may lead to retention of water, which may be condensed into water-damp. The spleen qi should ascend; if it fails to ascend, it will sink, leading to diarrhoea and prolapse of organs. The common symptoms for spleen dysfunction are abdominal distension, bloating or pain, poor appetite, loose stool, oedema, feeling of body heaviness, prolapse of organs, lassitude, bleeding etc. The stomach receives food and the stomach qi should descend, but if the function of the stomach is impaired, stomach qi will go upward and lead to counterflow of stomach qi. The common symptoms for stomach dysfunction are epigastric distension or epigastric pain, nausea, vomiting, belching, hiccoughs and acid regurgitation (Table 11-18).

Table 11-18 Physiology, pathology and common symptoms of the spleen and stomach

Physiology	Pathology	Common symptoms
The spleen governs transportation and transformation	Failure of transportation and transformation	Abdominal distension and pain, poor appetite, loose stool
	Failure to transform and transport may cause retention of fluid	Fluid retention, oedema, diarrhoea
The spleen governs raising of *qing* qi	Failure to transport the refined essence upward to the heart and lung to produce blood, and qi	Fatigue, lack of strength, shortage of qi, dislike of speaking
	Failure to keep the organs in normal position	Prolapse of internal organs, prolapse of the rectum or uterus
The spleen controls the blood	Failure to control the blood	Blood in the stools and urine, epistaxis, excessive menstrual flow, metrorrhagia
The spleen controls muscles and limbs	Failure to transform and transport, unable to form sufficient qi and blood	Thin body, flaccidity of muscles, weakness of the limbs
The spleen opens into the mouth	Failure to harmonise	A bland taste in the mouth, absence of taste, sweet or greasy sensation in the mouth
The stomach governs intake and controls the "rotting and ripening" of food	Stomach qi fails to descend	Poor appetite, fullness and distension of the epigastrium
	Stomach qi counterflows upward	Nausea, vomiting, hiccoughs, belching
	Retention of food in the stomach	Anorexia, foul belching, acid regurgitation
	Heat in the stomach	Constant hunger

Patterns of the spleen can be classified into two types: deficiency type and excess type. The former is mainly caused by improper diet, overstrain and fatigue, excessive thinking and worrying or improper nursing care in chronic diseases. Deficient types include:
- spleen qi deficiency,
- spleen qi sinking,
- spleen yang deficiency and
- failure of the spleen in controlling blood.

The excess type is mainly due to improper diet, invading of damp-heat or cold-damp, delayed treatment or incorrect treatment. Excess types include:
- cold-damp encumbering the spleen
- accumulation of damp-heat in the spleen.

Patterns of the stomach can also be classified into two types: deficiency type and excess type. The deficiency type is caused by improper diet or overeating, improper nursing care in chronic diseases, excessive vomiting or diarrhoea, damage of fluids in the late stage of warm diseases or blood and fluids deficiency in the elderly. The excess type is due to overeating, improper food or cold or heat pathogens invading the stomach, etc. (Fig. 11-27).

Spleen Qi Deficiency Pattern

Concept: This pattern is due to spleen qi deficiency and failure of transportation and transformation. It is also called spleen failing to transform and transport.

Clinical manifestations: Abdominal distension or bloating especially after meals, poor appetite, lack of ability to taste foods, loose stool, lassitude of the body and limbs, fatigue, lack of strength, shortage of qi, laziness in speaking, emaciation, sallow complexion, or obesity, oedema, a pale tongue with a white coating, a moderate and weak pulse.

Analysis: This pattern is usually caused by irregular diet, overstrain fatigue damage, over-thinking and over-worrying impairing the spleen, hereditary weakness, deficiency with old age, or improper nursing care in severe diseases (Fig. 11-28).

> **Key symptoms:** Abdominal distension, poor appetite, loose stool along with a qi deficiency pattern.

Sinking of Spleen Qi Pattern

Concept: This is due to spleen qi deficiency failing to raise qi upward leading to qi sinking. It is also called middle *jiao* qi sinking pattern.

Clinical manifestations: These include a bearing down sensation in the abdomen, distension in the epigastrium and abdomen especially after meals, frequent and urgent defaecation, and chronic diarrhoea, a bearing down sensation of the anus, prolapse of the rectum or uterus and turbid urine. These symptoms usually are accompanied by shortness of breath, lack of strength, lassitude, and laziness in speaking, dizziness, lustreless whitish complexion, poor appetite, loose stool, a pale tongue with a white coating and a moderate and weak pulse.

Analysis: This pattern is mainly caused by further development of spleen qi deficiency, by chronic diarrhoea or chronic dysentery, overstrain fatigue damage or by excessive childbearing and improper nursing care after childbirth, all of which consume the spleen qi (Fig. 11-29).

224 Diagnostics in Chinese Medicine

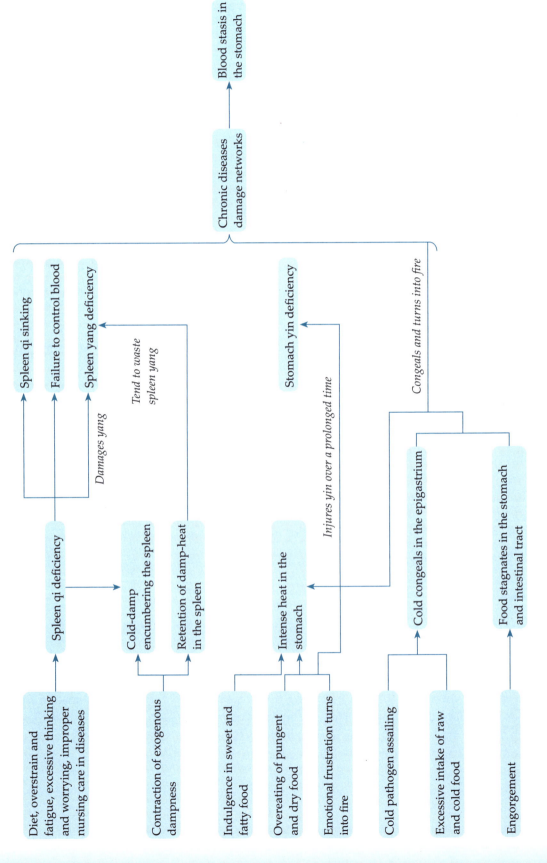

Fig. 11-27 Causes of stomach and spleen patterns

Chapter 11 Differentiation of Patterns According to the *Zang-Fu* Organs Section 3

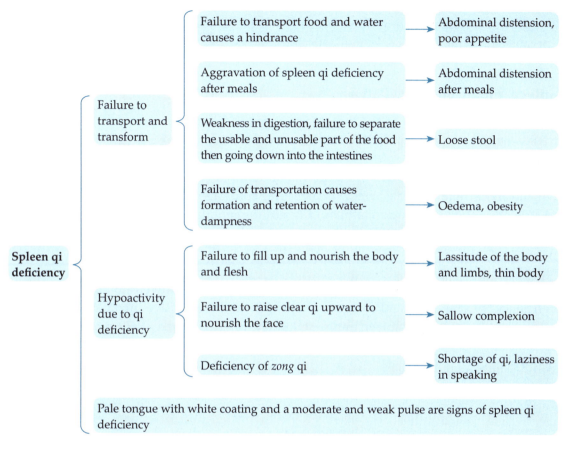

Fig. 11-28 Analysis of a spleen qi deficiency pattern

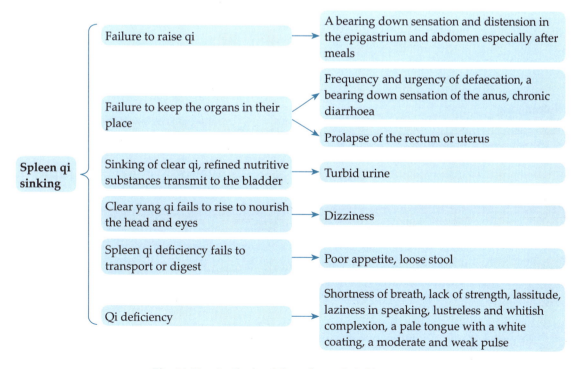

Fig. 11-29 Analysis of the spleen qi sinking pattern

Key symptoms: Bearing down sensation in the abdomen, and prolapse of internal organs with symptoms of spleen qi deficiency.

Spleen Yang Deficiency Pattern

Concept: This is due to spleen yang deficiency failing to warm and transport and transform and generating interior cold symptoms. It is also called a deficiency-cold pattern of the spleen.

Clinical manifestations: Poor appetite, abdominal distension, abdominal dull pain which can be relieved by warmth or pressure, cold limbs, shortage of qi, fatigue, lack of strength, white complexion, a bland taste in the mouth, no thirst, loose stool, general oedema, scanty urine, or profuse dilute and white leucorrhoea, a pale and plump tongue with or without teeth prints, a white and slippery coating, and a deep, slow and weak pulse.

Analysis: This pattern is mainly caused by the further development of spleen qi deficiency, by excessive intake of raw and cold food, by excessive intake of cold or cool medicines damaging the spleen yang, by kidney yang deficiency failing to promote the spleen or by insufficient *mingmen* (life gate) fire leading to failure of generating fire in earth (Fig. 11-30).

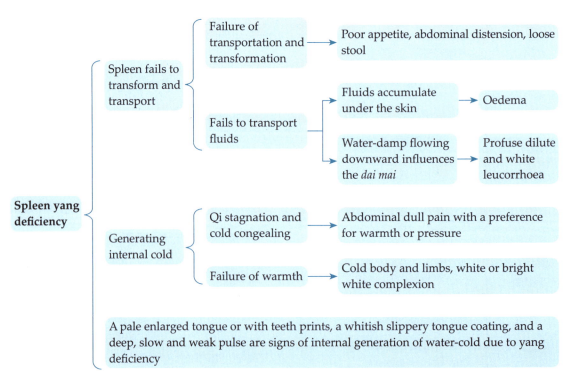

Fig. 11-30 Analysis of a spleen yang deficiency pattern

Key symptoms: Qi deficiency symptoms and deficiency-cold symptoms.

Spleen Failing to Control Blood Pattern

Concept: This is due to spleen qi deficiency failing to hold the blood in the vessels and causing extravasation of blood and haemorrhage. It is also called qi unable to hold the blood.

Clinical manifestations: Haemafaecia (blood in stools), haematuria (blood in the urine), gingival bleeding, epistaxis (nose bleeding), petechiae (haemorrhage into the skin), menorrhagia (excessive menstrual flow), metrorrhagia (bleeding from the uterus that is not associated with menstruation), uterine bleeding that is often accompanied by a pale complexion, lustreless skin, a poor appetite, loose stool, fatigue, lack of strength, shortness of breath, laziness in speaking, a pale tongue, a white tongue coating, and a thready and weak pulse.

Analysis: This pattern is usually caused by weakness of the spleen after a chronic disease, or by overstrain, which damages the spleen (fatigue damage), both of which lead to failure of the spleen in controlling blood (Fig. 11-31).

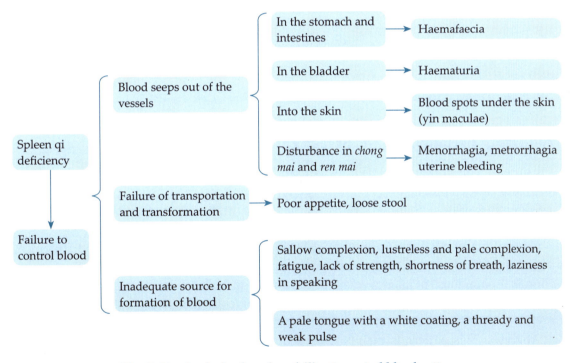

Fig. 11-31 Analysis of a spleen failing to control blood pattern

Key symptoms: Haemorrhage and spleen qi deficiency symptoms at the same time.

Identification: Four patterns of spleen deficiency (Table 11-19).

Table 11-19 Comparison of four patterns of spleen deficiency

Pattern	Common symptoms	Different symptoms	Tongue	Pulse
Spleen qi deficiency	Abdominal distension which is worse after eating, poor appetite, loose stool, short breath, lassitude of the limbs, laziness in speaking, a sallow complexion	Oedema, thin body	Pale tongue with a white coating	Moderate and weak
Spleen yang deficiency		Abdominal pain which is relieved by warmth or pressure, cold limbs, scanty urine, or heaviness of the body and limbs, or general oedema, or clear watery leucorrhoea	Pale enlarged tongue with a whitish slippery coating	Deep, slow and weak
Sinking of spleen qi		A bearing down sensation and distension in the epigastrium and abdomen, or frequency and urgency of defaecation, a bearing down sensation of the anus, or chronic diarrhoea, or even prolapse of the rectum or uterus, turbid urine	Pale tongue with a white coating	Weak
Spleen failing to control blood		Haemafaecia (blood in the stools), haematuria, petechiae (blood spots under the skin), epistaxis (nasal bleeding), menorrhagia, or metrorrhagia and metrostaxis	Pale tongue with white coating	Thready and weak

Cold-Damp Encumbering the Spleen Pattern

Concept: This is due to interior exuberance of cold-dampness encumbering the spleen and disturbs the spleen yang. It is also called dampness encumbering spleen yang, or cold-dampness obstructing the middle *jiao*. It is seen at the *taiyin* stage of the six channel patterns.

Clinical manifestations: Fullness and distending pain in the epigastrium and abdomen, a bland but slimy taste in the mouth, poor appetite, nausea, vomiting, absence of thirst, abdominal pain, loose stool, heaviness of the head and body, oedema, scanty urine, smoky yellow skin and yellow sclera, profuse leucorrhoea, an enlarged tongue with a white-greasy or white-slippery coating, a soft or deep and thready pulse.

Analysis: This pattern is mainly caused by improper diet, excessive intake of raw or cold foods, by exposure to a cold and damp environment like living in a damp or rainy place, or by other excessive endogenous dampness (Fig. 11-32).

Key symptoms: Symptoms of functional impairments of the spleen and stomach in transforming and transporting with manifestations of interior exuberance of cold-dampness at the same time.

Identification: Cold-dampness encumbering the spleen, and spleen yang deficiency (Table 11-20).

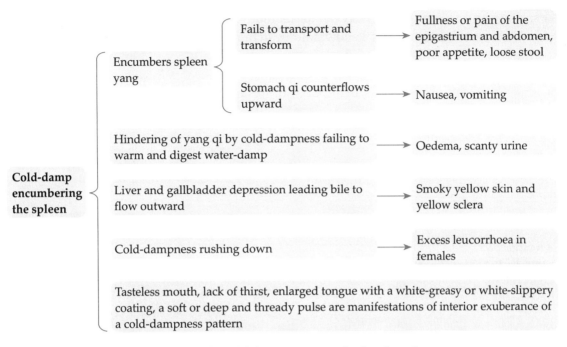

Fig. 11-32 Analysis of a cold-dampness encumbering the spleen pattern

Table 11-20 Differentiation of cold-dampness encumbering the spleen, and spleen yang deficiency

Pattern	Nature	Pathology	Onset and course	Clinical manifestations	
				Common	Different
Cold-dampness encumbering the spleen	Invasion of cold-dampness; excess-cold	Exuberance of cold-damp encumbering the spleen yang and irregularity in ascending and descending	An excess pattern, sudden onset, short course	Cold pain in the epigastrium, poor appetite, loose stool, oedema, abnormal leucorrhoea, etc.	Abdominal pain with a preference for warmth but reluctance for pressure, or smoky yellow skin and eyes, an enlarged tongue with a white-slippery coating, a soft or deep and thready pulse
Spleen yang deficiency	Interior formation of cold-dampness; deficiency-cold	Spleen yang deficiency failing to warm and transport and generating interior deficiency-cold	A deficiency pattern, moderate onset, long course		Abdominal dull pain which is relieved by warmth or pressure, a pale enlarged tongue with teeth prints and a white-slippery coating, a deep, slow and weak pulse

Retention of Damp-Heat in the Spleen Pattern

Concept: This is due to accumulation of damp-heat in the middle *jiao* leading to disturbances of the functions of the spleen and stomach in transporting and transforming. It is also called damp-heat in the middle *jiao* or damp-heat in the spleen and stomach.

Clinical manifestations: Fullness in the abdomen, poor appetite, nausea, loose stools with a foul odour, heaviness of the body and limbs, thirst with desire for drinking in small sips, rising and falling fever which cannot be relieved after sweating, jaundice of the skin and sclera with a fresh bright yellow colour, itching, a red tongue with a yellow-sticky coating and a soft and rapid pulse.

Analysis: This pattern is caused by invasion of a damp-heat pathogen, or excessive intake of acrid, warm, fatty, sweet foods, or alcoholic drinks which produces damp-heat (Fig. 11-33).

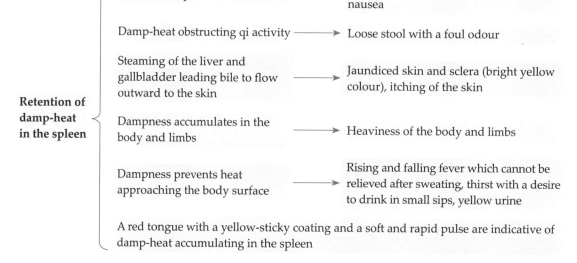

Fig. 11-33 Analysis of damp-heat in the spleen pattern

Key symptoms: Functional impairment of the spleen and stomach in transporting and transforming along with retention of damp-heat at the same time.

Identification: Damp-heat in the spleen and cold-dampness encumbering the spleen (Table 11-21), damp-heat in the spleen and damp-heat in the large intestine (Table 11-22).

Table 11-21 Differentiation of damp-heat in the spleen, and cold-dampness encumbering the spleen

Pattern	Similarities		Differentiation	
	Pathology	Clinical manifestations	Pathology	Clinical manifestations
Retention of damp-heat in the spleen	Interior exuberance of dampness encumbers the spleen which fails to transport and transform	Fullness or pain in the epigastrium and abdomen, poor appetite, nausea, yellow colour of the skin and sclera, loose stools, a feeling of heaviness, a greasy tongue coating, and a soft pulse	Damp-heat accumulation, failure to transform and transport	Fresh yellow skin and yellow sclera, itching of the skin, loose stools with a foul odour, thirst with a desire to drink in small sips, fever which cannot be relieved after sweating, a red tongue with a yellow sticky coating, and a soft and rapid pulse
Cold-dampness encumbering the spleen			Interior exuberance of cold-dampness encumbering the spleen yang	Smoky yellow skin and sclera, oedema, scanty urine, abdominal pain with preference for warmth, profuse leucorrhoea, enlarged tongue

Table 11-22 Comparison of damp-heat in the spleen, and damp-heat in the large intestine

Pattern	Common Symptoms	Location	Different Symptoms
Retention of damp-heat in the spleen	Fever, loose stools, yellow urine, red tongue with a white sticky coating, and a soft and rapid pulse	Middle *jiao*	Fullness or pain in the epigastrium and abdomen, poor appetite, nausea
Damp-heat in the large intestine		Large intestine	Abdominal pain, flooding diarrhoea, diarrhoea with pus and blood (dysentery)

Stomach Cold Pattern

Concept: This is due to a cold pathogen invading the stomach and manifests as cold pain in the epigastrium with excess-cold symptoms. It is also called cold invading the stomach.

Clinical manifestations: Sudden epigastric pain which is aggravated by cold and alleviated by warmth, nausea, vomiting, pain which is relieved temporarily after vomiting, a bland taste in the mouth and lack of thirst, or clear drooling (excess salivation), pale or blue complexion, cold limbs, a pale tongue with a white-moist and slippery coating, and a wiry or deep, slow and tight pulse.

Analysis: This pattern is mostly ascribed to an excessive intake of raw and cold food, or an attack on the stomach by cold, which leads to cold stagnation in the epigastrium (Fig. 11-34).

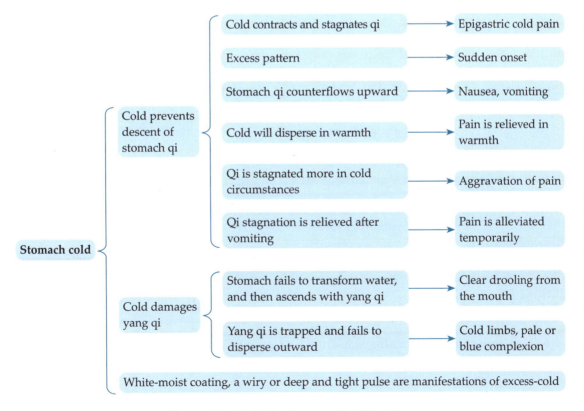

Fig. 11-34 Analysis of a stomach cold pattern

Key symptoms: Presence of epigastric pain and cold patterns at the same time.

Stomach Heat Pattern

Concept: This is due to scorching exuberance of stomach heat and stomach fails to descend. It is also called scorching exuberance of stomach heat, or flourishing of stomach fire.

Clinical manifestations: A burning sensation and pain in the epigastrium, dislike of pressure, thirst with preference for cold drinks, constant hunger, vomiting after eating, halitosis (foul breath odour), or inflammation, painful and bleeding gums (gingival haemorrhage), constipation, scanty dark urine, red tongue with yellow coating, and smooth and rapid pulse.

Analysis: This pattern results from an excessive intake of acrid, spicy, warm, greasy or dry food which turns into fire, from emotional frustration which leads to depression of qi that turns into fire or from invasion by endogenous heat-pathogens, all of which can lead to scorching exuberance of stomach heat (Fig. 11-35).

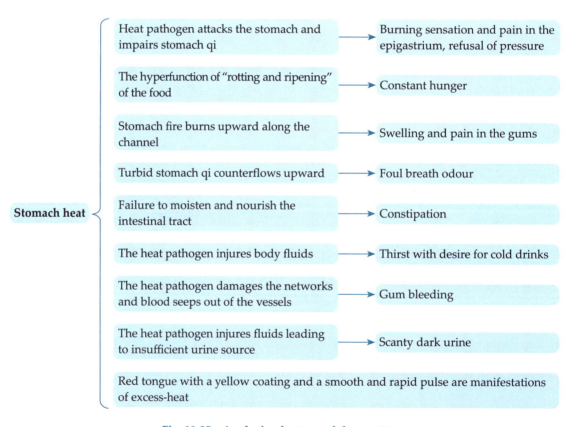

Fig. 11-35 Analysis of a stomach heat pattern

Key symptoms: A burning sensation and pain in the epigastrium with excess-heat symptoms.

Identification: Stomach heat and heat obstructing the large intestine (Table 11-23).

Table 11-23 Differentiation of stomach heat, and heat obstructing the large intestine

Pattern	Position	Nature	Pathology	Clinical manifestations	
				Specific Symptoms	General Symptoms
Stomach heat	Stomach	Interior excessive heat pattern	Scorching exuberance of stomach heat and stomach qi fails to descend	A burning sensation and pain in the epigastrium, refusal of pressure, constant hunger, foul breath odour, swelling and pain in the gums, gum bleeding	Thirst with desire for cold drinks, constipation, yellow urine, a red tongue with a yellow coating, and a smooth and rapid pulse
Heat obstructing the large intestine	Large intestine		A dry heat pathogen and stool bind internally and obstruct the large intestine	Distension, fullness, hardness and pain of the abdomen or around the umbilicus, refusal of pressure, constipation	High fever, or late afternoon tidal fever, sweating, thirst, constipation, possibly even coma and delirium, mania, scanty dark urine, a rigid tongue with a thick yellow coating, and a forceful, deep and rapid pulse

Stomach Yin Deficiency Pattern

Concept: This is due to the insufficiency of stomach yin failing to moisten and nourish the stomach. If a deficiency-heat pattern is not obvious, it is also called a stomach dryness pattern.

Clinical manifestations: Dull pain in the epigastrium, anorexia, fullness in the epigastrium, no appetite or intake of food (but yin deficiency with stomach heat results in swift digestion with increased appetite), retching, hiccoughs, dryness of the mouth and throat, dry stool, scanty urine, a red tongue with little moisture and diminished or no coating, and a thready and rapid pulse.

Analysis: This pattern is mainly caused by the consumption of stomach yin by febrile diseases, by emotional frustration leading to depression of qi, which then turns into fire to injure stomach yin, excessive vomiting or diarrhoea consuming body fluids, by excessive intake of acrid, spicy or hot foods, by eating too late in the evening, or by taking too many warm herbs consuming stomach yin (Fig. 11-36).

Key symptoms: Common symptoms of stomach diseases and the symptoms of yin deficiency.

Identification: Stomach yin deficiency, and dryness of the large intestine (Table 11-24).

Diagnostics in Chinese Medicine

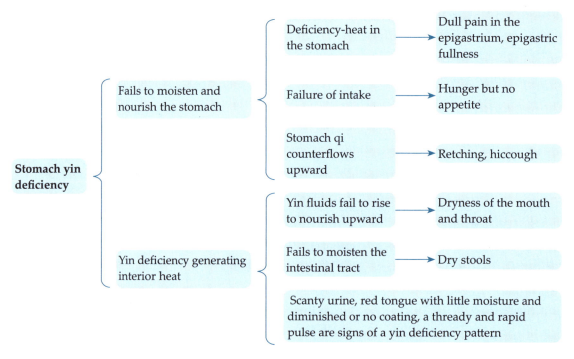

Fig. 11-36   Analysis of stomach yin deficiency pattern

Table 11-24   Comparison of stomach yin deficiency, and dryness of the large intestine

Pattern	Location	Pathology	Clinical manifestations	
			Common Symptoms	Different Symptoms
Stomach yin deficiency	Stomach	Insufficient stomach yin fails to moisten and nourish the stomach and prevents stomach qi from descending	Dryness of the mouth and throat, dry stools, a red tongue with little moisture	Dull pain in the epigastrium, hunger but no appetite, epigastric fullness, retching, hiccough, diminished or no tongue coating, a thready and rapid pulse
Dryness of the large intestine	Large intestine	Deficiency of fluids in the large intestine fails to moisten the intestines		Constipation, dry stools and difficult defaecation, defaecation once every several days, a dry mouth, or foul breath odour, a yellow dry coating, a thready and rough or choppy pulse

Retention of Food in the Stomach Pattern

Concept: This is due to food stagnation in the stomach and manifests as fullness, distension and pain in the epigastrium.

Clinical manifestations: Fullness, distension and pain in the epigastrium, refusal of abdominal pressure, anorexia, rotten or foul belching, acid regurgitation, vomiting of sour and undigested food, distension and pain which can be relieved after vomiting, or intestinal flatus, abdominal pain, diarrhoea with a sensation of incomplete defaecation and with a foul odour, or constipation, thick and sticky tongue coating, and slippery pulse.

Analysis: This pattern is mainly caused by irregular diet, voracious eating and drinking or by intrinsic stomach qi deficiency, which halts the digestion and transit of the food (Fig. 11-37).

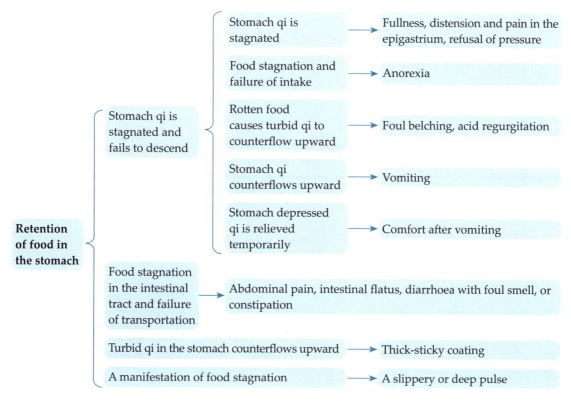

Fig.11-37　Analysis of food retention in the stomach

Key symptoms: Fullness, distension and pain in the epigastrium, foul belching, acid regurgitation, sour vomiting and a history of improper or voracious food intake.

Blood Stasis in the Stomach Pattern

Concept: This is caused by long-term spleen and stomach diseases, cold pathogen congestion or qi stagnation, all of which lead to blood stasis in the epigastrium.

Clinical manifestations: Epigastric stabbing pain, which is fixed in one place, pain aggravated by pressure and more severe after meals, poor appetite, emaciation, haematemesis (vomiting which contains blood), haemafaecia (blood in the stool), a dark purple tongue, and a choppy pulse.

Analysis: The newly acquired disease appears in the channel, and the chronic disease enters into the networks or collaterals (Fig. 11-38).

Key symptoms: Epigastric stabbing pain, purple tongue and choppy pulse.

Identification: Various differentiations of stomach patterns (Table 11-25).

Table 11-25 Comparison of stomach patterns

Pattern		Pain feature	Taste & thirst	Appetite	Vomit	Urine & stool	Other manifestations	Tongue	Pulse
Stomach cold		Sudden cold pain in the epigastrium, aggravated by coldness, preference for warmth	Tasteless mouth and no thirst	Pain is relieved after taking hot foods	Clear water	Loose stool	Borborygmus, cold body and limbs, fatigue, lack of strength	Pale tongue with a white-slippery coating	A slow or wiry and tight pulse
Stomach heat		Burning sensation and pain in the epigastrium	Thirst with preference for cold drinks	Constant hunger, vomiting after eating	Acid regurgitation	Constipation, yellow urine	Swelling and pain in the gums which may bleed when cleaned	Red tongue with yellow dry coating	A slippery and rapid pulse
Stomach yin deficiency		Dull pain in the epigastrium	Dryness of the mouth, thirst	Hunger but no appetite	Retching, hiccoughs	Dry stool	Epigastric fullness, emaciation	Red tongue with diminished or peeled coating	A thready and rapid pulse
Excess patterns	Retention of food in the stomach	Distension and pain in the epigastrium	Foul belching	Aversion to food smells	Acid and undigested food	Recurrent flatus, diarrhoea with foul smell, or constipation		Thick sticky coating	A slippery pulse
	Blood stasis in the stomach	Epigastric stabbing pain, fixed in one place, dislike of pressure, more severe after meals	Dry mouth without desire for drinks	Poor appetite	Vomiting blood	Stool with blood	Emaciation	Dark purple tongue	A choppy pulse

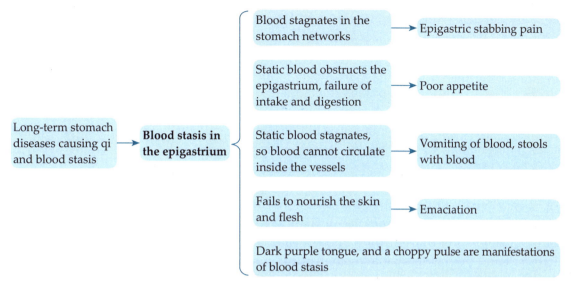

Fig. 11-38 Analysis of blood stasis in the stomach pattern

Section 4
Liver and Gallbladder Pattern Differentiation

The liver resides in the right costal region, and the gallbladder is attached to the liver. There is an extremely close association between the liver and gallbladder, which have great similarities and great differences; this association reflects how relationships really function. The liver and gallbladder have an exterior-interior relationship via the channels. The liver channel curves around the genitalia and runs up into the lower abdomen and then branches out in the hypochondriac and costal region. From here, it ascends to the throat and reaches the eye; running further upwards it reaches the top of the head. The gallbladder channel connects with the liver channel and also travels to the head; it ascends to the forehead and curves downwards to the region behind the ear.

The liver opens into the eyes, controls the sinews and manifests in the nails. The main function of the liver is to ensure the smooth flow of qi, its structure is yin but its function is yang, it is linked with responsibility for spreading and various discharges and needs to be moist and supple to carry out these activities. The liver likes the smooth flow of qi and dislikes being constrained or depressed downwards. The normal direction of liver qi movement is upward and outward, in all directions, to ensure the smooth and unimpeded flow of qi throughout the body. The liver has a deep influence on the emotional state and is easily injured by strong emotions. The moving and spreading function of the liver also ensures the flow of bile and assists digestive function of the stomach and spleen and transportation of qi and blood. In addition, the liver governs the storing of blood and its function is to store blood and regulate the blood volume according to physical activity.

The gallbladder is classified as both a *fu* organ and an extraordinary *fu* organ and is the only yang organ that stores a clear substantial fluid in the form of bile; it stores and secretes bile when needed during digestion. It controls judgment and gives an individual courage and initiative, so there is a saying "the gallbladder is the upright official that makes decisions" (*Yellow Emperor's Inner Classic*).

According to the physiological functions and characteristics of the liver and gallbladder, the liver diseases may manifest as depression, irritation, outbursts of anger, distending pain in the chest, hypochondrium, lower abdomen and head, dizziness, tremor of the limbs, convulsions of the limbs, eye diseases, abnormal menstruation, testicular disorders, etc. The gallbladder diseases may manifest as a bitter taste in the mouth; jaundice; palpitations due to fright; hesitation with a lack of courage and momentum; and disturbances in digestion, etc. (Table 11-26).

The patterns of liver diseases can be summarised into two types: excess types and deficiency types, although the former is more common. The former is usually caused by emotional problems which may result from: the liver failing to maintain the normal flow of qi; qi stagnation transforming into fire and later this fire rising upward; fire injuring liver yin and yin being unable to control yang, subsequently the hyperactive yang may transform into wind; or cold, heat or damp-heat pathogens invading the interior. The deficiency type is caused by chronic diseases, by the influence of other organ diseases

Table 11-26 The physiological function, pathological changes and common symptoms of the liver and gallbladder

Physiological function	Pathological changes	Common symptoms
Ensures the smooth flow of qi	Disharmony of emotions, depression or overexcitement	Depression, sighing, irritation, outbursts of anger
	Liver yang rising	Dizziness, tinnitus, deafness, red complexion, apoplexy (extreme anger), distending pain of the head, especially the temporal regions
	Qi stagnation and blood stasis	Distending pain in the chest and hypochondrium, lower abdomen or testes, distension of the breast, abdominal masses, abnormal menstruation
Stores blood	Blood seeps from the vessels	Vomiting of blood, gingival bleeding, hypermenorrhoea, metrorrhagia and metrostaxis
Controls the sinews and manifests in the nails	Failure to nourish the sinews	Tremor, numbness, disturbance in joint movements, convulsions, opisthotonos, withered and brittle nails
	Spasm of the sinews due to retention of cold	Contraction and pain of the scrotum and testes, hernia, tongue contraction
Opens into the eyes	Failure to nourish the eyes	Dryness of the eyes, night blindness
	Liver fire blazing upward	Red and painful eyes
The gallbladder stores and excretes bile	Bile counterflows upward	Bitter taste in the mouth
	Bile flows outward	Jaundice
The gallbladder manages decision making	Gallbladder qi deficiency	Panic, lack of courage, insomnia

or by blood loss; all of which may lead to liver yin or blood deficiency. The gallbladder diseases include: depressed gallbladder with phlegm harassing, damp-heat in the liver and gallbladder (Fig. 11-39).

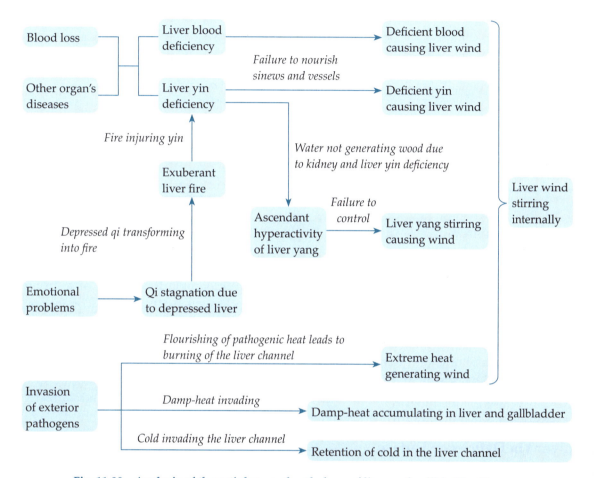

Fig. 11-39   Analysis of the aetiology and pathology of liver and gallbladder diseases

Liver Blood Deficiency Pattern

Concept: This is due to liver blood being unable to nourish the liver system.
Clinical manifestations: Dizziness, pale and lustreless complexion, withered and brittle nails, blurred vision or night blindness, numbness of the limbs, disturbance in joint movements, tremor of the limbs and muscular twitching, hypomenorrhoea, pale menstrual flow, amenorrhoea, with a pale tongue, and thready pulse.
Analysis: This pattern is usually caused by weakness of the spleen and kidney leading to insufficient production of qi and blood. Alternatively, it may be due to excessive bleeding (external or internal), chronic diseases which injure liver blood or a deficiency of nutrients (Fig. 11-40).

Diagnostics in Chinese Medicine

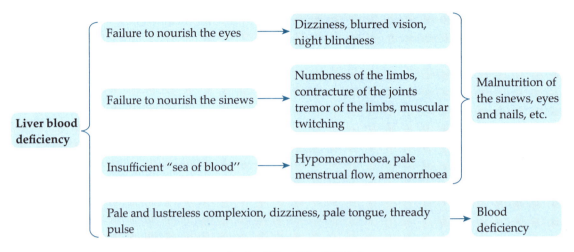

Fig. 11-40 Analysis of liver blood deficiency pattern

Key symptoms: Malnutrition of the sinews, eyes, nails and general symptoms of a blood deficiency pattern.

Although liver blood and heart blood deficiency have common signs of a blood deficiency pattern such as pale complexion, lips, nails and tongue with a thready or choppy pulse, there are quite a few differences between them. The former liver blood deficiency has particular emphasis on liver pathology such as failure to nourish and moisten the sinews resulting in numbness and tremors of the limbs; failure to nourish and moisten the eyes leading to blurred vision and floaters; and sea of blood deficiency in females leading to hypomenorrhoea and amenorrhoea. While the latter heart blood deficiency reflects directly on heart blood pathologies such as irritability and palpitations.

Liver Yin Deficiency Pattern

Concept: This is due to yin deficiency failing to moisten and nourish the liver. The pattern of deficiency of liver yin results from consumption of yin-fluids in the liver; further development of liver yin deficiency will fail to restrain yang, leading to a deficient-heat pattern affiliated with liver yang hyperactivity.

Clinical manifestations: Dizziness, tinnitus, dryness of the eyes, blurred vision, tidal fever, red cheeks, dry mouth and throat, feverish sensation in the chest, palms and soles, night sweating, creeping of the limbs (small involuntary movements of the limbs), a dull burning pain in the costal and hypochondriac regions, red tongue with little fluid, and a taut, thready and rapid pulse.

Analysis: This pattern is mainly caused by emotional frustration, which leads to qi stagnation, which then transforms into fire, followed by injury to the liver yin. Alternatively, the heat of warm diseases reduces liver yin in the later stages or insufficient kidney yin is unable to enrich and nourish the liver yin (Fig. 11-41).

Key symptoms: Malnutrition of the head, eyes, sinews and vessels. The liver channel complicated by yin deficiency generating a deficient-heat pattern.

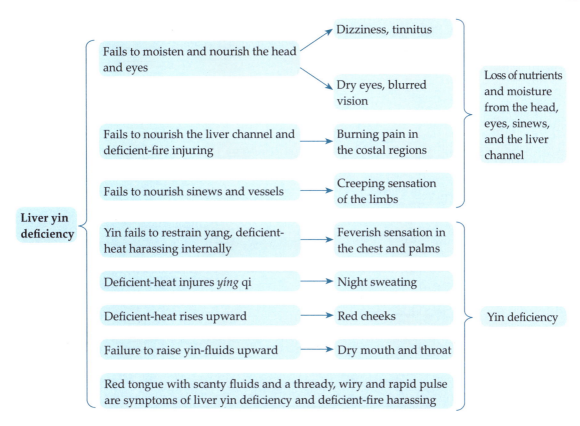

Fig.11-41   Analysis of liver yin deficiency pattern

Liver Constraint (Depression/Depressed/Stagnated) Pattern

Concept: This is due to a deficient condition of the liver function; leading to wood not controlling earth. Lack of liver function leads to stagnation, which may lead to internal heat and if this affects blood then blood stasis may also result.

Clinical manifestations: Stuffiness and suffocating feeling in the chest and hypochondrium or lower abdomen; depression and unhappiness; dysmenorrhoea, abnormal menstruation, amenorrhoea; sighing; globus hystericus or plum-stone throat (subjective feeling of a lump or obstruction in the throat); goitre; abdominal masses; digestive problems; stabbing intense pains if blood stasis is involved.

Analysis: Often caused by depressed emotions, which leads to stagnation of qi or blood (Fig. 11-42).

Key symptoms: Stuffiness in the chest, depression and menstrual problems.

Identification: Liver constraint and transverse invasion of hyperactive liver qi (Table 11-27).

Diagnostics in Chinese Medicine

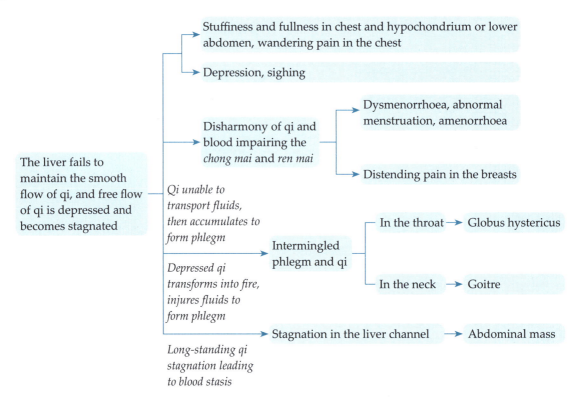

Fig.11-42　Analysis of liver constraint pattern

Table 11-27　Comparison of liver constraint and transverse invasion of hyperactive liver qi

Pattern	Similarity	Differential points	
		Pathogenesis	Clinical manifestation
Liver constraint	Distending pain along the liver channel, and emotional changes	A breakdown of the smooth flow of qi	Depressed emotions, sighing
Transverse invasion of hyperactive liver qi		Hyperactive flow of liver qi. Firstly affects the liver channel then invades the spleen and stomach	Irritability, propensity to outbursts of anger, scurrying pain in the chest and hypochondrium, symptoms of spleen and stomach failing to transform and transport such as distending pain of the epigastrium and abdomen, hiccough, nausea, vomiting

Reference:
Transverse Invasion of Hyperactive Liver Qi Pattern
Concept: Due to an excess condition of the liver function; leading to wood overacting on earth.

Clinical manifestations: Distending and wandering pain in the chest and hypochondrium; distension and pain in the breasts; anger and irritability; digestive symptoms such as belching, vomiting and bowel changes; wiry (bow-string) pulse.

Analysis: Usually caused by sudden anger or irritation. The excess liver qi brings about adverse horizontal movement of qi negatively affecting the spleen and stomach.

Liver Fire Blazing Upward Pattern

Concept: This is due to excess fire in the liver having a natural tendency to flare upward and many of the symptoms reflect the rising of liver fire upward. It is also simply called a liver fire pattern.

Clinical manifestations: Dizziness, severe distending pain in the head, flushed face, red eyes, bitter taste in the mouth, dry mouth, irritability, propensity to outbursts of anger, tinnitus, sudden deafness, or pus and swelling pain in the ear (antrum auris), insomnia, or dream-disturbed sleep with vivid dreams, burning pain in the costal and hypochondriac regions, haematemesis (vomiting of blood), epistaxis (nose bleeding), constipation, scanty yellowish urine, red tongue with a yellow coating, a wiry (taut) and rapid pulse.

Analysis: This pattern is mainly caused by emotional frustration making qi stagnate in the liver, which transforms into fire, or by a heat pathogen invading interiorly, or by fire of other organs invading the liver leading to liver and gallbladder fire flaring upward (Fig. 11-43).

Key symptoms: Excess-heat pattern along the liver channel.

Identification: Four fire-heat patterns (Table 11-28).

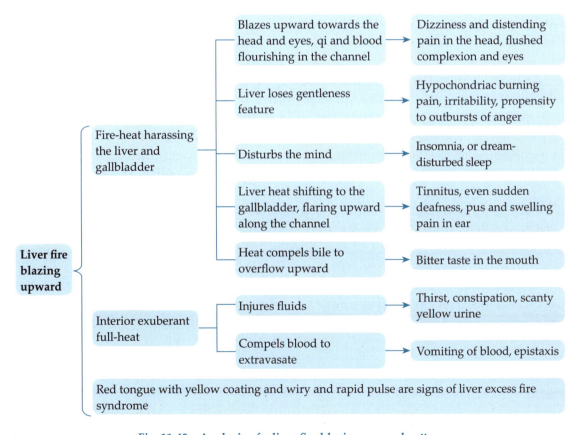

Fig. 11-43 Analysis of a liver fire blazing upward pattern

Table 11-28 Differentiation of the four fire-heat patterns

Pattern	Identical symptoms	Distinct symptoms
Heart fire hyperactivity	Aversion to heat and preference for cold, red complexion and eyes, thirst with a desire for cold drinks, restlessness, scanty-dark urine, constipation, red tongue with dry yellow coating, a powerful and rapid pulse	Mental restlessness, coma or delirium, red-crimson tip of the tongue, tongue ulcers
Retention of heat in the lung		Cough, wheezing, flaring nares, yellow thick sputum, chest pain, or throat pain, red tongue with yellow coating
Flourishing of stomach fire		Epigastric burning pain, polyorexia (extreme hunger), Halitosis (foul breath), pain and ulcers in the gums
Blazing of liver fire		Dizziness, tinnitus, distending pain in the head, hypochondriac burning pain, a wiry or bow-string pulse

Hyperactivity of Liver Yang Pattern

Concept: This is due to liver yin and kidney yin deficiency failing to control liver yang which leads to excessive rising of liver yang, the result is that it manifests as a pattern of upper excess and lower deficiency.

Clinical manifestations: Dizziness, tinnitus, distending pain of the head and eyes, red complexion and eyes, irritability, propensity to outbursts of anger, insomnia, dream-disturbed sleep, weakness and aching of the back and knees, heaviness of the head, red tongue with scanty fluid, a wiry pulse or wiry, thready and rapid pulse.

Analysis: This pattern is mainly caused by long-standing anger making qi stagnate which transforms into fire. The subsequent fire injures liver yin and kidney yin; by excessive sexual activity consuming yin; or by kidney yin deficiency in old age, leading to water not generating wood, with the consequence of deficiency of yin of the liver and kidney. These patterns then result in a failure to restrain liver yang. Therefore, deficiency of yin of the liver and kidney gives rise to hyperactivity of liver yang (Fig. 11-44).

> **Key symptoms:** Dizziness, distending pain in the head and eyes, heaviness of the head and a floating feeling of the feet (feelings of instability), weakness and aching of the back and knees.

Identification: Hyperactivity of liver yang and liver fire blazing upward (Table 11-29), liver constraint, liver fire blazing upward, liver yin deficiency, and hyperactivity of liver yang pattern (Table 11-30).

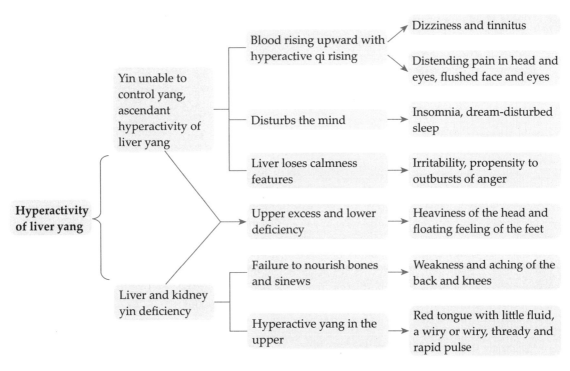

Fig.11-44　Analysis of a hyperactivity of liver yang pattern

Table 11-29　Comparison of hyperactivity of liver yang and liver fire blazing upward

Pattern	Identical symptoms	Key points for differentiation	
		Features	Clinical manifestation
Liver fire blazing upward	Symptoms in the head and eyes are obvious due to fire having a natural tendency to flare upward and excessive rising of liver yang: dizziness, tinnitus, distending pain of the head and eyes, a flushed red complexion and eyes, irritability, propensity to outbursts of anger	Short course, acute onset, excess pattern	*Excess fire pattern*: flushed complexion and eyes, severe distending headache, or hypochondriac burning pain, bitter taste, thirst, constipation, yellow urine, etc. Without yin deficiency symptoms
Hyperactivity of liver yang		Long course, chronic onset upper excess and lower deficiency; simultaneous excess and deficiency	*Upper excess pattern*: distending pain of the head and eyes, heaviness of the head, dizziness, etc. *Lower deficiency pattern*: weakness and aching of the back and knees, tinnitus, etc. Yin deficiency pattern

Table 11-30 Comparison of liver constraint, liver fire blazing upward, liver yin deficiency, and hyperactivity of liver yang patterns

Pattern	Property	Symptoms	Tongue features	Pulse tracings
Liver constraint	Mixed deficient and excess pattern	Stuffiness and fullness in the chest and hypochondrium or lower abdomen, wandering pain, sighing, propensity to mental depression and despondency, abnormal menstruation etc.	White tongue coating	Wiry pulse
Liver fire blazing upward	Heat pattern	Dizziness, severe distending headache, tinnitus, bitter taste, dry mouth, flushed complexion and eyes, irritability, propensity to outbursts of anger, insomnia, or dream-disturbed sleep, or hypochondriac burning pain, constipation, yellow urine, pus and swelling pain in the ear, haematemesis (vomiting with blood), epistaxis (nose bleeding)	Red tongue with yellow coating	Wiry and rapid pulse
Liver yin deficiency	Deficiency pattern	Dizziness, tinnitus, hypochondriac pain, dry eyes, red cheeks, feverishness in the chest, palms and soles, tidal fever, night sweating, dry mouth and throat, muscular twitching	Red tongue with little fluid	Thready and rapid pulse
Hyperactivity of liver yang	Deficiency in the root and excess in the branches	Dizziness, tinnitus, distending pain of the head and eyes, flushed complexion and eyes, irritability, propensity to outbursts of anger, palpitations, insomnia, dream-disturbed sleep, weakness and aching of the back and knees, heaviness of the head	Red tongue	Powerful and wiry pulse or thready, wiry and rapid pulse

Liver Wind Stirring Internally Pattern

There are four distinct types of liver wind pattern according to different causes:
- hyperactivity of liver yang causing wind;
- extreme heat generating wind;
- liver yin deficiency leading to liver wind; and
- liver blood deficiency leading to liver wind.

The common signs and symptoms of a liver wind pattern are: tremor, tic, numbness, dizziness and convulsions or paralysis.

Each of the four types of liver wind will be discussed separately.

1. Hyperactivity of liver yang causing wind

Concept: This is due to liver yin being unable to control liver yang, leading to liver yang transforming into wind.

Clinical manifestations: Dizziness that upsets balance, fainting, involuntary shaking of the head, headache, tremor of the limbs, rigidity of the neck, dysphasia, numbness of the limbs, floating feet sensations, red tongue with white or greasy coating, thready, wiry but powerful pulse. Possibly sudden fainting, unconsciousness, deviation of the eyes and mouth, hemiplegia, aphasia with a stiff tongue, wheezy phlegm in the throat.

Analysis: The pattern is mainly caused by depressed emotions leading to qi stagnation transforming into fire and injuring yin, or by innate deficiency of liver and kidney yin and yin failing to control yang, the hyperactive yang transforming into wind. Therefore this pattern also belongs to deficiency in the root and excess in the branches or a pattern of upper excess and lower deficiency (Fig. 11-45).

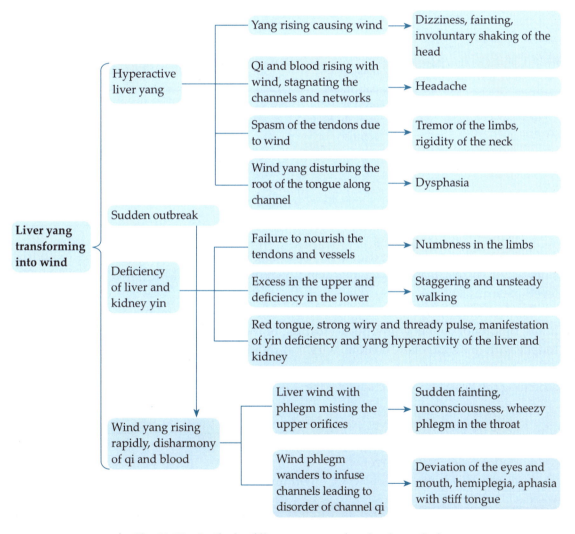

Fig. 11-45 Analysis of liver yang transforming into wind

Key symptoms: Dizziness, sudden unconsciousness or sudden fainting, hemiplegia.

Identification: Hyperactivity of liver yang causing wind, and hyperactivity of liver yang (Table 11-31).

Table 11-31 Identification of hyperactivity of liver yang causing wind, and hyperactivity of liver yang

Type of pattern	Similarity		Distinction	
	Pathogenesis	Symptoms	Pathogenesis	Symptoms
Hyperactivity of liver yang causing wind	Pattern of upper excess and lower deficiency, the former is the further development of the latter	Symptoms of excessive yang rising in the upper part, such as dizziness, tinnitus, distending pain in the head and eyes, flushed complexion and eyes, etc.	Liver yin unable to control liver yang, leading to liver yang transforming into wind	*Liver wind pattern:* sudden falling down, involuntary shaking of the head, tremor of the limbs, rigidity of the neck, numbness of the limbs, red tongue with white or greasy coating, thready wiry but powerful pulse, etc. or sudden fainting, unconsciousness, deviation of the eyes and mouth
Hyperactivity of liver yang			Liver yin and kidney yin deficiency failing to control liver yang and excessive rising of liver yang	*Upper excess:* dizziness, tinnitus, distending pain of the head and eyes, red complexion and eyes, irritability, propensity to outbursts of anger. *Lower deficiency:* insomnia, dream-disturbed sleep, weakness and aching of the back and knees, heaviness of the head, a red tongue with little fluid, a wiry or wiry, thready and rapid pulse

2. Extreme heat generating wind

Concept: This is due to extreme heat burning the fluids and being unable to nourish sinews and vessels, leading to a liver wind pattern. It is seen at the blood level of the four levels pattern.

Clinical manifestations: High fever, mental restlessness, mania, convulsions of the limbs, rigidity of the neck, an upward turning of the eyes, opisthotonos, coma, red-crimson tongue with dry and yellow coating, wiry and rapid pulse.

Analysis: This pattern is usually seen in warm diseases and is caused by exuberant heat scorching the heart and liver channels (Fig. 11-46).

Key symptoms: High fever and general symptoms of wind stirring pattern.

3. Deficient yin causing liver wind

Concept: This is due to deficiency of yin fluids being unable to nourish the sinews and vessels.

Clinical manifestations: Muscular twitching, dizziness, tinnitus, tidal fever, red cheeks, dry mouth and throat, thin body, red tongue with scanty fluids, thready and rapid pulse.

Analysis: This pattern is mainly caused by depletion of yin-fluids at the late stage of warm diseases, or chronic diseases leading to deficiency of yin fluids failing to nourish the sinews and tendons. See more specific analysis of the pattern in **Liver Yin Deficiency Pattern (P. 237)**.

Key symptoms: Wind stirring pattern such as muscular twitching, dizziness, etc., yin deficiency pattern.

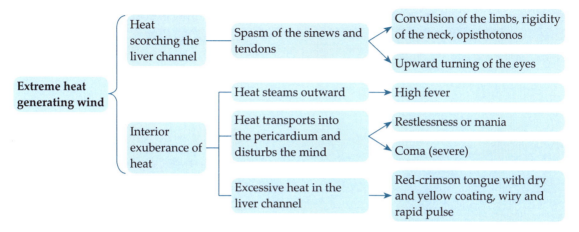

Fig. 11-46 Analysis of extreme heat generating wind

4. Blood deficiency causing liver wind

Concept: This is due to blood deficiency failing to nourish sinews and vessels.

Clinical manifestations: Tremor of the limbs, muscular twitching, numbness of the limbs, dizziness, tinnitus, pale face, withered and brittle nails, pale tongue, thready and weak pulse.

Analysis: This pattern is chiefly caused by internal diseases, chronic blood deficiency, or acute and chronic blood loss, all of which lead to blood deficiency with failure to nourish the sinews and vessels. See more specific analysis of the pattern in **Liver Blood Deficiency Pattern** (P. 239).

Identification: Four liver wind stirring patterns (Table 11-32).

Damp-Heat in the Liver and Gallbladder Pattern

Concept: This is due to damp-heat accumulating in the liver and gallbladder impeding the smooth flow of qi. It is seen in the middle *jiao* level of the *sanjiao* patterns. This pattern can lead to liver and gallbladder damp-heat accumulating and congealing.

Clinical manifestations: Distending and burning pain in the right hypochondrium, anorexia, abdominal distension, bitter taste, nausea, vomiting, irregular defaecations, scanty dark urine, or alternating chills and fever, jaundice (yellow skin and eyes). There may also be yellow and foul leucorrhoea, vaginal eczema with severe itching, papulovesicular rashes in the genital area, pruritus vulvae, or in males, eczema with unbearable itching of the scrotum, swelling and burning pain of the testes. In addition, a red tongue with a yellow greasy coating, and a wiry and rapid or slippery and rapid pulse.

Analysis: This pattern is due to the invasion of pathogenic damp-heat, or excessive consumption of warm, fatty or greasy, or sweet foods which produce dampness and heat, or spleen deficiency causing the formation of dampness which then turns into heat, followed by earth insulting wood, all of which lead to damp-heat accumulating in the liver and gallbladder (Fig. 11-47).

Table 11-32 Comparison of four liver wind stirring patterns

Pattern	Pathogenesis	Nature	Primary signs	Combined signs	Tongue	Pulse
Hyperactivity of liver yang causing wind	Liver yin unable to control liver yang leading to hyperactive yang rising causing wind	Upper excess and lower deficiency	Dizziness, fainting, involuntary shaking of the head, tremor of the limbs, dysphasia, or aphasia with a stiff tongue, or sudden fainting, unconsciousness, hemiplegia	Headache, rigidity of the neck, numbness of the limbs	Red tongue with white or greasy coating	Powerful, wiry pulse
Extreme heat generating wind	Extreme heat burning the fluids and inability to nourish the sinews and vessels leading to a liver wind pattern	Excess-heat pattern	High fever, convulsions of the limbs, rigidity of the neck, possibly even opisthotonos, an upward turning of the eyes	Coma, mania	Red tongue	Powerful wiry and rapid pulse
Deficient yin causing liver wind	Deficiency of yin fluids and blood being unable to nourish the sinews and vessels	Deficiency pattern	Muscular twitching, dizziness	Feverish sensation in the chest, palms and soles, tidal fever, dry mouth and throat, thin body	Red tongue with scanty fluids	Wiry, thready and rapid pulse
Deficient blood causing liver wind		Deficiency pattern	Tremor of the limbs, muscular twitching, numbness of the limbs, dizziness	Dizziness, tinnitus, pale face, withered and brittle nails	Pale tongue with white coating	Thready pulse

Key symptoms: Distending pain in the right hypochondrium, anorexia, abdominal distension, jaundice (yellowish colour of the skin and sclera of the eyes), vaginal itching, and signs of a damp-heat pattern.

Identification: Damp-heat in the liver and gallbladder and damp-heat (Table 11-33).

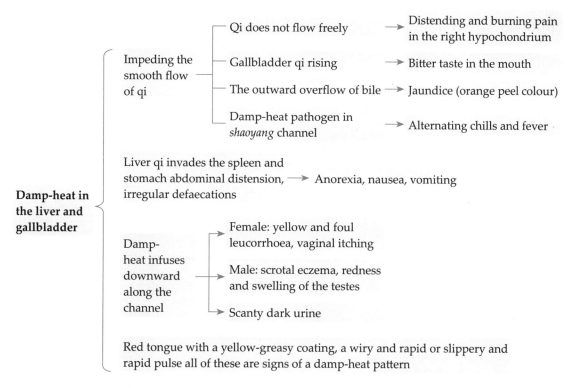

Fig. 11-47 Analysis of damp-heat in the liver and gallbladder

Table 11-33 Comparison of damp-heat in the liver and gallbladder and damp-heat accumulating in the spleen

Pattern	Pathogenesis		Location	Similar symptoms	Distinct symptoms
Damp-heat in the liver and gallbladder	Damp-heat accumulates in the middle *jiao*	Does not ensure the smooth flow of qi	Liver and gallbladder	Jaundice (like orange peel), poor appetite, abdominal distension, nausea, vomiting, red tongue with yellow greasy coating, a rapid pulse	Symptoms of impeding the smooth flow of qi such as, distending and burning pain in the right hypochondrium, a bitter taste, nausea, vomiting, or alternating chills and fever, vaginal itching, yellow and foul leucorrhoea, a wiry pulse, etc.
Damp-heat accumulating in the spleen		Abnormal function of the transformation and transportation	Spleen		Symptoms of the abnormal function of transformation and transportation such as stuffiness or pain of the epigastrium and abdomen, nausea, vomiting, poor appetite, loose stools with an offensive odour, unsurfaced fever, thirst with a desire to take sips of water, heaviness of the head and body, a soggy pulse, etc.

Cold Stagnation in the Liver Channel Pattern

This is due to a cold pathogen invading and congealing in the liver channel and manifests as a cold pain along the liver channel. It is also called liver cold pattern.

Clinical manifestations: Cold pain in the lower abdomen which refers to the scrotum and testes, alleviated by warmth, aggravated by cold, distension and bearing down sensation in the pudendal area or straining of the testes or contraction of the external genitalia or scrotum, a vertex headache, cold body and limbs, a pale tongue with a wet and white coating, and a deep and tight pulse, or wiry and tight pulse.

Analysis: See Fig. 11-48.

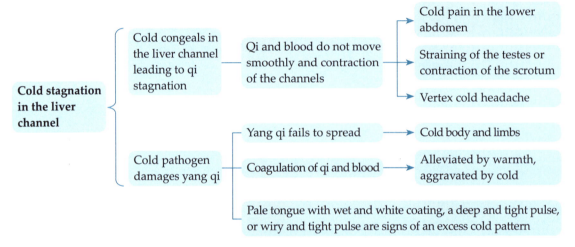

Fig. 11-48　Analysis of cold stagnation in the liver channel

Key symptoms: Cold pain in the lower abdomen and pudendum, vertex cold headache, a deep and tight pulse, or a wiry and tight pulse.

Depressed Gallbladder with Phlegm Harassing Pattern

Concept: This is due to phlegm and heat harassing interiorly in the gallbladder and then interfering with the smooth flow of liver qi.

Clinical manifestations: Lack of courage, palpitations due to fright, insomnia, dream-disturbed sleep, vexing heat, restlessness, fullness in the chest and distension of the hypochondrium, sighing, dizziness, tinnitus, bitter taste, nausea, vomiting, red tongue with a yellow-greasy coating, a wiry and rapid pulse.

Analysis: This pattern is mainly caused by emotional frustration or depressed emotions leading to liver constraint, creating stagnation, then turning into fire and injuring the fluids to form phlegm, then along with heat, harassing the heart and gallbladder (Fig. 11-49).

Key symptoms: Fright palpitations, insomnia, dizziness, yellow-greasy coating.

Identification: Depressed gallbladder with phlegm harassing and phlegm-fire harassing the heart (Table 11-34).

Chapter 11 Differentiation of Patterns According to the Zang-Fu Organs Section 4

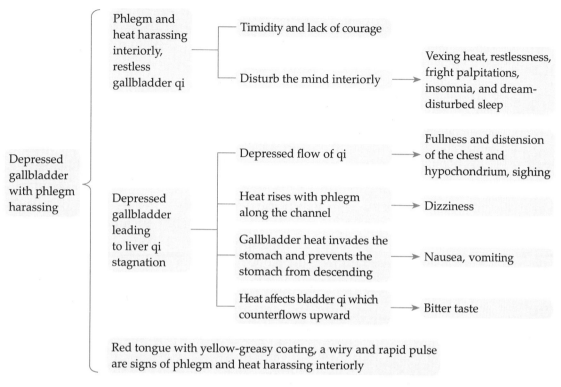

Fig. 11-49 Analysis of depressed gallbladder with phlegm harassing

Table 11-34 Comparison of depressed gallbladder with phlegm harassing and phlegm-fire harassing the heart

Pattern	Aetiology	Pathogenesis	Location	Clinical manifestations	
				Identical	Distinct
Depressed gallbladder with phlegm harassing	Excessive seven emotions affect qi flow and depressed qi transforms into fire	Heat injures the fluids to form phlegm, then on combining with heat, harasses interiorly	Mainly in the gallbladder	Dizziness, insomnia, mental restlessness, palpitations, chest stuffiness, red tongue with yellow greasy coating, a slippery and rapid pulse, or wiry and rapid pulse	The heat pattern is not obvious, palpitations, insomnia, fullness and distension of the chest and hypochondrium, combined with timidity and lack of courage, sighing, bitter taste, nausea, vomiting, etc.
Phlegm-fire harassing the heart	Besides emotional problems, heat pathogen invades and combines with phlegm harassing interiorly		Mainly in the heart		The symptoms of fire heat are obvious, mental disorders such as mania, rash behaviours etc.

Section 5
Kidney and Bladder pattern Differentiation

The kidney resides in the lumbar region. The kidney is related to the bladder in both the interior and the exterior via the channels and collaterals. Kidney dominates bones, produce marrow and fill up the brain, open into the ears, control the lower orifices, and manifest in the hair. They store essence and govern growth, development and reproduction. The kidney yin and kidney yang are the fundamentals of the yin and yang of the whole body, thus the kidney is regarded as the foundation or root of the congenital constitution. Storage is the kidney's nature; that is to say, primary yin and primary yang should be stored not used for consumption exorbitantly. Furthermore, the kidney also dominates water metabolism and the receiving of qi. The bladder, the water's officer, functions to store and discharge urine.

The primary pathological characteristics of kidney diseases manifest as abnormality in growth, development and reproduction and governing water and failing to grasp qi. The pathological changes also include abnormality of brain, marrow, bones, hair, ears, stool and urine (Table 11-35).

The kidney does not have excess patterns only deficient ones; so all kidney patterns are of the deficiency type. The commonly encountered patterns are:
- deficiency of kidney yang,
- deficiency of kidney yin,
- insufficiency of kidney essence and qi in childhood with hereditary insufficiency, or
- declining kidney essence in old age or with excessive sexual activity, etc.

As the kidney does not have a pattern of excess, all the excess patterns pertaining to the urinary system fall under the category of bladder patterns. Damp-heat in the bladder pattern is the primary excess type (Fig. 11-50).

Kidney Yang Deficiency Pattern

Concept: This is a type of deficient-cold pattern and is due to kidney yang deficiency leading to abnormality in warming and qi transformation.

Clinical manifestations: Bright white or dark complexion, cold soreness of the lumbar region and knee joints, cold body and cold limbs especially worse in the lower limbs, mental fatigue, lassitude, impotence, premature ejaculation and coldness in the perineal region in males, cold uterus leading to infertility, low libido, diarrhoea at dawn, maybe clear frequent urination, nocturia, possibly scanty urine, oedema of the whole body, pale tongue with white coating, and a deep, thready, and weak pulse.

Analysis: This pattern is due to innate yang deficiency, *mingmen* fire deficiency in old age, or chronic diseases impairing kidney yang, or excessive sexual activity gradually declining kidney yang (Fig. 11-51).

> **Key symptoms:** Hypofunctional sexual activity and reproduction, failing to control discharge of stool and urine, and symptoms of a deficient-cold pattern such as cold soreness of the lumbar region and knees, cold body and limbs.

Table 11-35 Physiological function, pathological changes, and symptoms of the kidney and bladder

Physiological function	Pathological changes	Common symptoms
Stores essence, governs growth, development and reproduction	Insufficient kidney essence	Five kinds of tardy growth in childhood, five kinds of flaccidity in childhood, premature senility in adults
	Hypofunctional reproduction	Male: scanty semen leading to sterility Female: hypomenorrhoea, amenorrhoea, infertility
	Kidney yang deficiency	Cold pain of the lumbar region, aversion to cold, impotence, cold uterus
	Kidney yin deficiency	Tidal fever, night sweats, spermatorrhoea, nocturnal emissions, irregular menstruation, low lumbar region pain
Governs water, controls discharge of stool and urine	Abnormal water metabolism	Oedema
	Not able to control discharge of stool and urine	Diarrhoea, faecal incontinence, dribbling after urination, enuresis, urinary incontinence
Governs receiving qi	Kidney failing to absorb qi	Panting or dyspnoea, hasty breathing, increased exhalation and decreased inhalation
Dominates bones and produces marrow	Failure to produce enough marrow to fill the brain	Dizziness, poor memory, absent-mindedness
	Failure to nourish the bones	Loose bones, loose teeth, soreness and weakness of the lumbar region and knee joints
Opens into the ears, manifests in the hair	Failure to nourish the hair and ears	Tinnitus, deafness, loss of hair, white hair
Bladder governs storing and expelling urine	Abnormal qi transformation of the bladder	Frequent, urgent, painful, and profuse urination

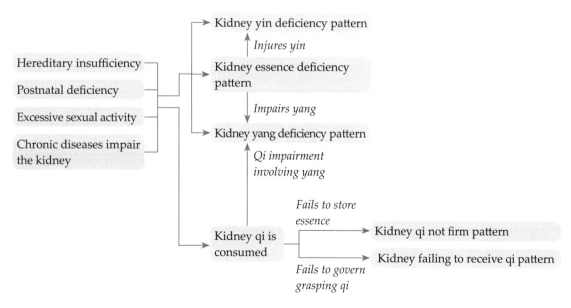

Fig. 11-50 Pathological factors and pathogenesis of the kidney patterns

Diagnostics in Chinese Medicine

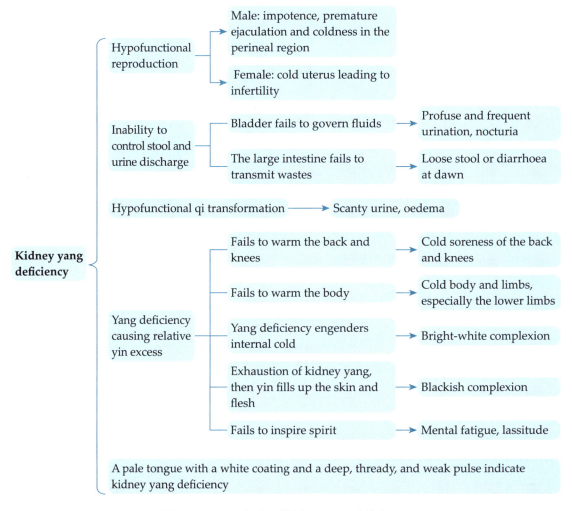

Fig. 11-51 Analysis of kidney yang deficiency

Kidney Yin Deficiency Pattern

Concept: This is due to consumption of kidney yin failing to nourish the *zang-fu* organs and engendering internal heat.

Clinical manifestations: Soreness and weakness of the lumbar region and knees, dizziness, tinnitus, loose teeth, alopaecia (hair loss), spermatorrhoea, premature ejaculation, hypomenorrhoea or amenorrhoea, possibly metrorrhagia (irregular inter-menstrual cycle bleeding) and metrostaxis (continuous blood loss from the uterus), insomnia, poor memory, dry mouth and throat, vexing heat in the chest, palms and soles, tidal fever (afternoon fever), night sweating, red cheeks in the afternoon, thin body, scanty yellowish urine, a red dry tongue with diminished coating or without coating, a thready and rapid pulse.

Analysis: This pattern is due to chronic illness consuming body fluids, or plundering of fluids after a warm heat disease, or excessive sexual activity tending to deplete kidney essence (Fig. 11-52).

Chapter 11 Differentiation of Patterns According to the *Zang-Fu* Organs Section 5

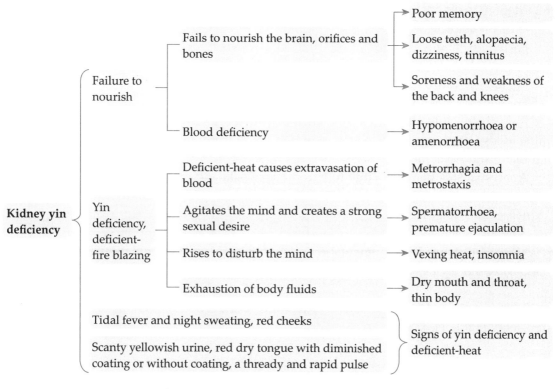

Fig. 11-52 Analysis of kidney yin deficiency

Key symptoms: Soreness and weakness of the lumbar region and knees, dizziness, tinnitus, spermatorrhoea in males and irregular menstruation in females combined with a deficient-heat pattern.

Identification: Four yin deficiency patterns (Table 11-36).

Table 11-36 Differentiation of four yin deficiency patterns

Patterns	Common symptoms	Different symptoms
Heart yin deficiency	Tidal fever and night sweats, red cheeks, vexing heat in the chest, palms and soles, dry throat, thin body, dark urine and dry stool, a dry red tongue with diminished coating, a thready and rapid pulse	Palpitations, insomnia, poor memory
Lung yin deficiency		Cough with scanty sputum, or dry cough, even haemoptysis, hoarseness
Liver yin deficiency		Dizziness, dry eyes, tinnitus, blurred vision, involuntary wriggling of hands and feet, hypochondriac pain
Kidney yin deficiency		Soreness and weakness of the lumbar region and knees, dizziness, tinnitus, loose teeth, alopaecia, spermatorrhoea, hypomenorrhoea or amenorrhoea

Kidney Essence Deficiency Pattern

Concept: This is due to kidney essence insufficiency and manifests as developmental retardation, hypofunctional reproduction and early senility.

Clinical manifestations:

<u>For children:</u> developmental retardation, dwarfism, delayed closure of the fontanel, mental retardation, weak bones, flaccidity of the bones.

<u>For males:</u> scanty semen leading to sterility.

<u>For females:</u> amenorrhoea leading to infertility.

<u>For adults:</u> low libido, early senility, tinnitus, deafness, poor memory, absent-mindedness, weakness of the feet, loss of hair, loose teeth, mental retardation, pale tongue, a thready and weak pulse.

Analysis: This pattern is due to hereditary weakness, or postnatal deficiency leading to *yuan* qi insufficiency, or chronic diseases, or excessive sexual activity gradually impairs kidney essence (Fig. 11-53).

> **Key symptoms:** Developmental retardation in children, hypofunctional reproduction and early senility in adults, but without an obvious cold or heat pattern.

Identification: Kidney essence deficiency, kidney yin deficiency, and kidney yang deficiency (Table 11-37).

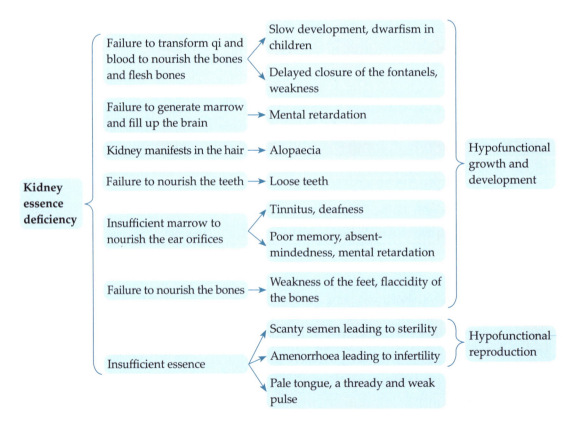

Fig. 11-53 Analysis of kidney essence deficiency

Table 11-37 Comparison of kidney essence deficiency, kidney yin deficiency, and kidney yang deficiency

Patterns	Pathogenesis		Clinical manifestations	
			Common	Distinction
Kidney essence deficiency	Deficiency pattern	Kidney essence deficiency	Soreness and weakness of the lumbar region and knees, poor memory, hypofunctional reproduction	Developmental retardation, dwarfism in children; hypofunctional reproduction and early senility in adults; scanty semen leading to sterility; amenorrhoea leading to infertility; pale tongue, a thready and weak pulse, without an obvious cold or heat pattern
Kidney yin deficiency		Kidney yin deficiency, failure to nourish, deficient-fire blazing		Yin deficiency and deficient heat pattern such as vexing heat in the chest, palms and soles, tidal fever and night sweats, red cheeks in the afternoon, thin body, scanty yellowish urine, a red dry tongue with diminished coating or without coating, a thready and rapid pulse
Kidney yang deficiency		Kidney yang deficiency leading to abnormality in warming		Combined with a deficient-cold pattern such as cold body and limbs especially lower limbs, cold soreness of the lumbar region and knees; chronic diarrhoea, diarrhoea at dawn, clear frequent urination, profuse nocturia, a pale tongue, a deep, thready and weak pulse

Kidney Qi Deficiency Pattern

Concept: This is due to kidney qi deficiency and abnormal function of sealing and storing.

Clinical manifestations: Soreness and weakness of the lumbar region and knees, mental fatigue, lassitude, tinnitus, deafness, clear frequent urination, dribbling after urination, enuresis (involuntary voiding of urine), nocturia (abnormally large or frequent urination at night), urinary incontinence, nocturnal emissions without dreams, or spermatorrhoea and premature ejaculation in males, metrorrhagia, profuse clear leucorrhoea, stirring of the foetus (foetal distress) in women, pale tongue with white coating, a weak pulse.

Analysis: Kidney qi deficiency is due to hereditary weakness, excessive sexual activity, chronic disease and occurs with the aging process (Fig. 11-54).

Key symptoms: The symptoms are related to dysfunction in storing of the kidney and bladder.

Identification: Kidney qi deficiency, and kidney yang deficiency (Table 11-38).

Diagnostics in Chinese Medicine

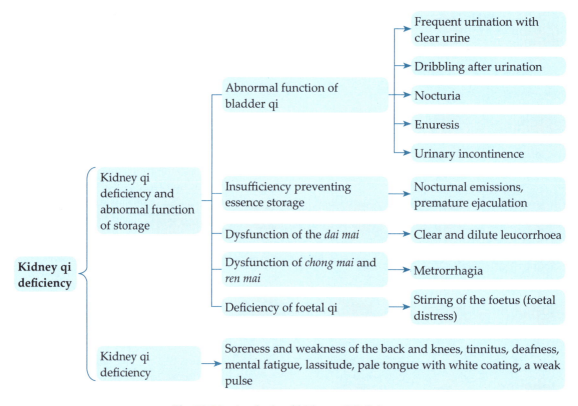

Fig. 11-54 Analysis of kidney qi deficiency

Table 11-38 Differentiation of kidney qi deficiency and kidney yang deficiency

Patterns	Pathogenesis	Common symptoms	Different symptoms
Kidney qi deficiency	Kidney qi deficiency and dysfunction of storing	White complexion, soreness of the lumbar region, tinnitus, urinary disturbances, hypofunctional reproduction, etc.	Symptoms of failing to store urine, essence, and a foetus etc. resulting in: frequent urination, dribbling after urination, nocturnal emissions, premature ejaculation, clear profuse leucorrhoea, metrorrhagia, stirring of the foetus, no cold pattern
Kidney yang deficiency	Kidney yang deficiency and dysfunction of warming and qi transformation		Symptoms of deficient yang generating internal cold such as: soreness of the lumbar region and lower limbs, impotence, premature ejaculation, cold uterus leading to infertility, diarrhoea at dawn, scanty urine, oedema, etc.

Kidney Failing to Receive Qi Pattern

This pattern which is also called deficiency of lung qi and kidney qi, is due to failure of the kidney in grasping or receiving qi and mainly manifests as panting and shortness of breath.

Clinical manifestations: Panting, shortness of breath on exertion, difficulty in inhaling, severe panting on exercise, lethargy in speaking, spontaneous sweating, fatigue, soreness of the lumbar region and knee joints, pale tongue, a large but forceless pulse, or weak breathing, cold profuse sweating, cold limbs, cyanosis (blue colouration) of the complexion, a weak and deep pulse.

Analysis: This pattern may be due to chronic cough damaging lung qi. Alternatively the problem may be with the kidneys such as chronic diseases eventually affecting the kidneys, physical exertion over a long period of time weakening kidney qi, hereditary weakness of *yuan* (original) qi or kidney qi deficiency associated with the ageing process, any of these mechanisms can cause failure of the kidney in receiving qi (Fig. 11-55).

> **Key symptoms:** Chronic panting, shortness of breath, difficulty in inhaling. Severe panting aggravated on exertion, symptoms of lung and kidney qi deficiency.

Identification: Although both this pattern and the lung qi deficiency pattern have panting and shortness of breath, these symptoms are more severe in this pattern along with symptoms of kidney deficiency such as soreness of the lumbar region, etc. (Table 11-39).

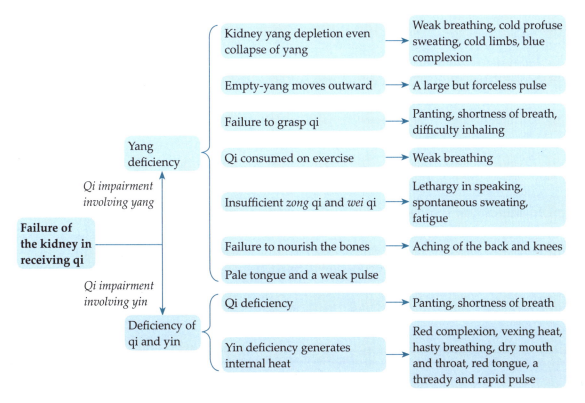

Fig. 11-55 Analysis of kidney failing to grasp qi

Damp Heat in the Bladder Pattern

Concept: This pattern is ascribed to the invasion of damp heat in the bladder. Damp heat impairs the function of the bladder. According to the *sanjiao* pattern differentiation it belongs to the lower *jiao*.

Clinical manifestations: Frequent and urgent urination, distending pain in the lower abdomen, burning pain on urination, scanty dark-yellow urine or turbid (cloudy) urine, haematuria (blood in the urine), stones in the urine, fever, distension and pain of the

Diagnostics in Chinese Medicine

Table 11-39 Differentiation of *zang* qi deficiency patterns

Pattern	Common symptoms	Different symptoms
Heart qi deficiency	Pale complexion, pale lips, shortness of breath, mental fatigue, lack of strength, dizziness, spontaneous sweating and severe sweating on exertion, pale and tender tongue, a deficient pulse	Palpitations, chest pain
Lung qi deficiency		Shortness of breath, cough with watery sputum, aversion to wind, propensity to catch colds
Spleen qi deficiency		Poor appetite, abdominal distension, loose stool, thin body, oedema
Kidney qi deficiency		Soreness of the lumbar region, tinnitus, frequent urination, dribbling after urination, enuresis, nocturnal emissions without dreams, clear profuse leucorrhoea, metrorrhagia, foetal distress
Kidney failing to receive qi		Chronic panting, shortness of breath, difficulty in inhaling, soreness of the lumbar region

lumbar region, red tongue, yellow and sticky tongue coating, a slippery and rapid pulse.

Analysis: This pattern may be due to exogenous pathogenic factors, or over eating and drinking without control generating internal damp-heat, both of which can cause damp heat brewing and binding in the bladder and lead to abnormal function of bladder qi transformation (Fig. 11-56).

Key symptoms: Frequent and urgent urination, burning pain on urination, stones or blood in the urine.

Identification: These patterns of bladder damp heat and the excessive heat in the small intestine pattern have common symptoms such as frequent and urgent urination and burning on urination. However, the latter is due to heart fire moving downward to the small intestine and includes heart vexation, thirst, insomnia and ulcers in the mouth and on

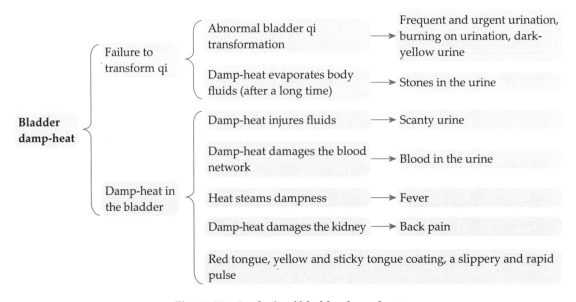

Fig. 11-56 Analysis of bladder damp-heat

the tongue, etc; while the former pattern is caused by bladder damp heat, accompanied by kidney disease manifestations such as fever, soreness of the lumbar region, etc, because the kidney is related to the bladder in both the interior and the exterior, and by the channels and collaterals.

SECTION 6
COMBINED PATTERNS OF ZANG-FU ORGANS

Clinically the combined or concurrent syndromes of the *zang-fu* organs refer to the patterns involving at least two *zang-fu* organs, which are very common and complicated, and we will discuss twelve kinds of the most common patterns.

Disharmony between the Heart and Kidney Pattern

Concept: This is caused by kidney yin deficiency, which fails to ascend to cool the heart fire; subsequently it will lead to hyperactivity of the heart fire. This leads to flaring up of heart deficiency fire and deficiency of heart yin.

Clinical manifestations: Heart vexation, insomnia, palpitations, dream-disturbed sleep, dizziness, tinnitus, forgetfulness, weakness and aching of the back and knees, or nocturnal emissions, feverishness in the chest, palms and soles, or tidal fever, night sweating, dry mouth and throat, red tongue with diminished coating or without coating, thready and rapid pulse.

Analysis: This pattern is mainly caused by apprehension and anxiety, or by emotional changes, which turn into fire and injure heart yin and kidney yin. It may also be due to prolonged illness or excessive sexual activity, which leads to consumption of kidney yin failing to control heart yang, then it causes hyperactivity of heart deficiency fire. In this case, the fire is hyperactive in the upper part, so rises upwards to disturb the mind (Fig. 11-57).

Key symptoms: Palpitations, insomnia, dream-disturbed sleep, nocturnal emissions, weakness and aching in the back and knee joints, and manifestations of a yin deficiency pattern.

Identification: Although this pattern and the heart yin deficiency pattern both have palpitations, insomnia and a yin deficiency pattern, this pattern includes the kidney yin deficiency pattern symptoms such as aching back, tinnitus, and nocturnal emissions while the heart yin deficiency pattern does not include it.

The difference between this pattern and the kidney yin deficiency is that this pattern is composed of both kidney yin and heart yin deficiency patterns.

Heart and Kidney Yang Deficiency Pattern

Concept: This pattern is caused by heart and kidney yang deficiency unable to warm the whole body and failing to move qi, blood, and fluids, leading to blood stasis and retention and stagnation of the body fluids and manifests as a deficiency cold pattern.

Clinical manifestations: Palpitations, cold body and limbs, oedema, urinary problems, mental fatigue, lack of strength, pale cyanosis of the lips and nails, light-dark or purple tongue with white and slippery coating, and deep, thready and faint pulse.

Analysis: This pattern can develop from a chronic condition of heart yang deficiency along with kidney yang deficiency failing to transform qi leading to water overflowing to the heart.

Key symptoms: Palpitations, oedema; symptoms of a deficiency cold pattern.

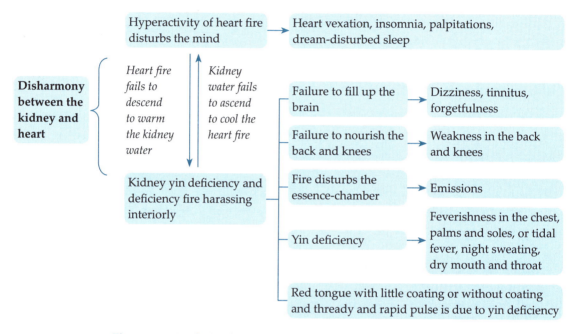

Fig. 11-57 Analysis of disharmony between the kidney and heart

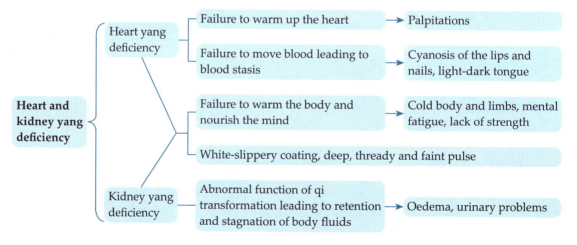

Fig. 11-58 Analysis of heart and kidney yang deficiency

Heart and Lung Qi Deficiency Pattern

This pattern is due to both heart and lung qi deficiency and manifests as palpitations, cough and panting.

Clinical manifestations: Chest stuffiness or an oppressed feeling of the chest, palpitations, cough, panting or asthma, shortness of breath which is aggravated on exertion, clear and dilute sputum, dizziness, mental fatigue and lassitude, weak voice, spontaneous sweating, lack of strength or listlessness, pale complexion, or light purple lips and tongue, deep and weak pulse or knotted and intermittent pulse.

Analysis: This pattern is caused by chronic illness, cough and laboured breathing, which damage the qi of the lung, and then the heart, or by a weak constitution with weakness of old age or excessive overexertion fatigue, which lead to inadequacy in the sources to generate qi (Fig. 11-59).

Key symptoms: Cough, laboured breathing, palpitations and manifestations of a qi deficiency pattern.

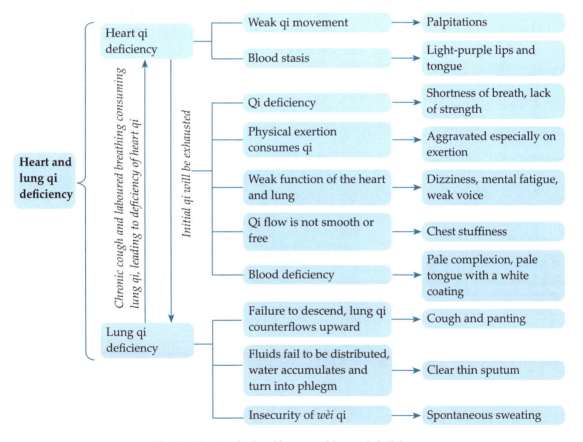

Fig. 11-59 Analysis of heart and lung qi deficiency

Deficiency of Both Heart and Spleen Pattern

Concept: This pattern is due to heart blood deficiency and spleen qi deficiency and manifests with heart blood deficiency symptoms such as abnormality of the heart mind, and deficiency of spleen qi, which may cause failure in the source for producing qi and blood, and failure in the control of blood.

Clinical manifestations: Palpitations, insomnia, dream-disturbed sleep, dizziness, forgetfulness (amnesia), poor appetite, abdominal distension, loose stool, shortness of breath, mental fatigue, lack of strength, sallow or pale complexion, pale lips and nails, bleeding spots under the skin, scanty pale menstruation, or amenorrhoea, pale and tender tongue, thready and weak pulse.

Analysis: This pattern is caused by chronic diseases, or worry and anxiety, or by irregular dietary habits damaging the spleen and stomach, or by chronic haemorrhage leading to both blood and qi deficiency (Fig. 11-60).

> **Key symptoms:** Palpitations, insomnia, poor appetite, abdominal distension, chronic haemorrhage, and symptoms of qi and blood deficiency.

Identification: Although both this pattern and the spleen not controlling blood pattern have both spleen qi deficiency and the blood loss pattern, there are some differences between them. The former has particular emphasis on an abnormal heart mind such as palpitations and insomnia. The latter has particular emphasis on haemorrhage but without heart blood deficiency.

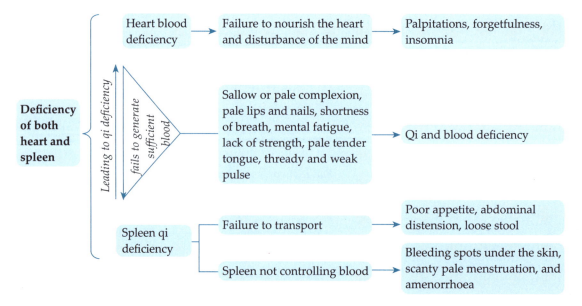

Fig. 11-60 Analysis of deficiency of both heart and spleen

Heart and Liver Blood Deficiency Pattern

Concept: This pattern manifests as an abnormal heart mind and failure of nourishment of the eyes and related organs with the blood deficiency pattern.

Clinical manifestations: Palpitations, forgetfulness, insomnia, dream-disturbed sleep, dizziness, dry eyes, blurred vision, or numbness of the limbs, tremor, cramps, or scanty light menstruation, amenorrhoea, dull pale complexion, withered and brittle nails, pale tongue, thready pulse.

Analysis: This pattern is caused by worry and anxiety injuring heart blood, by excessive loss of blood or by spleen deficiency failing to generate blood (Fig. 11-61).

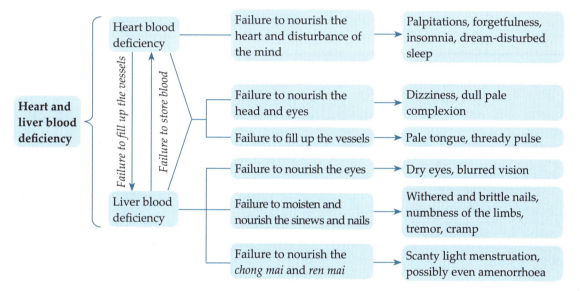

Fig. 11-61 Analysis of heart and liver blood deficiency

Key symptoms: Abnormality of the heart mind, failure of nourishment of the eyes, sinews and nails, and symptoms of blood deficiency.

Spleen and Lung Qi Deficiency Pattern

Concept: This pattern results from the spleen's failure to transform and transport and the lung failing to disperse, descend and depurate.

Clinical manifestations: Poor appetite, abdominal distension, loose stool, chronic cough, shortness of breath, panting, weak voice, laziness in speaking, lack of strength, shortage of qi, profuse clear dilute sputum, oedema, pale complexion, pale tongue with a white-slippery coating, thready and weak pulse.

Analysis: This pattern is caused by prolonged cough, which may cause deficiency of the lung and later affects the spleen (disorder of the child-organ affecting the mother-organ); or irregular eating and overstrain which may injure the spleen, leading to failure in transporting the essence to the lung (Fig. 11-62).

Diagnostics in Chinese Medicine

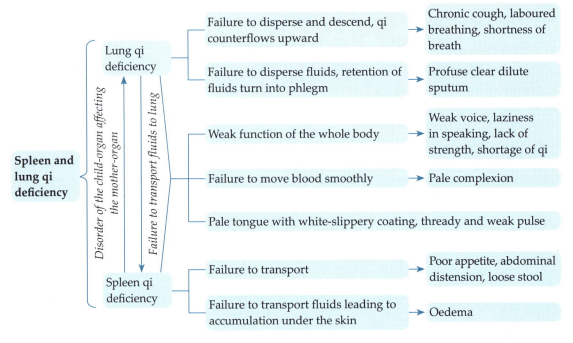

Fig. 11-62 Analysis of spleen and lung qi deficiency

Key symptoms: Poor appetite, loose stool, cough, panting, shortness of breath, and common manifestations of qi deficiency.

Kidney and Lung Yin Deficiency Pattern

Concept: This is due to lung and kidney yin deficiency generating deficient heat. The yin of the lung and kidney nourish each other. The dispersing and descending of lung fluid provides nourishment for the kidney and the rising of kidney yin nourishes the lung.

Clinical manifestations: Cough with scanty sputum or with blood-tinged sputum, dry mouth and throat, hoarse voice, soreness and weakness of the lumbar region and knee joints, tidal fever, night sweating, red cheeks, thin body, nocturnal emissions, irregular menstruation, red tongue with diminished coating, thready and rapid pulse.

Analysis: This pattern is caused by dry-heat or tuberculosis injuring lung yin or by chronic cough and panting damaging lung yin, and then further development of kidney yin deficiency, or by excessive sexual activities consuming kidney yin causing it to fail to rise to nourish the lung (Fig. 11-63).

Key symptoms: Cough with scanty sputum, aching back and knee joints, emissions and symptoms of a deficient-heat pattern.

Liver Fire Insulting the Lung Pattern

The liver is characterised by ascending and the lung is characterised by descending. When there is too much ascending of the liver qi, the liver fire will go upward to insult the

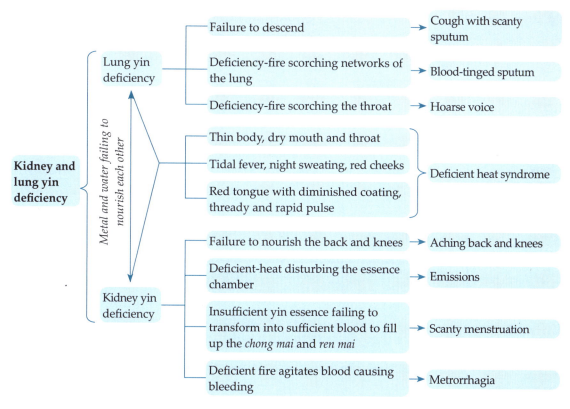

Fig. 11-63 Analysis of kidney and lung yin deficiency

lung. It is also called "invasion of the lung by liver fire".

Clinical manifestations: Oppressed feeling and burning pain in the chest and hypochondrium, irritability, outbursts of anger, distending headache, dizziness, red complexion and eyes, feverishness, bitter taste of the mouth, cough with sticky, thick, and yellow sputum, haemoptysis, red tongue with a diminished yellow coating, and a taut and rapid pulse.

Analysis: This pattern is caused by depression and anger that damage the liver leading to qi stagnation and then transforming into fire or by a heat pathogen blazing upward through the liver channel to insult the lung (Fig. 11-64).

Key symptoms: Cough, or haemoptysis, burning pain in the chest and hypochondrium, outbursts of anger and symptoms of an excess-fire pattern.

Disharmony between the Liver and Stomach Pattern

Concept: This pattern is caused by liver fire due to liver constraint and qi stagnation which attacks horizontally to the stomach leading to stomach failing to govern descending and manifests as distending pain in the epigastrium and hypochondrium. It is also called 'invasion of the stomach by liver'.

Clinical manifestations: Distending pain or wandering pain in the chest, epigastrium and hypochondrium, hiccoughs, belching, acid regurgitation, epigastric discomfort,

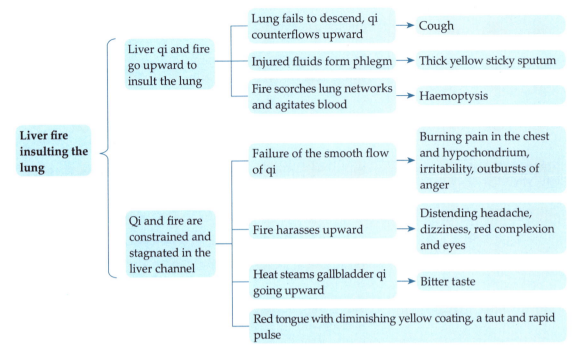

Fig. 11-64 Analysis of liver fire insulting the lung

depression, or irritability, outbursts of anger, sighing, poor appetite, thin white or yellow coating, taut (wiry) or taut and rapid pulse.

Analysis: This pattern is caused by depressed emotions leading to liver constraint and qi stagnation, which turns into liver fire and horizontally invading the stomach (Fig. 11-65).

Key symptoms: Distending pain or wandering pain in the chest, epigastrium and hypochondrium, hiccoughs, belching.

Liver Invading the Spleen Pattern

Concept: This pattern is due to liver failing to ensure the smooth (free) flow of qi, leading to dysfunction of the spleen in digestion and transportation, and manifests as distending pain in the chest and hypochondrium, abdominal distension, and loose stool. It is also known as "the wood overacting on the earth". It is also called the pattern of disharmony between the liver and spleen, or liver constraint and spleen deficiency pattern.

Clinical manifestations: Distending or wandering pain in the chest and hypochondrium, sighing, emotional frustration, or irritability, outbursts of anger, poor appetite, abdominal distension, loose stool with sensation of incomplete defaecation, flatulence, abdominal pain and diarrhoea, or alternating constipation and diarrhoea, pale tongue coating, and taut or weak pulse.

Analysis: This pattern is caused by depressed emotions especially repressed anger damaging the liver leading to a breakdown of the smooth flow of qi, or by irregular diet or overstrain and stress which injure the spleen leading to failure of the spleen in digestion and transportation (Fig. 11-66).

Chapter 11 Differentiation of Patterns According to the *Zang-Fu* Organs **Section 6**

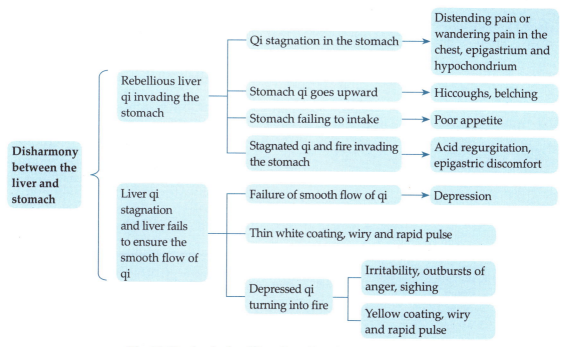

Fig. 11-65 Analysis of liver invading the stomach pattern

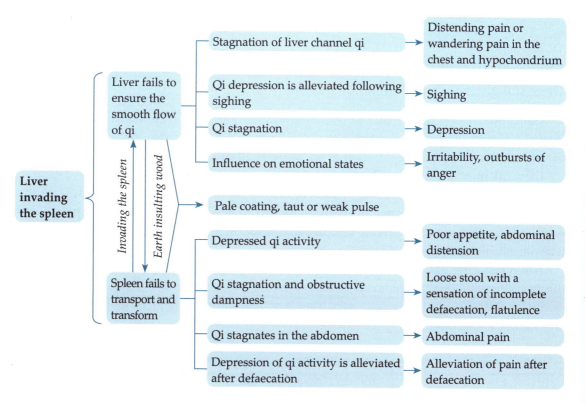

Fig. 11-66 Analysis of liver invading the spleen pattern

> **Key symptoms:** Distending pain in the chest and hypochondrium, abdominal distension, poor appetite, loose stool.

Identification: Liver invading the spleen and liver invading the stomach (Table 11-40).

Table 11-40 Differentiation of liver invading the spleen and liver invading the stomach

Pattern	Pathogenesis		Clinical manifestations	
			Common symptoms	Different symptoms
Liver invading the spleen	Liver fails to ensure smooth flow of qi	Invading the spleen	Depression, irritability, outbursts of anger, distending pain in the chest and hypochondrium, poor appetite	Symptoms of the spleen failing to transport and digest such as abdominal distension, loose stool with a sensation of incomplete defaecation, flatulence, or abdominal pain with a feeling of diarrhoea that is alleviated after defaecation, or intermittent constipation and diarrhoea, pale tongue coating, taut or weak pulse
Liver invading the stomach		Invading the stomach		Symptoms of the stomach failing to descend such as epigastric distension, nausea, vomiting, hiccoughs, belching, acid regurgitation, epigastric discomfort, thin white or yellow coating, taut or taut and rapid pulse

Liver and Kidney Yin Deficiency Pattern

Concept: This pattern is due to liver and kidney yin deficiency, which causes failure of yin in controlling yang, consequently a deficiency of yin gives rise to internal heat. This pattern is seen at the middle *jiao* level of the *sanjiao* patterns.

Clinical manifestations: Dizziness, tinnitus, forgetfulness, dry mouth and throat, insomnia, dream-disturbed sleep, hypochondriac pain, soreness and weakness of the lumbar region and knee joints, feverishness or burning sensation in the chest, palms and soles, night sweating, red cheeks, nocturnal emissions, scanty menstruation, red tongue with little coating, thready and rapid pulse.

Analysis: This pattern is caused by chronic diseases leading to consumption of yin fluids, or by emotional problems injuring yin, or by excessive sexual activity depleting yin essence, or chronic warm diseases impairing liver and kidney yin, all of which lead to liver and kidney yin deficiency (Fig. 11-67).

> **Key symptoms:** Weakness and pain of the back and knee joints, hypochondriac pain, tinnitus, nocturnal emissions, and dizziness. Symptoms of a deficiency-fire pattern.

Identification: Liver and kidney yin deficiency and excessive rising of liver yang (Table 11-41).

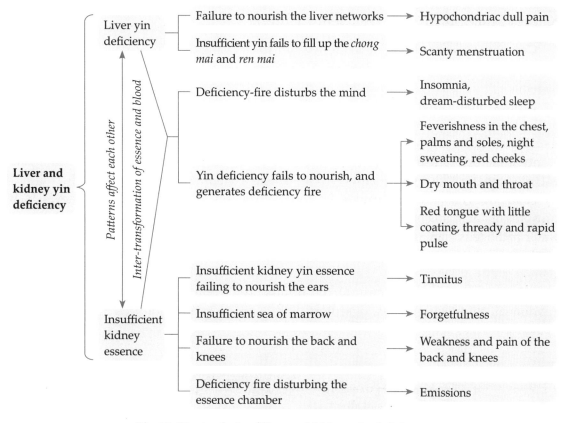

Fig. 11-67 Analysis of liver and kidney yin deficiency

Table 11-41 Differentiation of liver and kidney yin deficiency and excessive rising of liver yang

Pattern	Pathogenesis		Nature	Clinical manifestations	
				Common symptoms	Different symptoms
Liver and kidney yin deficiency	Liver and kidney yin deficiency and water not nourishing wood	Insufficient yin essence and deficiency fire harassing the interior	Deficiency	Dizziness, tinnitus, forgetfulness, dry mouth and throat, insomnia, dream-disturbed sleep, hypochondriac pain, weakness and aching in the back and knees	Yin deficiency pattern: feverishness in the chest, palms and soles, night sweating, red cheeks, emissions, scanty menstruation, red tongue with a thin coating, thready and rapid pulse
Excessive rising of liver yang		Excessive rising of liver yang and qi and blood counterflowing upward	Upper excess and lower deficiency		Distending pain in the head and eyes, red complexion and eyes, heaviness of the head, irritability, outbursts of anger, red tongue with scanty fluid, a taut or taut, thready and rapid pulse

Kidney and Spleen Yang Deficiency Pattern

Concept: This pattern is due to kidney and spleen yang deficiency, which fails to warm the interior and manifests as a deficiency cold pattern with symptoms such as diarrhoea or oedema.

Clinical manifestations: A bright-white complexion, cold body and limbs, cold pain of the lumbar region and knee joints or the lower abdomen, diarrhoea at dawn, chronic diarrhoea with undigested food, or chronic dysentery, watery diarrhoea, general oedema, scanty urine or profuse clear urine, abdominal distension like the surface of a drum, pale enlarged tongue with a white-slippery coating, and a deep, slow and weak pulse.

Analysis: This pattern is caused by chronic diseases of the spleen and kidney, which consume qi and damage yang, or by chronic diarrhoea, or by longstanding accumulation of water pathogens, damaging kidney yang which causes failure to warm the spleen yang, or by chronic spleen yang deficiency failing to nourish the kidney yang (Fig. 11-68).

> **Key symptoms:** Cold pain of the lumbar region and knee joints or the lower abdomen, chronic diarrhoea, dysentery, and oedema, in addition to a deficiency cold pattern.

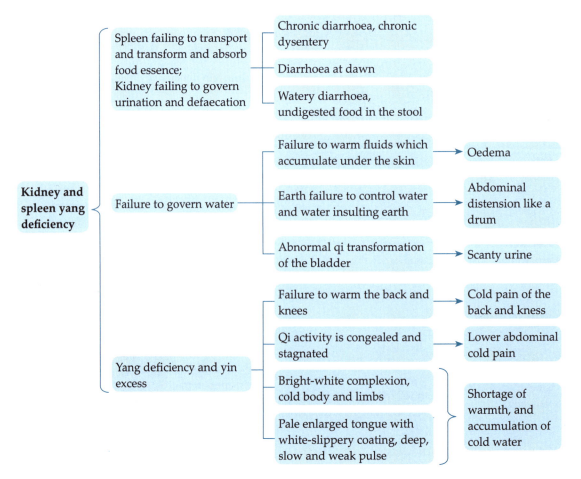

Fig. 11-68 Analysis of kidney and spleen yang deficiency

CHAPTER 12
Additional Patterns Differentiation

SECTION 1
PATTERN DIFFERENTIATION ACCORDING TO THE SIX CHANNELS/STAGES

General Introduction

This is a method by which the diseases caused by externally contracted pathogens are classified into three yang patterns: *taiyang* (greater yang), *yangming* (yang brightness), and *shaoyang* (lesser yang), and three yin patterns: *taiyin* (greater yin), *shaoyin* (lesser yin), and *jueyin* (reverting yin) according to their different stages of development. By means of this classification, we are able to recognise characteristics such as changes in the location of disease, nature, development, and severity of the disease; as well as the conditions of the pathogenic factor (pathogen) and *zheng* (healthy) qi, and then diagnosis and treatment are based on this classification. Pattern differentiation according to the theory of the six channels was formulated by Zhang Zhong-jing, an ancient CM doctor of the East *Han* Dynasty, on the basis of *Basic Questions-Discussion on Heat* (*Sù Wèn-Rè Lùn*, 素问·热论) of the *Yellow Emperor's Inner Classic* which discussed many types of externally contracted diseases.

The six channels are the principles of pattern differentiation discussed in the *Treatise on Cold Damage* (*Shāng Hán Lùn*, 伤寒论). In this classification *taiyang* corresponds to the exterior, *yangming* corresponds to the interior, and *shaoyang* is located between the exterior and interior; on the other hand the three yin channels all refer to the interior. For instance, if the pathogenic qi is located in the skin, flesh or channel, it is ascribed to an exterior pattern; if it enters interiorly and transforms into heat, it is ascribed to interior excess and heat patterns. The pattern of the three yang channels originate from the yang and are based on the disease of the six *fu* organs, which pertain to a heat pattern or an excess pattern, while the patterns of the three yin channels result from the yin and refer to the diseases of the five *zang* organs, and refer to a cold pattern or a deficiency pattern. This pattern differentiation applies not only for externally contracted diseases but also for interior disease, but mainly it is a method and guide for the pattern identification of externally contracted diseases.

Taiyang Pattern

The *taiyang* pattern is the beginning stage of the course of externally contracted disease. *Taiyang* dominates the exterior portion of the whole body, serving as the fence for the six channels. The foot *taiyang* channel travels along the neck and back of the body, and governs both the *ying* (nutrient) and *wei* (defensive qi). The *fu* organ of the *taiyang*, the bladder stores urine and discharges it by its qi-transformation action. When the exogenous pathogenic factors invade the body, the *taiyang* channel is the first to be affected. The *wei* qi rises to fight against the pathogenic factors and the struggle between the *wei* qi and the pathogenic factors in the exterior or skin results in the *taiyang* channel pattern and is due to an external wind-cold pathogen (exogenous pathogenic factor). If the pathogenic factors are not eliminated, the *taiyang* channel pattern is not relieved, and the pathogen penetrates into the *fu* organs along the channel, subsequently a *taiyang fu* organ pattern results, which is divided into the water-retention pattern and the blood-retention pattern (Fig. 12-1).

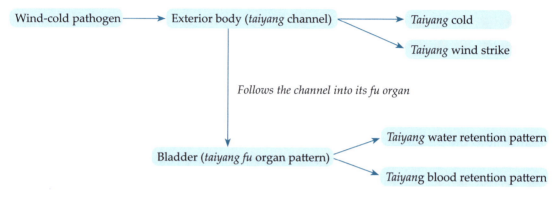

Fig. 12-1 Mechanism of the *taiyang* disease pattern

Physiology and pathology of the *taiyang* channel:
The *taiyang* channel includes the bladder channel of the foot *taiyang* and the small intestine channel of the hand *taiyang*. *Taiyang* governs the *ying* and *wei* systems and dominates the exterior portion of the whole body, serving as a barrier for the six channels.

The *taiyang* channel is rich in yang qi. The *taiyang* channel depends on the *mingmen* fire for warming and defending the body, because yang qi follows through its channel and collaterals to the exterior portion of the body and covers the whole body. Both the *taiyang* channel and lung govern the exterior portion of the body so they are closely related to each other. The *taiyang* channel disperses yang qi to the exterior of the body, while the lung disperses fluid to nourish the skin and hair; therefore they collaborate with each other and serve as the barrier for the body.

Taiyang disease is mainly due to two features: invasion of pathogens and inner disharmony; both of these influence and transform into each other. The first is due to insufficiency of *wei* qi and wind-cold invading the *taiyang* channel, causing disharmony between the *ying* and *wei*; the latter is a yin pattern transforming into a yang pattern or transmitting from the interior to the surface. *Taiyang* disease is mostly due to exuberance of the pathogenic qi, so belongs to exterior, excess (repletion), and yang patterns.

1. ***Taiyang* channel pattern**
Concept: This pattern is due to exterior wind-cold, which invades the skin or the exterior portion of the body leading to the struggle of pathogenic qi and *zheng* (healthy) qi and manifesting as a disharmony between the *ying* and *wei*. It is the initial stage of the course of externally contracted disease.

Clinical manifestations: Fever, aversion to cold, pain and stiffness in the head and neck, and floating pulse are the main symptoms of the *taiyang* channel pattern.

Analysis: This pattern is caused by wind-cold invading the *taiyang* channel. In order to resist the pathogen, the *wei* (defensive) qi collects in the exterior of the body, which causes fever and a floating pulse. Simultaneously the *wei* qi fails to defend the exterior portion of the body, and is unable to warm the flesh; consequently there is an aversion to wind and cold. Since the foot *taiyang* channel runs up to the forehead and vertex, down the neck and travels along the back of the body, when the *taiyang* channel qi contracts cold it constricts the exterior, and there is severe headache and neck pain. These are the channel signs that should be seen in a *taiyang* channel pattern. The *taiyang* channel pattern is divided into the two categories of wind stroke and cold damage, due to the strength or weakness of the body and the mild or strong nature of the contracted pathogen.

A. *Taiyang* wind strike pattern:

Concept: This pattern results from flaccidity of the pores allowing external invasion of wind-cold, then an attack of pathogenic wind-cold (with predominance of wind) on the *wei* qi, and disharmony between the *ying* system and the *wei* system results.

Clinical manifestations: Aversion to wind, fever, sweating, pain and stiffness in the head and neck, a floating, moderate pulse, sometimes nasal obstruction and retching.

Analysis: See Fig. 12-2.

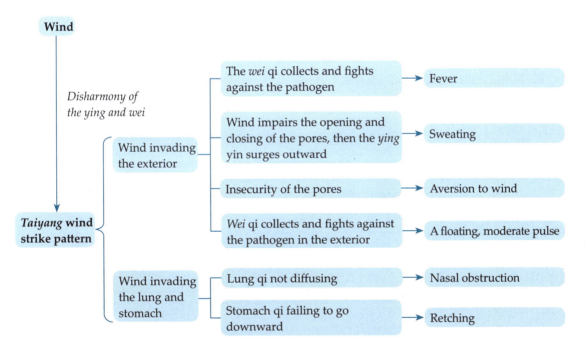

Fig. 12-2 Analysis of the *taiyang* wind strike pattern

Key symptoms: Aversion to wind, sweating, and a floating, moderate pulse.

B. *Taiyang* cold damage pattern:

Concept: This pattern is caused by wind-cold, with predominance of cold, invading the *taiyang* channel leading to constriction of the *wei* qi and stagnation of the *ying* yin.

Clinical manifestations: Aversion to cold, fever, lack of sweating, panting, severe pain and stiffness in the head and neck, general pain of the body, and a floating and tight pulse.

Analysis: See Fig. 12-3.

Diagnostics in Chinese Medicine

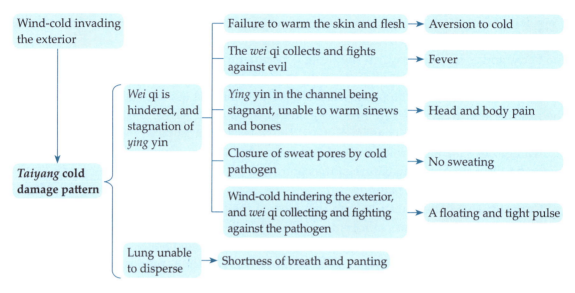

Fig. 12-3　Analysis of the *taiyang* cold damage pattern

Key symptoms: Lack of sweat, body pain, aversion to cold, and a floating and tight pulse.

Identification: *Taiyang* wind strike and *taiyang* cold damage (Table 12-1).

Table 12-1　Comparison of the *taiyang* wind strike and *taiyang* cold damage

Category of Six Channels	Type	Symptoms	Main Differential Points
Taiyang disease	Cold damage	Aversion to cold with fever, no sweat, laboured breathing, body pain, vomiting, a floating and tight pulse	Exterior excess pattern, no sweat, a floating and tight pulse
	Wind strike	Fever, sweat, aversion to wind, a floating and moderate pulse	Exterior deficiency pattern, sweat, a floating and moderate pulse

2. *Taiyang fu* organ pattern

If the *taiyang* channel pattern is not cured, external pathogens are not eliminated, and they penetrate into the *fu* organ along the channel, leading to the *taiyang fu* organ pattern, which is again divided into the *taiyang* water-retention pattern and the *taiyang* blood-retention pattern.

A. *Taiyang* water-retention pattern:

Concept: This pattern is generally due to failure of elimination of a *taiyang* channel pattern, allowing the external pathogen to follow through the channel and enter the related *fu* organ, resulting in dysfunction of the qi transformation of the bladder.

Clinical manifestations: Aversion to cold, fever, inhibited urination, distension and fullness of the lesser abdomen, thirst, and sometimes in severe cases there is thirst with a desire for water, but when the water is taken there is vomiting, and a floating or rapid pulse.

Analysis: See Fig. 12-4.

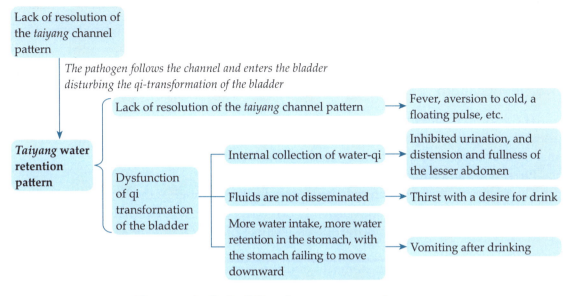

Fig. 12-4 Analysis of the *taiyang* water-retention pattern

Key symptoms: *Taiyang* channel pattern, accompanied by inhibited urination, and distension and fullness of the lesser abdomen.

B. *Taiyang* blood retention pattern:

Concept: This pattern is generally due to failure of elimination of a *taiyang* channel pattern, allowing the heat pathogen to follow the channel and enter the *fu* organ where the heat and the blood bind together and the blood amasses in the lesser abdomen.

Clinical manifestations: Hard fullness and pain in the lesser abdomen, incontinent urination, a sprit-mind that is manic and chaotic, forgetfulness, black stool with blood, a deep and choppy pulse, or a deep and knotted pulse.

Analysis: See Fig. 12-5.

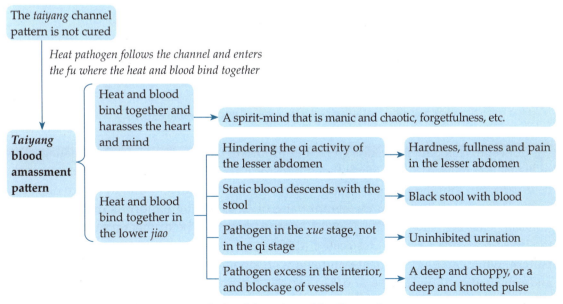

Fig. 12-5 Analysis of the *taiyang* blood retention pattern

Key symptoms: Hard, fullness and pain in the lesser abdomen, uninhibited urination, and a spirit-mind that is manic and chaotic.

Yangming Pattern

The *yangming* pattern refers to a stage of the extreme struggle between the vigourous *zheng* (healthy) qi and pathogenic qi, which is characterised by exuberant yang heat, and manifests as dryness and heat in the stomach and intestines.

Physiology and pathology of yangming channel:

The *yangming* channel includes the large intestine channel of the hand *yangming* and the stomach channel of the foot *yangming*; respectively they are associated with the lung channel of the hand *taiyin* and the spleen channel of the foot *taiyin* as the exterior and interior.

Food and drink enter the stomach, and the stomach, spleen, and intestines digest, transform, and absorb the food and drink, and then produce the essence of food, which in turn generates fluids and yang qi; therefore, the *yangming* is the channel with abundant yang qi, and the developmental peak of yang qi compared to the *shaoyang* and *taiyang* channel. The main function of this complex synthesis is to ensure the transformation of qi, blood and essence and coordinate the rising and falling of qi in the whole body (Fig. 12-6).

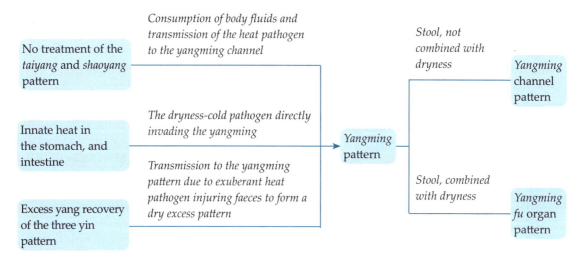

Fig. 12-6 Formation mechanism of the *yangming* pattern

Concept: This pattern results from inappropriate treatment or mistaken management of the *taiyang* pattern, injury of the fluids transforming into dryness, and penetration of the heat pathogen into the interior, or from direct attack of wind-cold due to innate depletion of the body fluids, but with exuberant yang qi. A *yangming* pattern is divided into the *yangming* channel pattern and *yangming fu* organ pattern. The exuberant heat pathogen in the intestines with a lack of desiccated (dry) faeces or constipation indicates the channel pattern, while binding of a heat-pathogen with stool and forming desiccated (dry) faeces and constipation indicates the *fu* organ pattern; both of these have the same nature as the interior, heat and excess patterns.

Clinical manifestations: Fever, lack of aversion to cold but aversion to heat, spontaneous sweating, and large pulse.

Analysis: This pattern is mostly due to an unrelieved *taiyang* channel pattern, which transmits to the interior *yangming* channel and transforms into heat; or inappropriate treatment of *shaoyang* disease, which causes the heat pathogen to be transmitted to the *yangming*, and then transforms into heat and dryness; or due to constitutional heat in the body; or inward penetration of exterior pathogens at the onset of a disease, leading to transformation of pathogens into heat (Fig. 12-7).

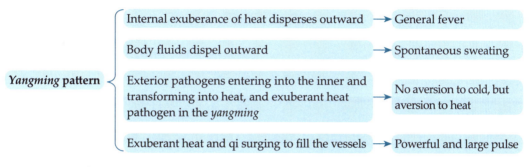

Fig. 12-7 Analysis of the *yangming* pattern

The main pathogenesis of *yangming* disease is an excess pattern of the stomach and intestines, which means an excess of pathogenic qi. The *yangming* channel is usually abundant in qi, blood, and yang qi; therefore when the exterior pathogen invades the *yangming* channel, it can easily be transformed into the dryness and heat.

The *yangming* pattern can be divided into the *yangming* channel pattern and *yangming fu* organ pattern.

1. *Yangming* channel pattern

Concept: The *yangming* channel pattern occurs when an exuberant heat pathogen fills up the *yangming* channel and suffuses throughout the whole body, while there are no dry stools in the intestine.

Clinical manifestations: High fever, profuse sweating, extreme thirst with desire for cold water, heart vexation and irritability, panting, flushed complexion, yellowish and dry tongue coating, large and surging pulse.

Analysis: See Fig. 12-8.

> **Key symptoms:** High fever, profuse sweating, extreme thirst, and a large and surging pulse

2. *Yangming fu* organ pattern

Concept: A *yangming fu* organ pattern occurs when an exuberant heat pathogen fills up the *yangming* channel, while a heat pathogen in the interior combines with stool thus forming desiccated (dry) faeces and constipation.

Clinical manifestations: Tidal fever in the afternoon; sweating of the palms and soles; abdominal fullness with distension and pain which is aggravated by pressure; delirium with floccillation in severe cases (floccillation is an aimless plucking at the bedclothes

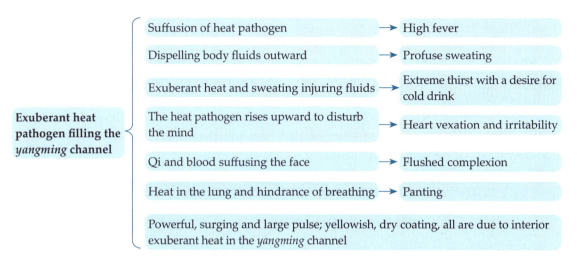

Fig. 12-8 Analysis of the *yangming* channel pattern

occurring especially in the delirium of a fever). There may even be loss of consciousness; insomnia; dry, thick, and yellowish tongue coating with prickles, possibly even a black burnt coating or dry fissured coating (in severe cases); and a deep and powerful or slippery and rapid pulse.

Analysis: See Fig. 12-9.

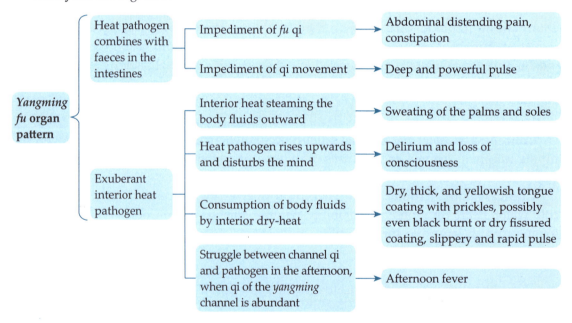

Fig. 12-9 Analysis of the *yangming fu* organ pattern

Key symptoms: Tidal fever, sweating, abdominal distending pain, constipation, dry and thick yellowish coating, deep and rapid pulse, etc.

Shaoyang Pattern

The *shaoyang* pattern represents a stage in the course of an externally contracted disease, in which the struggle between *zheng* qi and pathogenic qi is located between the exterior and interior, and pathogenic qi invades the gallbladder and *sanjiao*. The *sanjiao* governs regulation of the water passages and the gallbladder stores essential juices and governs coursing through and discharge. When an external pathogen attacks the *shaoyang*, the qi of the gallbladder becomes stagnated, then the stagnated qi transforms into fire. The nature of the fire is to blaze upward, and its rising dries the orifices and causes a bitter taste in the mouth, dry throat, and dizziness. When the functional mechanism of the *sanjiao* is impaired, the channel qi is inhibited, which further influences the spleen and stomach and so there may be alternating chills and fever, fullness in the chest and hypochondrium, loss of appetite, frequent retching, a wiry pulse, etc. These are the primary clinical manifestations of *shaoyang* disease.

In the course of an externally contracted disease, it can frequently be observed that the disease has already entered the *shaoyang* stage, yet the *taiyang* pattern is not finished, or, when a *shaoyang* pattern has not finished, a *yangming* pattern also may arise. Therefore the pattern of *shaoyang* is often combined, sometimes with *taiyang* exterior patterns or sometimes with *yangming* interior patterns.

Clinical manifestations: A bitter taste in the mouth, dry throat, dizziness, alternating chills and fever, fullness in the chest and hypochondria, no desire for food or drink, heart vexation or restlessness, frequent retching, wiry pulse.

Analysis: This pattern is due to an unrelieved *taiyang* pattern, causing invasion of the heat pathogen toward the gallbladder; or may result from a direct attack of pathogenic qi into the *shaoyang* due to insecurity of the pores and exuberant pathogenic qi; or is caused by the *jueyin* emerging into the *shaoyang* (Fig. 12-10).

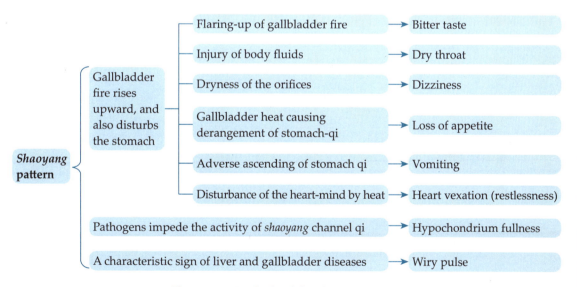

Fig. 12-10 Analysis of the *shaoyang* pattern

Key symptoms: Alternating attacks of chills and fever, fullness in the chest and hypochondrium, and wiry pulse.

Taiyin Pattern

The *taiyin* pattern is indicative of dampness and is regarded as the screen of the three yin channels. It is due to yang transforming into yin and the *zheng* qi beginning to become debilitated. When exterior pathogens attack the three yin channels, the *taiyin* channel is the first channel to be affected. The *taiyin* is the beginning of the three yin patterns, therefore, generally the severity of disease is not extremely critical and, if properly treated, then the prognosis will be very good. When disease enters the *taiyin*, the spleen yang is damaged. This pattern is caused by improper or mistaken treatment of the three yang channels, which injures spleen yang; or by direct attack on the *taiyin* by a cold pathogen due to deficiency of yang in the middle *jiao*, thus leading to weakness of the spleen yang, dysfunction of digestion and transportation, and retention of cold-damp, which manifests as abdominal fullness, vomiting, inability to swallow food, diarrhoea, occasional abdominal pain, white tongue coating, and a moderate, weak pulse.

The *taiyin* and *yangming* patterns may be transmitted to each other under certain conditions. For instance, excessive use of purgatives for a *yangming* disease may damage the spleen yang, changing the disease into a *taiyin* pattern; while extreme use of warm-dry medications or prolonged retention of cold-damp turning into heat, may transform the *taiyin* disease into a *yangming* disease. So there is a saying that "the *yangming* disease is an excess pattern while the *taiyin* disease is a deficiency pattern".

Clinical manifestations: Abdominal fullness, vomiting, loss of appetite, diarrhoea, no thirst, occasional abdominal pain, cold limbs, white tongue coating, and a moderate, weak pulse.

Analysis: This pattern may be caused by inappropriate treatment of the three yang channels, damaging spleen yang; or by direct attack on the *taiyin* by a cold-pathogen due to deficiency of yang in the middle *jiao* (Fig. 12-11).

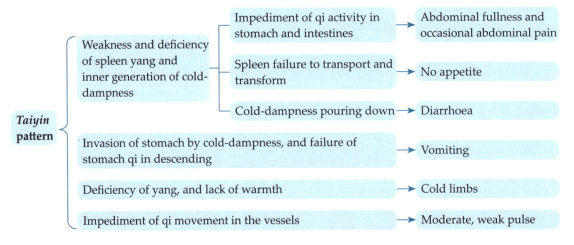

Fig. 12-11 Analysis of the *taiyin* pattern

Key symptoms: These include abdominal fullness and occasional abdominal pain, diarrhoea, absence of thirst, and other symptoms of a deficiency cold pattern.

Shaoyin Pattern

The *shaoyin* pattern represents the severe stage of externally contracted disease. When the disease enters the *shaoyin*, there is injury to the heart and kidney, in which kidney disease is regarded as the main pattern. The *shaoyin* pattern is ascribed to inappropriate treatment or lack of treatment of other channel patterns which injures the kidney yang, leading to transmission of the disease into the *shaoyin* channel, or to direct attack by pathogens due to innate deficiency of the heart and kidney; all may impair the functions of the heart and kidney, causing pathological changes of debility of the heart and kidney. Due to the different causes of the disease and differences in the body's constitution, the *shaoyin* pattern is divided into cold transformation and heat transformation. If the heart and kidney yang qi are deficient and debilitated, this manifests as a deficiency cold pattern. If the kidney yin is deficient, and the heart yang is hyperactive, this results in manifestations of internal heat due to yin deficiency. The former comes from the *shaoyin* cold pattern of yin transforming into cold. The latter comes from the *shaoyin* heat pattern of yang transforming into heat.

1. Cold-transformation pattern of the *shaoyin*

Concept: The cold transformation pattern of the *shaoyin* is caused by a direct attack on the *shaoyin* by cold due to deficiency of yang of the heart and kidney, or by injury to the yang qi of the heart and kidney due to excessive perspiration caused by improper treatment, which is a manifestation of a deficient cold pattern.

Clinical manifestations: Aversion to cold, no fever, preference for lying in a curled-up posture (or lying huddled), listlessness, cold limbs due to reverse flow of qi, diarrhoea with undigested food, vomiting and anorexia, no thirst, or preference for warm fluids, profuse and clear urine, a deep and faint pulse; or general fever but lack of aversion to cold, and possibly a red face.

Analysis: See Fig. 12-12.

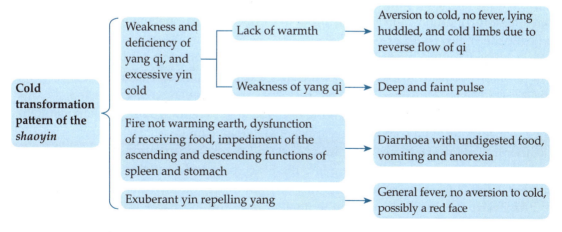

Fig. 12-12 Analysis of a cold transformation pattern of the *shaoyin*

Key symptoms: Aversion to cold, no fever, diarrhoea, cold of the four limbs due to reverse flow of qi, a faint pulse.

2. Heat transformation pattern of the *shaoyin*

Concept: This pattern is due to kidney yin deficiency of the *shaoyin* causing the heart fire to rise up excessively. The heat transformation pattern of the *shaoyin*, a manifestation of a deficient heat pattern, occurs when the yin deficiency is unable to control yang and then heat is generated by relative yang excess.

Clinical manifestations: Heart vexation (irritability), insomnia, dryness of the throat and mouth, red tip of the tongue, and a thready or fine and rapid pulse.

Analysis: See Fig. 12-13.

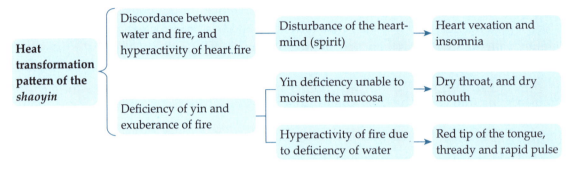

Fig. 12-13   Analysis of a heat transformation pattern of the *shaoyin*

Jueyin Pattern

Concept: *Jueyin* means that yin is on the verge of extinction, whilst yang is starting to rise, and that there is yang within yin. The *jueyin* pattern is the final stage of an externally contracted disease. When the *jueyin* is affected, the evolution of the febrile disease caused by cold to the six channels has reached the last stage, at which the pathological conditions are complicated. The *jueyin* includes the two viscera of the liver and the pericardium (primarily the liver); because the liver and the pericardium both store the fire, they are ascribed to yang within yin. This yang within yin remains under cover and does not grow. Under pathological conditions, this yang within yin can become pathogenic fire and manifests as a heat pattern. If it is dispersed and does not grow, it may manifest as a pattern of yin cold. The *jueyin* pattern is frequently the simultaneous presentation of a cold and heat pattern. If yin cold transforms from excess into deficiency and yang qi from weakness to recovery, the disease is relieved. However, if yin cold remains strong and yang qi is exhausted, the case is critical. If yin cold is exuberant, but yang qi is still able to fight against the pathogenic cold, the mixture of heat and cold patterns appears at the same time.

Clinical manifestations: Persistent thirst and excessive urination (wasting-thirst/*xiāo kě*), a feeling of qi rising and dashing into the heart, pain and sensation of heat in the heart, hunger with no desire to eat, and vomiting or vomiting of roundworms after eating.

Analysis: The *jueyin* channel is the final stage of the six channels, the *jueyin* pattern is mostly caused by transmission of other channels' patterns into the *jueyin* channel, among which the *shaoyang* pattern has the main role (Fig. 12-14).

Transmission of the Six Channel Pattern

The six channel pattern is based on the transmission of the diseases among the *zang*-

Chapter 12 Additional Patterns Differentiation Section 1

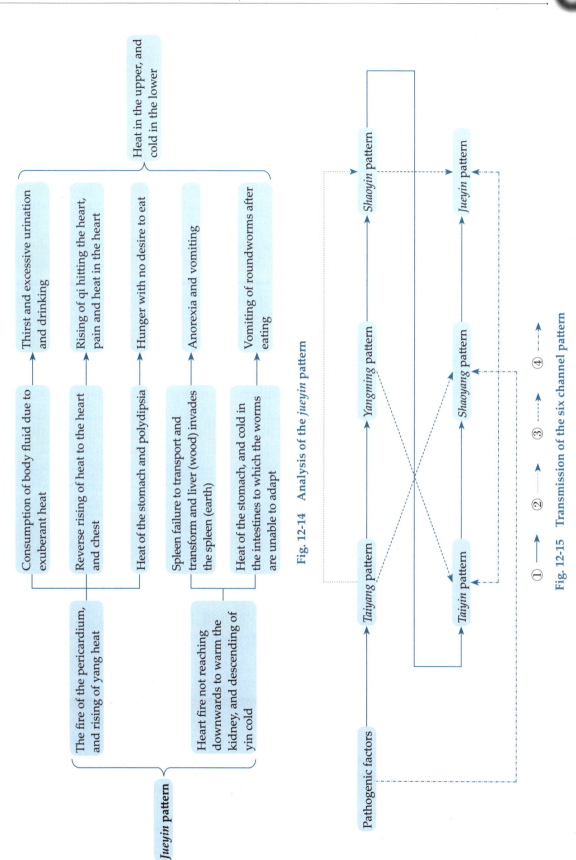

Fig. 12-14 Analysis of the *jueyin* pattern

Fig. 12-15 Transmission of the six channel pattern

fu organs and channels. Between these channels exists an interconnection; therefore, according to the transmission of diseases among the six channels, the pathogenesis of these patterns can be developed by various mechanisms, such as, transmission of diseases from one channel to another channel; or direct attack of a pathogen on a certain channel; or a combination of patterns; or complications and so on (Fig. 12-15).

① Transmission of disease along the order of channels, which may also occur as a channel-bypassing transmission.

② Inner-transmission of a superficial pattern, which may also occur as a direct attack.

The disease of one channel often affects another channel, therefore leading to mutual transmission and transformation. Transmission of the channel pattern indicates a certain tendency for pathological changes to develop.

Firstly, the exterior pathogenic factor invades the human body, and then it gradually develops into the interior from one channel to another one. If this transmission occurs in the order of the six channels as in: *taiyang* pattern → *yangming* pattern → *shaoyang* pattern → *taiyin* pattern → *shaoyin* pattern → *jueyin* pattern, it is called "transmission of disease along the order of the channels"; if it avoids one or two channels, it is called "channel-bypassing transmission"; if it transmits from an exterior channel into the interior channel, it is called "inner-transmission of a superficial pattern", such as *taiyang* pattern being transmitted into a *shaoyin* pattern. If during the onset of a cold-attack, the disease of the three yin channels is attacked directly by the pathogenic factors without the transmission of the three yang channels, it is called a "direct attack".

The "combination of patterns" refers to the patterns of two or three channels appearing at the same time, such as a combination of the *taiyang* and *yangming* pattern, or the *taiyang* and *taiyin* pattern.

The "complication" refers to the appearance of the pattern in another channel while the pattern in another channel has not yet been relieved, such as complication of the *taiyang* and *shaoyin* pattern, the *taiyin* and *shaoyin* pattern, etc.

Section 2
Pattern Differentiation According to the Wei, Qi, Ying, and Blood

Wei (defence) - qi - *ying* (nutrient) - blood pattern identification is the primary method of warm disease pattern identification (*wēn bìng*) presented by Ye Tian-shi, a famous CM doctor of the *Qing* Dynasty. This method is called pattern differentiation according to *wei*, qi, *ying* and blood system; or also called the four levels pattern differentiation, or the four aspect pattern identification. In this chapter we preferably use their original names as *wei*, qi, *ying*, and blood systems. Warm disease is the name for several types of acute heat diseases caused by different heat pathogens during the four seasons.

The *Yellow Emperor's Inner Classic* has a chapter about *wei*, qi, *ying* and blood, which refers to the physiological functions of the body and indicates that within the human body the four systems are divided into layers of different depths. Ye Tian-shi extended the meaning of these four concepts and used them to explain the occurrence of warm diseases, their course of development, and their transmission from superficial to deep and mild to severe, and classified them into *wei, qi, ying,* and blood systems. The *wei* system governs the exterior, so the pathological changes are located in the lung and the skin and body hair. The qi system governs the interior; so the pathological changes that occur in this system are in the lung, chest and diaphragm, spleen and stomach, intestines, gallbladder, etc. The *ying* system pattern occurs when a heat pathogen penetrates into the construction of the heart and the disease is in the heart (*ying*/construction) and pericardium. The blood system pattern occurs when a heat pathogen penetrates into the heart, liver and kidney with an emphasis on stirring and consumption of blood.

The clinical significance of this pattern is for differentiating the level of a warm disease pattern (*wēn bìng*); explanation of the rules of the pathological change of disease; determining a suitable diagnosis, and developing treatment principles.

Wei System Patterns

Concept: *Wei* system patterns occur when a warm heat pathogen invades the body surface and muscles and manifests as abnormalities of the *wei* qi. They are mostly seen at the onset of externally contracted heat diseases.

Clinical manifestations: Fever, slight aversion to wind or cold, red on the sides and tip of the tongue, a floating and rapid pulse, and possibly headache, cough, a dry mouth with slight thirst, swelling and pain of the throat.

Analysis:

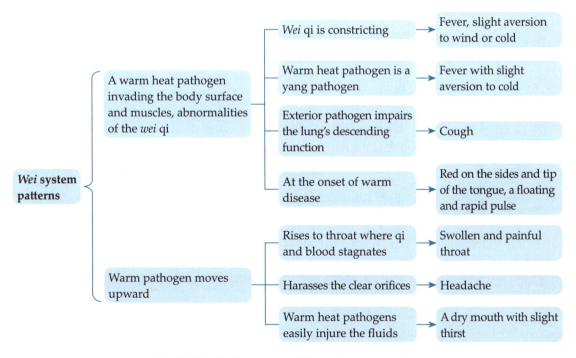

Fig. 12-16 Pathogenesis of the *wei* system patterns

Key symptoms: Fever, slight aversion to wind or cold, red on the sides and tip of the tongue, a floating and rapid pulse.

Diagnostics in Chinese Medicine

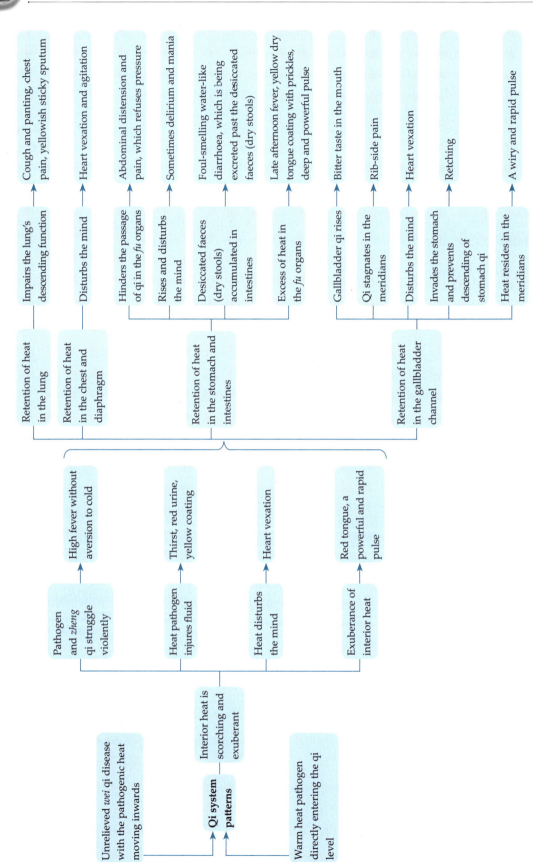

Fig. 12-17 Analysis of the qi system patterns

Qi System Patterns

Concept: The pattern of the qi system is an interior heat pattern in which the heat pathogen is transmitted inward to affect the *zang-fu* organs. The *zheng* (healthy) qi is energetic and strong and the pathogen is excessive, so the struggle between them is aggressive. When a pathogen enters the qi system, although there are some primary common signs that can be found, the range of the pattern of the qi system is very wide.

Clinical manifestations: High fever, copious sweating, thirst with a desire for cold drinks, heart vexation, red urine, a red tongue with a dry, yellow coating and a powerful and rapid pulse. Possibly accompanied by cough and panting, chest pain, yellow sticky phlegm that is difficult to expectorate; possible vexation and agitation, scorching heat of the chest and diaphragm; tidal fever, hardness and pain that refuses pressure, and in extreme cases there may be delirium, constipation or water-like diarrhoea, probably with a bitter taste in the mouth, rib-side pain, retching, heart vexation, yellow and dry tongue coating, and a rapid and powerful pulse or maybe a wiry pulse.

Analysis: This pattern is mainly due to unrelieved *wei* system disease with the pathogenic heat turning inside and entering the qi system, or by a warm heat pathogen directly entering the qi system (Fig. 12-17).

> **Key symptoms:** High fever without aversion to cold, a red tongue with a dry yellow coating, a powerful and rapid pulse are the important points in pattern identification. In addition, according to possible signs and symptoms we are able to judge the involvement of different *zang-fu* organs.

Ying System Patterns

Concept: The *ying* system pattern is a deeper and more serious stage of warm-heat disease that is marked by further penetration of the heat pathogen. The pattern of the *ying* system is characterised by injury of *ying* yin by heat pathogens, and its characteristic sign is pathological change caused by irritation of the mind.

Clinical manifestations: Severe fever at night, no thirst or a little thirst, heart vexation, restlessness and insomnia, sometimes there is delirious speech or coma, maculopapular skin eruptions, crimson and dry tongue and a thready and rapid pulse.

Analysis: This is due to unresolved qi system disease turning inwards to the *ying* system. It also can be due to counterflow turning of *wei* system disease toward the pericardium, which is called "abnormal passage to the pericardium"; and it can be due to an exuberant heat pathogen invading and entering directly into the *ying* system (Fig. 12-18).

> **Key symptoms:** Severe fever at night, heart vexation, delirium and loss of consciousness, a crimson tongue and a thready and rapid pulse.

Blood System Patterns

Concept: The blood system pattern is the last stage of all four levels' pathological changes. It is a more serious level in the course of development of warm heat disease. It is characterised by

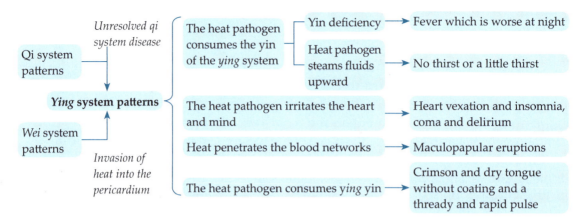

Fig. 12-18 Aetiological factors and pathogenesis of the *ying* system patterns

the consumption and stirring-up of the blood. It mainly damages heart, liver, and kidney.

Clinical manifestations: Fever that is worse at night, restlessness, insomnia, mania, clear dark purple maculopapular eruptions, haematemesis (vomiting of blood), epistaxis (nose bleeding), haematuria (urine with blood), haemafaecia (stool with blood), a deep crimson tongue and a thready and rapid pulse. Possibly, in extreme cases, clonic convulsions, neck rigidity, arched back rigidity, upward gazing eyes, tightly clenched jaw, cold limbs due to reverse flow of qi, possible lingering low fever, night fever abating at dawn, vexing heat in the five centres, mind fatigue, deafness, a thin body, a thready and moderate pulse; possible wriggling of the limbs, or convulsions etc.

Analysis: This is generally due to an unresolved *ying* system entering the blood system; or by direct invasion from the unresolved qi system; or by the stubborn persistence of the heat pathogen in the qi system complicated by the blood system heat pathogen already being exuberant, creating blazing of both qi and blood (Fig. 12-19).

To sum up, blood system patterns are mainly divided into three types:
- Extreme heat stirring the blood.
- Extreme heat generating wind.
- Extreme heat damaging yin.

Key symptoms: Severe fever at night, mania or delirium, clear eruptions of dark purple maculae and papulae, haemorrhage, a deep crimson tongue and a thready and rapid pulse are the important points in its pattern identification. Possible symptoms may be seen according to different pathogenesis. In extreme cases collapse of yang and collapse of yin emerges.

Transmission of the Four Systems Patterns-Warm Heat Patterns

Wei, qi, *ying* and blood summarise the four categories of warm heat patterns (*wēn bìng*). They also represent the four stages of the depth of the development of warm heat diseases. Transmission of the four system patterns is divided into two types: Ordinary transmission and reverse transmission.

① Ordinary transmission

When a warm pathogen invades the body, in general it goes from exterior to interior,

Chapter 12 Additional Patterns Differentiation Section 2

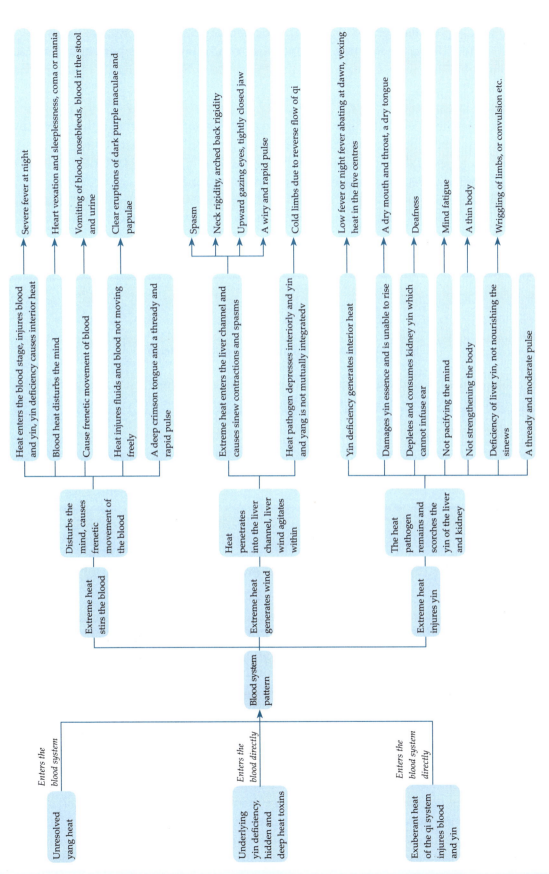

Fig. 12-19 Analysis of the blood system patterns

beginning in the *wei* system, gradually, and in order, advances to the qi system, *ying* system and blood system. It penetrates from a superficial condition to a deeper condition and becomes stronger. This represents a turn in the disease conditions from mild to severe and from excess to deficiency.

② Reverse transmission

When a warm heat pathogen invades the body, it does not pass through the qi system, but instead abnormally passes through and enters the *ying* or blood system directly. This is called ordinary transmission. In fact, reverse transmission is only a special type of ordinary transmission, but is more severe and more dangerous (Fig. 12-20).

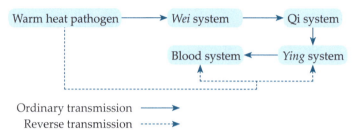

Fig. 12-20 Transmission of the four system patterns

In addition, the rules of the transmission of warm disease are not fixed and unchanging in proportion to specificity of the pathogen and body constitution. For example, beginning in the qi or *ying* systems directly; or if a *wei* system pathogen is not fully resolved but is combined with the qi system, this indicates simultaneous disease in the *wei* and qi, and also there is simultaneous disease in the qi and *ying* or qi and blood. In short, the transmission of warm disease is complicated.

Section 3
Pattern Differentiation According to the Sanjiao Theory

Sanjiao pattern differentiation is also one of the methods for identification of warm diseases and can be very useful for differentiation of diseases associated with heat and damp together. It was set forth by Wu Ju-tong of the *Qing* Dynasty corresponding to the concept of the *sanjiao* in the *Yellow Emperor's Inner Classic*. The *sanjiao* is composed of upper *jiao*, middle *jiao*, and lower *jiao*. This theory is based on identification according to the theory of *wei*, qi, *ying*, and blood. Wu Ju-tong used the *sanjiao* as the principle in the pattern identification of warm diseases, and used the *wei*, qi, *ying*, and blood patterns to elucidate how the *sanjiao* was attributed in the pathological changes that occur to the *zang-fu* over the course of warm heat diseases. He took this as the groundwork to recognise the depth of the pathogens in order to explain the different stages in the course of a disease and the mutual transformation of the patterns, thus determining the principle of treatment.

Pathological changes and clinical manifestation of the *zang-fu* organs related to the *sanjiao* theory indicate different stages over the course of warm heat diseases. The upper *jiao* disease pattern includes the symptoms of the lung channel of the hand *taiyin* and the pericardium channel of the hand *jueyin*, and the initial stage of disease starts from the upper *jiao*. If the disease of the upper *jiao* is not relieved, the pathogenic factors may penetrate to the middle *jiao*, corresponding to the spleen and stomach, where the disease transmits deeper and thus is more severe. The stomach (*yangming*) is easily affected by dryness while the spleen (*taiyin*) is easily affected by dampness. If the disease of the middle *jiao* is not relieved, it will transmit to the lower *jiao*, corresponding to the kidney channel of the foot *shaoyin* and the liver channel of the foot *jueyin*, where the pathogens go still deeper inward; this is the last stage of a warm disease.

This is the general law of transmission, but as the exterior pathogens vary in nature, there are some exceptions. For instance, some diseases may appear not only in the lower *jiao*, but also in the middle *jiao* and upper *jiao*.

Upper *Jiao* Patterns

Concept: This pattern is due to a warm-heat pathogen invading the lung channel of the hand *taiyin* and the pericardium channel of the hand *jueyin*.

Clinical manifestations:

Attack of the lung by a warm pathogen: Headache, fever, mild aversion to wind and cold, sweating, cough, thirst, red tip and sides of the tongue, a floating and rapid pulse.

Retention of heat in the lung: Fever, no aversion to cold, sweating, thirst, cough, panting, yellow tongue coating, and a rapid pulse.

Attack on the pericardium by heat: High fever, loss of consciousness, delirium, cloudy mind and an inability to speak; cold limbs, a stiff and red-crimson tongue.

Analysis: See Fig. 12-21.

Middle *Jiao* Patterns

Concept: This pattern is due to a warm-heat pathogen invading the spleen and stomach. It indicates disorders of the hand *yangming*, and foot *taiyin* channels. The *yangming* governs dryness while the *taiyin* governs dampness. The warm pathogen penetrates into the *yangming* transforming into dryness, which manifests itself as an excess pattern of interior heat-dryness, excess of non-substantial heat, or accumulation of substantial heat, similar to excess of heat in the stomach and retention of heat in the intestinal tract in the qi stage pattern of warm disease. If the pathogen penetrates into the *taiyin*, it transforms into dampness, usually manifesting itself as warm diseases caused by dampness.

Clinical manifestation:

Excess heat in the *yangming* (*yangming* warm disease): High fever often described as tidal fever which may be worse at dusk, flushed face, abdominal fullness, constipation, loss of consciousness, delirium, thirst with a desire for cold drinks, burnt dry mouth and lips, dark and scanty urine, yellow and dry or dark-yellow tongue coating with prickles, a deep, and powerful pulse.

Damp-heat in the middle *jiao*: Slight fever which is worse in the afternoons and is only temporarily relieved by sweating, heaviness of the limbs, body, and head, distension and fullness in the chest and epigastrium, nausea and vomiting, loose stool with a sensation of incomplete defaecation, or sloppy stools, a yellow and greasy coating, a soggy (soft) and rapid pulse.

Diagnostics in Chinese Medicine

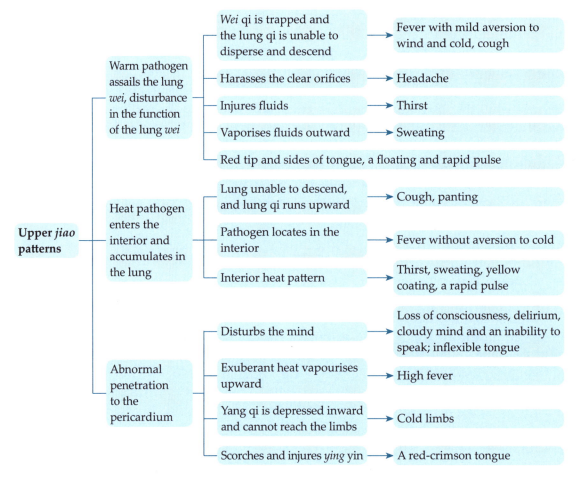

Fig. 12-21   Pathogenesis of the upper *jiao* patterns

Analysis: See Fig. 12-22.

Lower *Jiao* Patterns

Concept: This pattern indicates transmission of the disease into the kidney channel of foot *shaoyin* and liver channel of the foot *jueyin*. The warm diseases, after penetrating to the lower *jiao*, manifest as kidney and liver yin deficiency. The sustaining heat will damage yin essence, leading to a deficient-heat pattern due to kidney yin deficiency. Once the kidney yin is consumed, the water is unable to nourish the wood, resulting in malnutrition of the liver and the tendons, consequently the stirring-up of wind.

Clinical manifestations:

<u>Kidney yin deficiency</u>: Fever with malar flush (red cheeks), feverish sensation in the chest, palms, and soles that is more severe than that on the dorsum of the hands and feet, dry mouth and throat, spirit fatigue (listlessness), deafness, a rapid and deficient pulse.

<u>Stirring-up of the wind</u>: Wriggling of the hands and feet, clonic convulsions, stirring of the heart (violent palpitations), spirit fatigue (listlessness), crimson tongue with diminished coating, and a deficient pulse.

Analysis: See Fig. 12-23.

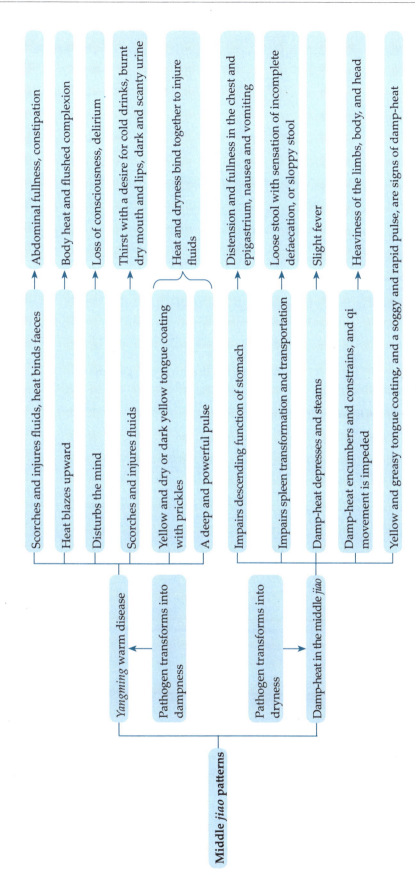

Fig. 12-22 Pathogenesis of the middle *jiao* patterns

Diagnostics in Chinese Medicine

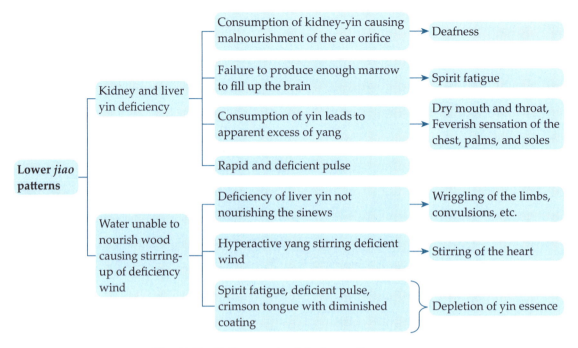

Fig. 12-23 Pathogenesis of the lower *jiao* patterns

Transmission of *Sanjiao* Patterns

Transmission of the *sanjiao* patterns usually occurs via two ways: ordinary transmission and reverse transmission.

① Ordinary transmission

Warm heat diseases initiate from the upper *jiao*, where the disease is shallow in depth and mild in severity. If the upper *jiao* disease is not resolved, this results in transmission of pathogens to the middle *jiao*, and then the disease of the middle *jiao*, if not relieved, will transmit to the lower *jiao*. This represents a transmission of disease from superficial condition to a deeper condition and from mild to severe.

② Reverse transmission

When a heat pathogen invades the body, if the disease is adversely transmitted from the lung to the pericardium, the pathological condition will be worse. This is called reverse transmission, and the disease is more severe and dangerous.

In addition, the rules of the transmission of warm disease are not absolute and unchanging. If the upper *jiao* disease is resolved, the transmission is stopped; but sometimes the upper disease is not resolved. Consequently, upper *jiao* disease can then be combined with middle *jiao* disease; and also sometimes a pathogen can directly transmit from the upper *jiao* to the lower *jiao*. The case is the same for simultaneous disease in the middle and lower *jiao*. Occasionally it can start from the lower *jiao*. In short, the transmission of warm disease is complicated and should be analysed systematically.

Section 4
Pattern Differentiation According to the Twelve Channels

Channel and network pattern identification is a diagnostic method in which the theory of channels and networks is applied to analyse clinical manifestations so as to determine the involved channels. Principally, this method of pattern identification allows us to distinguish symptoms and signs according to the involved channel. Problems of the internal organs can affect the associated channels, and on the contrary, symptoms, which initiate as channel problems can penetrate into the interior and be transmitted to the organs. The twelve channels are related internally to the *zang-fu* organs and externally to the limbs and exterior portion of the body, and they transport qi, and nourish the whole body. Therefore, pathological manifestations of the twelve channels internally appear in dysfunction of the associated *zang-fu* organs, and externally manifest in disorders of the areas connected to the channel. This pattern identification is a complementary and assisting method for identification of patterns according to the theory of *zang-fu* organs. This method is widely used in acupuncture, moxibustion and tuina treatments.

The twelve principal channels are composed of the three yin channels of the hand, the three yin channels of the foot, the three yang channels of the hand, and the three yang channels of the foot. Each channel pattern includes disease of the channel pathway and its related organ. Channel problems can appear in three ways:

① When exterior pathogenic factors, such as cold, wind, damp or heat invade the channels, the channel-qi cannot move freely, and signs and symptoms will emerge along the channel pathway.

② Signs and symptoms of the channels and their related organs emerge simultaneously.

③ Several channels are invaded at the same time. Channel and network pattern identification primarily explains the signs and symptoms that appear along the course of the channels and networks, and then among these signs and symptoms, some will be closely related to the *zang* and *fu* organs.

Table 12-2 Pattern differentiation according to the twelve principal channels

Channel Pattern	Clinical manifestation		
	Dysfunction of the associated *zang-fu* organ	Impediment of the channel qi	Reactions to the pathogen
Lung channel of the hand *taiyin*	Distension and fullness of the chest, cough and panting	Pain of the supraclavicular fossa, shoulders, back, and anterior border of the medial aspect of the arm	Aversion to cold with fever due to wind-cold attack; sweating due to wind attack; shortage of qi due to lung qi deficiency

Continued

Channel Pattern	Clinical manifestation		
	Dysfunction of the associated *zang-fu* organ	Impediment of the channel qi	Reactions to the pathogen
Large intestine channel of the hand *yangming*	Yellowing of the eyes, dryness of the mouth, constipation or loose stool	Pain or dysfunction of the shoulders, lateral aspect of the upper arm, the thumb, and the index finger	Toothache, neck swelling, inflammation of the throat, epistaxis (nose bleeding)
Stomach channel of the foot *yangming*	Abdominal distension and fullness, mania, borborygmus, swift digestion with rapid and frequent hungering	Pain around the breasts, around the ST 30 (*qì chōng*), ST 32 (*fú tù*) areas, pain of the groin, swelling and pain of the knees, the anterolateral aspect of the lower limbs, the dorsum of the foot, or motion impairment of the middle toe	Dry sores on the lips, epistaxis, deviation of the mouth, inflammation of the throat, neck swelling; if qi is exuberant, there is heat along the front portion of the body
Spleen channel of the foot *taiyin*	Vomiting, epigastric pain, abdominal distension, belching, heaviness of the body, susceptibility to vomiting, heart vexation, acute pain below the heart, sloppy diarrhoea, difficulty with urination, jaundice	Pain or dysfunction of the knee, thigh, and big toe	Stiffness and pain in the root of the tongue
Heart channel of the hand *shaoyin*	Cardiac pain, dryness of the throat, thirst with a desire to drink	Hypochondriac pain, pain in the posterior border of the medial aspect of the upper limbs, and heat sensation in the palms	Yellowing of the eyes
Small intestine channel of the hand *taiyang*		Deafness, yellowing eyes, cheek swelling, pain in the nape of the neck, shoulders, posterior border of the lateral aspect of the elbows and arms	Sore throat, swelling of the jaw, inability to turn the head, severe pain of the shoulder and arm
Bladder channel of the foot *taiyang*		Puffy swelling, or distension and pain of the eyes; stretching pain in the nape of the neck, extreme pain of the spinal column and lumbus; pain or dyskinesia of the thigh, popliteal fossa; tearing pain of the calf, and impaired movement of the small toe	Cold and heat patterns; aversion to cold with fever, surging headache, nasal obstruction

Continued

Channel Pattern	Clinical manifestation		
	Dysfunction of the associated *zang-fu* organ	Impediment of the channel qi	Reactions to the pathogen
Kidney channel of the foot *shaoyin*	Sallow complexion, lassitude, feeling of hunger, haemoptysis, shortness of breath, panting, heart vexation and chest pain, propensity to fright, a predilection for lying down	Pain in the posteriomedial aspect of the thigh, soreness of the lumbar region and knee joints, flaccidity of the lower limbs, and burning pain in the soles	Feeling of heat in the mouth, sore throat, dryness and swelling of the tongue and throat, qi rising counterflow with panting cough
Pericardium channel of the hand *jueyin*	Palpitations, heart vexation, cardiac pain, and mental disorders	Pain and fullness of the chest and hypochondrium, heat sensation in the palms	Hypertonicity or contracture of the arms and elbows, swelling and pain of the axillary fossa, flushed face
Sanjiao channel of the hand *shaoyang*		Pain of the outer canthus, swelling and pain of the cheeks, pain in the retroauricular region, pain and dyskinesia (lack of voluntary movement) on the lateral aspect of the shoulder, arm and the elbow, and impaired movement of the little finger	Deafness, tinnitus, swelling and pain of the throat, sweating, pain of the chest and hypochondrium
Gallbladder channel of the foot *shaoyang*	A bitter taste in the mouth, a tendency to sigh, pain of the chest and hypochondrium, inability to rotate, twist or turn to the lateral side	Headache, pain of the mandible, swelling and pain in the supraclavicular fossa, swelling below the axilla; pain and dyskinesia along the lateral aspect of the chest and hypochondrium, the thigh and knee to the lower leg, in front of the external malleolus; and impaired movement of the small toe	The face has a slightly dusty complexion, phlegm nodes and sabre (curved and smooth) lumps in the neck, lustreless skin, heat on the lateral side of the feet, sweating, alternating chills and fever
Liver channel of the foot *jueyin*	Fullness and pain in the chest and hypochondrium, vomiting due to counterflow of qi, swill diarrhoea	*Hú shàn* (狐疝, foxy mounting, scrotum hernia) or mounting qi pain (acute pain in the lesser abdomen referring to the testicles), enuresis or dribbling urinary block	Pain of the lumbus that inhibits stretching, swelling of the lesser abdomen in women, dry throat

CHAPTER 13
The Case Record

Keeping track of the medical encounter through the documentation of a case record is a fundamental aspect of clinical work and an integral part of the entire process of patient care. Case record taking is a particular type of knowledge construction that aims to represent a patient and their illness. By gathering and condensing information, the practitioner aims to reconstruct the information into a written record and thus help to transform the patient's condition into a manageable problem. In constructing a case record, the practitioner needs to transform/translate the information into evidence in a structured, linked and formal manner.

- Principles and Priorities for Recording a Case Record
    - The Personal Record - general information
    - Chief Current Condition (complaint/concern)
    - Present Illness History
        - The occurrence of disease
        - The development of disease
        - Procedure of diagnosis and treatment prior to the initial consultation
        - The present symptoms
    - Past Medical History
- Signs, Symptoms, and Aetiologies
- Diagnosis, Interpretation and Analysis
- Treatment Principle and Strategy
- Treatment Plan
- Treatment i.e. Point Prescription or Herbal Prescription
- Outcome Measures, Action and Advice
- Storage, Access and Retrieval

Principles and Priorities for Recording a Case Record

The case record (also referred to as a medical record or patient record) is the written account that is made by the practitioner of the clinical encounter and should be patient-centred. In order to achieve a high level of care it is essential to have good systematic, accurate records not only of patients' wishes and thoughts but also of all the actions taken and outcomes arrived at. The case record needs to document the initial consultation and any follow up appointments, as well as all treatments given; keeping a complete treatment record benefits both practitioner and patient.

It is important to remember that the case record may be read by the patients and their families. In light of this, there must be a clear process confirming that patients know their right of access to their case record, and that they know who else might have access and who will not.

In light of the semi-public scope of access to case records, how they are written is extremely important. All case records should be complete. Every entry should be legible, written in permanent ink, dated and signed by the practitioner (alternative methods must be designed and used if computer technology is used for case record taking). The language used should be succinct and easy to understand by others, and the use of acronyms and abbreviations should be avoided. The language used should not contain humour or irony, nor should it be in any way disparaging.

One of the aims of a good case record is to seek to reveal the patient's perspective on their experiences of illness. Therefore, the language used in case records should be appropriately sensitive to the patient's concerns and express things from the patient's point of view. These considerations establish the need for recording the patient's narratives, quotes, metaphors, symbols, and anecdotes, as these all give support to the patient/practitioner dialogue and help explore it. All these forms of information when used by the patient should be included in the case record. In order to reliably gather the important issues, it is essential that the consultation establishes rapport between the patient and the practitioner and builds the patient's trust in the practitioner. Any problems of communication or other difficulties arising in this therapeutic relationship should be documented.

(1) The personal record - general information

As well as being a clinical document the case record is a legal document and must contain full information about the patient. In non-emergency situations, the first information or data gathered is that of the personal profile. This profile might include:
- The person's name, address, date of birth and contact details e.g. telephone numbers, email, etc.
- The person's primary physician/general practitioner (GP) and whether permission to contact the primary physician/GP has been given.
- How the person was referred or who recommended you to them.
- An 'In Case of Emergency' (ICE) contact's telephone number.

To facilitate the capturing and recording of this preliminary information it may be written into a pre-prepared form and may be completed either by the practitioner or by support staff. Patients are often allocated a reference code number, and either this or their name should be on every sheet and each sheet should be numbered.

Throughout treatment, the patient's informed consent and its documentation is the on going responsibility of the practitioner; in addition, if the notes in the case record are to be used for other purposes such as teaching, research, and audit, there also must be documentation of the patient's knowledge and consent for this.

The preliminary information in the case record is usually followed by a general description of the individual:
- The patient's age and sex
- The patient's occupation and home situation
- The patient's general appearance, bearing and disposition
- The habits and customs in the patient's life
- The patient's relationships, family and work context
- The patient's diet and his/her activities
- The patient's mental state
- Any special factors of a general nature, like pregnancies etc.

(2) Current condition (complaint/concern)

It is necessary to appreciate that, for the patient, the important thing will undoubtedly be their reason for coming, and therefore this must be suitably highlighted in the case record. Traditionally this reason for coming has been referred to as the "main complaint" or "chief complaint" but the term "patient's chief concern" is now preferred.

(3) Present illness history

It is important to document:
   a. The occurrence of disease: How long this concern has been present, and the circumstances of the onset (the emergence of the illness)
   b. The development of disease and (later) transformations of the illness and the symptoms and effects as experienced by the patient (the "subjective patho-conditions").
   c. Procedure of diagnosis and treatment prior to this first consultation, including the results of any tests that have been carried out
   d. The present symptoms
      Moreover, any secondary or further concerns should also be documented. All case records must contain this concise aspect of the patient history, and include not only the initial presentation but also the practitioner's initial reaction to the patient. Furthermore, it is essential that the practitioner respects the patient's understanding of their illness, his/her health beliefs, feelings and expectations and reflect on relevant factors in the patient's circumstances and profile.

(4) Medical history

Following identification of the patient's main concern, the case record should document a general medical history, including individual life history, family history and so on. This might include, for example, accidents and operations, and, for women, a broad gynaecological history. Also documented as a high priority is all medication currently being taken; if this list is substantial, it may be written on a separate sheet. In addition, contact details of all the other people and professionals involved in the patient's care should be documented.

It is perhaps appropriate here to note that it may not be possible to obtain information from a patient in a structured manner. Information will need to be gathered when provided, and if necessary written again in the correct order after the consultation. Also, important to note is that the practitioner should aim to select only that information which is pertinent to the case.

Signs, Symptoms, and Aetiologies

Chinese medicine employs the methods of *sì zhěn* 四诊 (inspection, listening and smelling, inquiry, pulse reading and palpation) which are used to gather information. Consequently, any signs and symptoms attained through these practices should be recorded. No one method should hold precedence over any other, and one of the strengths of Chinese medical diagnosis is its ability to assimilate multiple diagnostic indicators. In order to provide sufficient information for later, it is necessary to document all information collected; not just from the inquiry examination but also from observation, from listening and smelling, and from the palpatory examinations.

Information is perhaps best recorded on a mixture of printed patient note forms (see Table 1) and blank sheets of paper. The printed forms ensure that all major areas have been addressed, and the practitioner can use this template for writing up the first consultation. The plain sheets of paper allow the practitioner to ensure that not only the information that they wish to elicit is gathered but also any information that the patient wishes to express is noted. The plain sheets of paper can stimulate the practitioner to uphold the richness of the case history and to elaborate where necessary.

Diagnosis, Interpretation and Analysis

Recorded during and after the data collection should be the entire diagnostic picture, which should include *biàn bìng*[1] 辨病, and *biàn zhèng*[2] 辨證 (证) differential diagnostic labels. The signs and symptoms need to be organised to support the conclusions, and the whole pathological process needs to have transparency. Emphasis should be on identifying the possible aetiology or causes of the disease, and the pathways of transmission. The case record should make the decision-making process clear and easy to follow.

The case record should also make note of the management of contradictions; of possible alternative diagnoses; of the significance of biomedical factors; and of the relevance of psycho-social factors.

Additional printed forms may be used to record such instances as when summaries and reviews are carried out; for discharge summaries; for a change of diagnosis; or for reviews of the patient's progress at the conclusion of each agreed cycle of treatment.

Also referenced or included in the case record should be all literature consulted in the management of the case and that supports any decisions made.

Treatment principle and strategy

The treatment principles and strategies recorded in the case record outline how the practitioner aims to go about treatment to rectify the patient's situation. An indication needs to be provided as to the priorities of treatment, and the discussion of the thinking behind these decisions. Methods used to treat as well as descriptions and explanations given ought to include the features of the process or the *lǐ* 理 (principles, orientations or ability to grasp); *fǎ* 法 (strategies and methods), and *yì* 意 (intentions, reason or signification). Finally, detailed explanations of the *běn* 本 (root) and *biāo* 标 (branch) of the case should be recorded, as well as the reasons behind the priorities for treatment, fully showing the rationale for proceeding. It is essential to make careful use of language in this respect, giving due consideration to the fact that many of these terms are translated and imbibed with their own cultural significance is imperative.

Treatment plan

The records made at the first visit should include a treatment plan, which reflects the contract made with the patient and the rationale for these choices. The records should suggest how often the patient will attend for treatment, and what number of treatments might be carried out. In addition, the treatment plan should state:
- What the practitioner will do; for example: write a referral letter, write a letter to the patient's GP or primary physician.
- What the patient will do; for example: carry out the practitioner's advice and/or any

---

[1] *biàn bìng* 辨病 refers to disease identification. Patients may have a biomedical diagnosis that also needs to be recorded.

[2] *biàn zhèng* 辨證 (证) refers to pattern identification.

recommended lifestyle changes.
- What might be achieved and by what stage.
- Any factors that will alert a change to the plan; for example: changes of personal circumstances, accidents etc.

It is essential that the practitioner constantly check there is a consistency of theory and method throughout the case record; reflection is an imperative throughout this process. The practitioner's ability to reflect over time is supported by accurate documentation of any difficulties and contradictions in the case; of any alternative diagnosis; of observations about the dynamics between practitioner and patient; and the practitioner's thoughts and feelings about the case.

At each follow-up session, notes should include any new, unusual or key features for the day; priority in this is given to patient's own words. They should also include any new information and impressions relating to any of the sections mentioned earlier in this chapter. It is important to describe and critically assess any change in diagnosis, treatment principle or strategy, point prescription, treatment or prognostic evaluation. It is recommended that the practitioner record any of his or her ideas for follow-up, connections or research, including discussion with peers, and that they record conclusions drawn.

Point Prescription or Herbal Prescription

A detailed point prescription must be recorded at every session. Many of the details to include in the case record might be appropriately similar to those set out by MacPherson et. al. (2002) in the Standards for Reporting Interventions in Controlled Trials of Acupuncture (STRICTA) guidelines. These guidelines suggest recording the following:
- Firstly, the specific points used (ideally, both in numerical form and named); the type and size of needles used; and the angle of insertion and depth of needling in the proportional measurement of *cun*.
- Secondly, the treatment methods, such as the technique used on each needle; the total number of needles used in the prescription and the amount of time the needles are left in.
- Finally, any adjuncts used, such as moxibustion, cupping or plum blossom needling.

In addition, it can be argued that it can be useful for future reflection to include: Any reactions observed; sounds heard like stomach gurgling; and any sensations described by the patient such as tingling, like water trickling down, like electricity shooting, or spreading aches.

Moreover, to demonstrate the academic and critical thinking behind these prescriptions, case notes should also include point classifications and the reasoning behind why points were chosen.

Any herbal prescription should include all the details and quantities of the herbs prescribed. Current advice is to type this information so as to reduce the possibility of mistakes being made.

A printed form can be used to record each treatment and details of the patient's progress.

Outcome Measures, Action and Advice

Outcome measures (OM) cover both those measures of treatment that are carried out by clinicians in the treatment room, and those that would be carried out in hospitals and other assessment centres. In order for the practitioner to obtain reliable measures of treatment outcomes a variety of methods should be considered. These OM can include the use of a subjective measure, such as Measure Yourself Medical Outcome Profile (MYMOP) (Paterson, 2010), as well as other validated outcome measures[1] identified for specific situations as appropriate.

In addition, in Chinese medicine OM need to take into consideration not only measures of pain and of functionality but also the energy levels or the feelings of health and well-being experienced by the patient. Also, valid measurements of treatment outcome can include such factors as improved self-esteem, greater confidence, return to work and change in behaviour. The collection of long-term outcome measures is essential to reflect the general aims of long-term changes to health, even after treatment has finished. Some of these relatively new dimensions of measurement equate more closely with the patient experience providing another valid reason to use them to measure treatment success.

Storage, Access and Retrieval

For legal reasons, the storage and transmission of patients' case records must be taken seriously and given due consideration. All the sheets and forms used will need to be kept neatly together in a file. Records can be kept either as a hard copy in a file and stored in a filing system or kept in computerised form. It is very important to demonstrate confidentiality in respect of case records, as befits the principles and the values of confidential professional relationships. In addition, records should be used only for the purposes for which they were intended, and no information should ever be passed on to any commercial organisation of any kind.

Whether records are kept in manual or electronic form, they must be kept according to the Data Protection Act in the country of practice. Manual files may need to be stored in fireproof cabinets, under lock and key; electronic files may need to be password-protected. Whatever means of storage is used, considerations of security are paramount. Patient's case notes and records are the property of the practitioner, who is responsible for keeping or disposing of them. There is often a legal requirement that patient records are kept for a minimum of seven years.

For ease of retrieval, patient notes are best filed systematically, usually alphabetically. It may be useful for audit purposes to be able to identify easily any information that might be considered suitable for collective management, and separate data collection forms may be used for this purpose.

Conclusion

Creating and keeping good case records is a serious endeavour and requires self-discipline from the practitioner. However, case records are a legal requirement and the value of good case records does support the effort. Good case records enhance good clinical decision–making and help to communicate information to others as and when required.

---

1 Examples of valid and reliable OM's: McGill's pain questionnaire (1975 & 1987). Delighted-Terrible Faces Scale (Andrews and Witney 1976); The Visual Analog Scale (VAS) (Huskisson 1974); Headache Disability Inventory Self-completed disability scale; Headache-specific Locus of control scale (HSLC), etc.

Finally, it is worth considering that case records are an important way to contribute to our knowledge and understanding, and to help to benefit patients, practice and the profession.

Table 1   Sample Case Record Form

Practitioner taking initial case:

Date of 1st Consultation:

Patient Reference Code: DOB:

PRACTITIONER RECORD

Practitioner Name	From	To	Practitioner Name	From	To

RECORD OF INITIAL CONSULTATION	
PRESENTING CONCERN	DURATION
PRESENTING CONCERN	DURATION
PRESENTING CONCERN	DURATION

ONSET AND CLINICAL MANIFESTATION OF PRESENTING CONCERN

OTHER CLINICAL MANIFESTATION

Continued

MEDICATION	FAMILY MEDICAL HISTORY
MEDICAL HISTORY	WORK, HOME, RELATIONSHIPS & SUPPORT **(if appropriate)**

EENT/ HEADACHE
CHEST/ RESPIRATION
DIGESTION / APPETITE
THIRST
BOWELS
URINATION
SWEAT
SLEEP
ENERGY/WELL BEING
PAIN
HOT/ COLD
MENTAL/ EMOTIONAL/ SHEN **(if appropriate)**
MENSTRUATION

DIET		FACE
BREAKFAST		BODY/ POSTURE
LUNCH		BLOOD PRESSURE
DINNER		
TEA/COFFEE	ALCOHOL	
TOBACCO	OTHER	

Continued

TONGUE

PULSE
        R   L

Patient Reference:

Diagnosis
- with supporting Signs & Symptoms (list patterns in order of importance; include contradictions)

Consideration of Alternative Diagnostic Approach - with rationale

Key Aetiological & Pathological Factors - that led to syndromes and to major symptoms (use extra sheet for development)

Treatment Principle and Strategy

Points Prescription - with explanation for use of points

Continued

Treatment Plan	
Number of visits agreed:	Frequency of treatments:
Referral:	Letter to GP:

Recommendations to patient - including diet, exercise, relaxation, smoking, etc.

	Signature

References:

MacPherson, H., White, A., Cummings, M., Jobst, K.A., Rose, K., Niemtzow, R.C., (2002). Standards for Reporting Interventions in Controlled Trials of Acupuncture: The STRICTA Recommendations. *The Journal of Alternative and Complementary Medicine.* 8(1): 85-89.

Paterson, C., (2010). Quality of Life Measures. *British Journal of General Practice.* 60(570): 53-57.

CHAPTER 14
Examples of Traditional Chinese Medical Records

EXAMPLE OF HOW TO WRITE AN OUTPATIENT MEDICAL RECORD

First visit record

Name: ×× **Sex:** Male **Age:** 35 years **Record Number:** 69428
Divisions: Internal Medicine March 9, 1990

Inquiry examination:

Chief complaint:

Stomach pain, broke out 15 years ago but has had repeated episodes, recurred 4 days ago, aggravating 1 day.

Case History:

The patient experienced stomach pain due to hard work and irregular diet fifteen years ago. The condition was relieved after taking Chinese medicine, but it always recurrently attacks. A fibergastroscopy indicated GA (Gastric Antrum) Superficial Gastritis and a duodenobulbar ulcer in one hospital, in August 1988.

At this time, the disease recurred four days ago, because the patient was dissatisfied with his job and drank too much alchohol. Taking painkillers has no effect. At present, the patient has burning pain in the stomach and anorexia, hypochondriac distension, restlessness of emotions, which is accompanied by acid regurgitation, epigastric upset, hiccough, dry stool and normal urine.

Examinations of Inspection, Palpation, Listening and Smelling:

Strong physique and body, normal mental status, red margins of the tongue with a thin yellow coating, a wiry and thready pulse, and tenderness of the stomach.

Analysis of Pattern Differentiation:

Due to the history of stomach pain, the negative emotions and over-consumption of alchohol, the condition transformed to fire-heat and then invaded the liver and stomach. Liver-stomach disharmony leads to the above symptoms.

Diagnosis:

Diagnosis of CM: Stomach pain (pattern of liver-stomach disharmony)
Diagnosis of Western Medicine: 1. Acute gastritis 2. Gastrelosis

Treatment:

Calming liver qi and harmonising the stomach, regulating qi and relieving pain.

Prescription:

白芍	bái sháo	30 g	Radix Paeoniae Alba
柴胡	chái hú	6 g	Radix Bupleuri
法半夏	fǎ bàn xià	10 g	Rhizoma Pinelliae Preparatum
川芎	chuān xiōng	12 g	Rhizoma Ligustici Chuanxiong
香附	xiāng fù	10 g	Rhizoma Cyperi

陈皮	chén pí	10 g	Pericarpium Citri Reticulatae
枳壳	zhǐ qiào	10 g	Fructus Aurantii
郁金	yù jīn	12 g	Radix Curcumae
吴茱萸	wú zhū yú	4 g	Fructus Evodiae
黄连	huáng lián	6 g	Rhizoma Coptidis
甘草	gān cǎo	6 g	Radix Glycyrrhizae

Decoct one dose every day and divide in two, to take warm, twice a day. Take three doses in total (over three days).

Alternatively, or in addition, acupuncture at PC 6 (*nèi guān*), LV 14 (*qī mén*), LV 3 (*tài chōng*) and Ren 13 (*shàng wǎn*) to smooth and move the liver; descend the stomach qi; or for the fire-heat, clear heat with: LI 4 (*hé gǔ*) or LI 11 (*qū chí*), ST 44 (*nèi tíng*) or ST 40 (*fēng lóng*).

Advice:

It was suggested that he take an upper gastrointestinal contrast examination or fibergastroscopy and change to a soft foods diet, avoid pungent foods, alchohol and rage.

Full name of the doctor: ××

CHAPTER 15
Diagnosis Methods Training and Case Analysis

SECTION 1
DIAGNOSIS METHODS TRAINING

The Methods of the Inspection Examination

Guidelines for the inspection examination

In "inspection", there are three aspects that should always be addressed. Firstly, it is important that the light should be sufficient. Ideally, the inspection examination should be performed in light that is adequate, natural and soft. However, if there is insufficient natural light, a fluorescent lamp can be used, but examination may need to be rechecked later as necessary. It is especially important to avoid any coloured light. Secondly, ensure that the temperature of the clinic room is suitable. If the temperature of the clinic room is suitable, the patient's skin and muscles will naturally be relaxed, qi and blood will flow smoothly and the signs of disease can be accurately determined. If the temperature is too cold, the skin and muscles of the patient will be contracted, with inhibited flow of qi and blood. This will not only influence the authenticity of the obtained data, but may also subject the patient to the possibility of catching cold, on top of their original illness. Thirdly, the areas to be inspected should be exposed thoroughly, thus allowing the practitioner to inspect and observe every location completely and carefully.

The contents of the inspection of spirit

The emphasis of the inspection of spirit: In inspecting the spirit, the expression of the eyes, facial expression, facial complexion, mental status, and movement of the body should be inspected, but especially the expression of the eyes.

1. Eye spirit: this means the appearance of the spirit in the aspects of the colour, lustre and form of the eyes. The vital essences of the five *zang* and six *fu* are all concentrated in the eyes. The eyes are linked with the brain; they are also the orifices of the liver, messenger of the heart, and dormitory of the spirit; so the eyes can precisely reflect the strength or weakness, deficiency or excess of the *zang-fu*'s function. For this reason, the practitioner should observe the eyes first when inspecting the spirit, especially in serious or critical situations. Just through observing the eyes alone, the practitioner can make an initial diagnosis of the condition of the patient's spirit. The eye spirit can be reflected mainly in the appearance of bright or dull eyes and the flexibility or lack of vitality in the activity of the eyeballs.

2. Spirit-affect: this relates to the person's mind, level of consciousness and their facial expressions. The specific performance of spirit-affect relates to how lucid or cloudy the mind is and how methodical or confused the thought process is. This also relates to the sensitivity or dullness of a person's reactions and the expressiveness or indifference of the

facial expression. It is the external display of the exuberance or decline of the heart-mind and *zang-fu*'s vital essence.

3. Complexion: this is the colour of a person's skin and surface tissue; however, it is mostly based on the facial colour. The manifestation of primary importance in the complexion is the difference between how lustrous or withered it appears and this can reflect the *zang-fu*'s exuberance or decline of qi and blood, as well as strength or weakness of the *zang-fu*'s function.

4. Posture: this is the body shape and how the person sits or stands. For example: Fat or thin body, freely moving or abnormal positions of the body, both of these aspects of posture are important markers for the bodily functions.

Inspection of the Superficial Vein of the Index Finger

1. The practitioner instructs the parents to hold the child facing a place with sufficient light, and then the practitioner faces the child.

2. When observing the superficial vein of the right index finger of the child, the practitioner holds the end of the finger with the thumb and forefinger of the left hand, and then pushes and scrapes, two to three times, with the lateral margin of the right thumb, from the tip to root of the child's index finger with moderate strength, till the superficial vein appears in order to allow inspection. When observing the superficial vein of the child's left hand, the actions of the practitioner are the mirrored opposite to this i.e. child's left index finger is held with the practitioner's right hand and so forth.

3. The emphasis of inspecting here is focused on the three passes of the child's finger, the vein there reflects the changes between floating or deep; the colouration - red or purple, lightness or density; length or shortness, thickness or thinness.

Inspection of the skin and lower orifices

Depending on the age of the patient and the type of examination, one should ensure that the patient is accompanied by a suitable person, such as a chaperone, relative or health practitioner, to help avoid any disputes between the practitioner and the patient.

Method and Guidelines of the Tongue Examination

The tongue diagnosis mainly refers to the tongue observation, but is also listening to the construction of words; associated smells; inquiring; and scraping or wiping the tongue may also be combined for the overall diagnosis.

The position for tongue observation and posture of tongue extending

For tongue examination, the patients may take a sitting or supine position. A bright and clear, preferably natural, light is required for the observation of the tongue surface. The patient should extend the tongue out of the mouth easily, with a relaxed tongue body, a flat tongue surface and a slightly downward tongue tip; thus fully exposing the tongue body. Over-exertion on extending the tongue, tension or twisting of the tongue body and holding it out for a long duration may all affect the qi and blood circulation of the tongue and lead to changes in tongue colour, tongue coating and changes in dryness or wetness.

The method of tongue observation

The order of tongue observation: the tongue tip is first, then the middle part of the tongue and edges of the tongue and finally the root of the tongue; tongue coating is observed first and then the tongue body. The practice of tongue observation should be done quickly but carefully and comprehensively. The patient should, as far as possible, reduce the length of time the tongue is extended for. If unable to quickly diagnose the tongue manifestation, ask the patient to have a rest for about three to five minutes and then observe once more.

As stated, apart from the observation, other methods are combined to get the most information regarding the character of the tongue when necessary. For instance, the method of testing the coating by scraping the floating coat and observing the bottom of the coating, is an important aspect in differentiating the tongue. Any remaining tongue coating after scraping, or dirt left behind, indicates an excess pattern. Alternatively, any tongue coating that is easy to remove with scraping or a clean and smooth tongue body left after scraping indicates a deficient pattern. By using a sterilized tongue-depressor the practitioner may scrape the tongue surface from back to front, three to five times, with moderate force. For wiping out the tongue coating, the practitioner needs to wrap sterilized gauze on the finger and dip it in a little normal saline solution and then wipe several times. The above methods can all be used for the differentiation of tongue coating with or without root or a dyed coating from such things as food or medications.

Furthermore, the practitioner should inquire about the ability to taste and about any new or unpleasant tastes such as sweetness or bitterness and if there is either numbness, pain, or any hot or burning sensation of the tongue body.

The guidelines for tongue examination

Tongue examination is an important diagnostic tool in clinical practice, and some confounding factors have to be excluded in order to ensure accurate information.

1. **Influence of the light**

The observation of the tongue should be done in sufficient and soft natural light during the daytime, with the light shining directly onto the tongue surface. Coloured light should be avoided, as strong, weak or coloured light may affect the correct judgment. Lack of light or illumination may cause a dark tongue colour; a fluorescent lamp may cause a purple tongue colour and an incandescent lamp may cause a yellow tongue colour. In addition, reflection of surrounding coloured objects may also cause some changes to the tongue colour.

2. **Influence of food, drinks or medications**

Food, drinks or some medications may cause tongue changes. For example, the tongue coating may change from thick to thin after food because of the chewing friction and self-cleaning of the oral cavity; the tongue coating may change from dry to moist after drinking water; tea or fruit juices may change the colour of the coating, a relatively red tongue may occur after hot and spicy food; a thick and greasy coating may occur after overeating sweets, or sweet and greasy food and administration of narcotics; and a dark and greasy coating or mouldy and curdy coating may occur after long-term administration of antibiotics.

Some food or medications may colour the tongue coating, which is also called a stained coating. For instance, a white and thick coating may occur after drinking milk or soybean milk; a yellow coating may occur after eating egg yolk, orange and lactochrome (E20 colouring), and a grey coating may occur after eating black-coloured food, such as olives and dark plums, after some medications, as well as from long-term smoking. The stained coating will naturally emerge and disappear within a short period of time or can be wiped out easily. Generally the stained coating is not evenly stuck on the tongue surface and not consistent with any disease condition. If during inspection these colours are noticed then some questions can follow, the practitioner may inquire about the patient's intake of food and medications, or attempt to identify it by using the wiping-out method.

3. Influence of the oral cavity

Loss of teeth may cause a relatively thick tongue coating on the same-side, inserting artificial teeth may leave teeth marks on the tongue, and mouth breathing (possibly due to a blocked nose) may cause a dry tongue coating.

The above abnormal tongue changes need to be differentiated clinically to avoid confusing the whole diagnostic picture.

The sublingual veins

The sublingual veins refer to the big vertical vessels on the two sides of the frenulum on the under-surface of the tongue. The sublingual veins are pale purple, less than 2.7 mm in diameter and less than 3/5 of the distance from the sublingual fleshy attachment of the tongue to the tongue tip in length. The observation of sublingual vessels includes the observation of the changes in length, shape, colour, thinness or thickness and also the small sublingual vessels.

The method of observing the sublingual veins: ask the patient to open the mouth and curl the tongue body up to the palate, with the tongue tip slightly touching the palate and the tongue body naturally relaxed for the full exposure of the sublingual veins. Firstly, observe the changes of the big veins in thinness or thickness, colour, varicosity and curvature; and then observe the changes of the small and thin peripheral veins in colour, shape and whether or not there are dark purple bead-like nodules or purple veins present.

The Guidelines for Inquiry and History of the Present Disease

The guidelines for inquiry

1. Avoid the possibility of being disturbed, use a quiet and suitable environment

The communication of the practitioner and the patient must be in a quiet and suitable clinical room, which will not only help the practitioner focus on the task in hand, but will also be of benefit for the patient to open his thoughts and describe all kinds of sensations of the disease sufficiently. In this way, the practitioner can obtain the true disease data opportunely and exactly. This is most important to support the patient when they are reluctant to talk about their problems.

2. Be careful, kind, patient, empathic and attentive

The practitioner should have compassion and aim to comprehend the patient's suffering, with a kind, solemn, empathic and careful attitude. The practitioner should not only ask and listen to the patient's pathogenic condition and their concerns patiently and carefully, but also make the patient feel comfortable and want to actively engage in a discourse about their problems. Furthermore, the practitioner should pay attention to the patient's facial expression, body language and posture, and so on, giving timely and appropriate feedback, either verbally or by their general demeanour.

3. Use simple and easy language and react appropriately

During inquiry, the practitioner should use simple and easy words, avoiding using unnecessarily complicated medical terms. In the course of inquiry, the practitioner should not react to the patient's pathogenic conditions with language or facial expression that is pessimistic or shocked, for it may increase the patient's burden and be harmful to the recovery of the disease.

4. Inquire with emphasis; exhaustively, meticulously and in depth

Inquiry not only should emphasise the important, but also should be detailed and complete. The practitioner should focus on and grasp the patient's chief complaint or concern and inquire about it purposefully, in depth and with care. Although it is expected that the practitioner should give priority to the chief complaint, they must also gather the information regarding the general accompanying signs, while extensively collecting all the data of the pathogenic conditions. This process will reduce the possibility of missing the disease and unnecessarily, and incorrectly, affecting the diagnosis.

Consequently, during the inquiry examination, the practitioner should pay attention to, and listen out for, the chief complaint/concern of the patient and make an inquiry with this aim, but also meticulously inquire in sufficient depth. For example, if the practitioner understands the patient's chief symptom is a headache, one should further ask the position, characteristics, degree, time, triggers and other accompanying symptoms. At the same time, one should give consideration to other areas, such as sleep, emotion, or any disease in the whole body, which can assist in reaching the correct diagnosis and avoid missing the offending pathogenic conditions.

5. Encourage appropriately but avoid suggestive hints

When the patients fail to describe their disease conditions clearly, the practitioner should ask with an objective focus. When the patients are reluctant to describe some conditions in the presence of other people, the practitioner should ask in private. The practitioner should not suggest or induce the patients to describe their disease conditions according to the practitioner's subjective assumptions. By avoiding and abstaining from one-sided discourse, engaging in narrative discourse and keeping the inquiry patient centred, the practitioner can avoid distortion of the data of disease.

6. Make the treatment a priority for critical and emergency patients

When faced with patients in critical conditions, the practitioner should make a brief inquiry of the major symptoms and a quick examination to give time for the treatment.

In critical and emergency cases the practitioner should not hold up urgent treatment for questioning.

Definite identification of the chief complaint/concern

The chief complaint refers to the main symptoms and the duration of these ailments; such as, four limbs and joint migratory pain, lasting for one month; or cough with recurrent asthma attacks for twenty years and becoming more serious, accompanied by palpitations for one week.

The chief complaint is mostly the primary reason that prompted the patient to visit the clinic. It is also the primary symptom of the disease and an important clue and foundation for investigating, analysing and treating the disease. According to the chief complaint, the practitioner can estimate the category of the disease and the severity of the condition.

The chief complaint is often seen as the main diagnosis guide. However, the patient may complain about symptoms in any order and regardless of primary and secondary importance. Thus, the practitioner should firstly be adept at grasping the chief complaint through inquiring in depth. The practitioner should also inquire into the position, character, degree, triggers and time of the symptoms. If the pathogenic condition is complicated, the course of disease is long, multiple *zang* and *fu* are affected and there are many symptoms, and the chief complaint is difficult to identify, the practitioner should solve this by taking the most painful and urgent symptoms as the chief complaint.

The chief complaint may be summed up in concise and refined medical terminology. If this is the case then it should not use the patient's words and generally not be over twenty words. However, many Western practitioners of Chinese diagnostic methods use the patient's own words to describe the chief complaint/concern with the practitioner's explanations and descriptions coming later.

History of Present Illness (HPI)

The history of present illness (HPI) means inquiring about the whole course from the onset, and development, to changes of the illness and the treatment progress from its occurrence to the time that the patient visits the doctor. It includes four parts:
- The occurrence of the disease
- The development of the disease
- The procedure of the diagnosis and treatment
- The present symptoms.

1. The occurrence of the disease

The occurrence of the disease includes information on: when the symptoms began, what time of year/day; the degree of urgency; any reasons for its occurrence; the primary symptoms and characteristics; and any initial treatment received. When inquiring about the occurrence of the disease, it is very important to distinguish the cause, location and nature of a disease.

Generally, when the onset of a disease is acute and the duration is short, this usually belongs to an excess pattern. Alternatively, if the duration of the disease is chronic and there are recurrent attacks, with a prolonged time passing without healing, this mostly belongs to an internal injury disease, deficiency pattern or pattern of intermingled deficiency and excess.

The order of the occurrence of symptoms also gives a great deal of information e.g. if the disease presents with rib-side distension and pain following irascibility due to emotional dissatisfaction, this commonly belongs to the pattern of stagnation of liver qi; if the disease presents with distension in the stomach, with belching and lack of appetite and can be seen as due to voracious eating and drinking, this usually belongs to food stagnating in the stomach.

2. The development of the disease

The development of the disease means the changing conditions of the patient's disease from onset up to visiting the clinic. It is usually inquired of in the order of: time of onset, including characteristics and degree of the symptoms at the onset of the disease; when it took a favourable turn or became more serious; when new symptoms appeared; whether or not there is a regular pattern to the pathogenic conditions, and so on. Inquiring into the development of the disease is helpful to understand its pathogenic changes and trends.

3. The procedure of the diagnosis and treatment

The procedure of the diagnosis and treatment informs on the diagnosis and treatment conditions of the patient prior to this visit. For the initial visit, the practitioner should inquire carefully, in accordance with the order of time, such as which tests had been taken, the results, what diagnosis and treatment has been undertaken, and about the effect and reaction of any treatment, etc. Understanding the past conditions of the diagnosis and treatment can be used as reference in the current diagnosis and treatment.

4. The present symptoms

The present symptoms mean all the painful and uncomfortable symptoms of the patient, when visiting the clinic. The present symptoms are the most important evidence in differentiating disease and patterns, and are the most important findings of the inquiry examination. The collection of the present symptoms is a part of HPI but may be extensive and the reader is directed to the specific section on this in the inquiry examination in chapter five.

The Method and Guidelines of the Pulse Examination

The time

Morning is the best time for pulse examination, for it is easy to feel the true pulse condition without food or exercises influencing the yin-yang, qi, blood and meridians. The pulse examination should be done in a quiet internal and external environment.

The pulse taking requires one to three minutes and the practitioner should have even respiration to count the pulse beats of the patients' and to fully concentrate on the sensations from the fingers.

The posture

In either sitting or supine position, the patients are asked to place their arm at the same level as the heart, with the palm tilted upward and with a small pulse pillow under the dorsum of the wrist joint. This position allows for easy circulation of the qi and blood, not only making it easy for taking the pulse, but also for reflecting the true pulse of the body.

The fingers
The practitioner should be face-to-face with the patient, and should palpate the patient's right hand with their left hand and the patient's left hand with their right hand (although some practitioners will use their dominant hand for both sides, and some palpate simultaneously on both sides for comparison).

1. Location

The practitioner is supposed to locate the *guān*-region with their middle finger first, on the medial aspect of the styloid process, over the radial artery, and then to locate the *cùn*-region with their index finger and the *chǐ*-region with their ring finger. For children, the practitioner can use one thumb for the three regions because of their shorter and smaller *cùnkǒu* area.

2. The arrangement of the fingers

The three fingers are arched so the fingertips are at the same level, and the practitioner should feel the pulsation with the area between the fingertips and the belly of the tip (or pad), because this is the most sensitive area. The arrangement of fingers needs to be proportionate with the patient's body height, spreading fingers out for those who are tall with longer arms and keeping fingers closer together for those who are short with shorter arms.

3. Individual-finger palpation or simultaneous palpation with three fingers

Individual-finger palpation refers to palpating one region with one specific finger to experience the characteristic of one region, and the simultaneous palpation with three fingers refers to palpating the three regions together with even force to experience the overall pulse conditions of three regions and nine locations. Clinically the practitioner always combines the two ways.

4. Touching, pressing and searching

These three methods use the force of the fingers for the pulse examination to explore and distinguish the pulse manifestation. To press the finger gently and lightly on the skin is called touching, it is also called palpating by superficial or light touch. To press the finger in to the muscles and bones is called pressing, which is also called palpating by deep or heavy pressing. To investigate the most obvious characteristic of the pulsation using alternately gentle to heavy force, heavy to light force and pressing around to the left, right, back and front, is called searching. The practitioner should carefully experience the changes between touching, pressing and searching.

The body posture of palpation examination
Generally, the patient can be in a sitting position, supine position or side lying position, to sufficiently expose the areas for palpation. If the patient is sitting, the practitioner should stand or sit facing the patient, gently supporting the body with their left hand and palpate and press each area with the right hand. This posture is mostly used in the palpation of the

skin, hands and feet, and acupuncture points.

As for palpating the chest and abdomen, the patient should be in a supine position, relaxing the body, with the arms naturally lying at the sides of the trunk, and the legs naturally straightened. The practitioner should be standing to the right hand side of the patient, palpating areas of the patient's chest and abdomen, with the right or both hands. When palpating a lump in the patient's abdomen or testing abdominal tension, the practitioner may ask the patient to bend the knees and thus relax the abdominal muscles, or take a deep breath to assist the palpation examination.

In palpating the skin, the patient can choose suitable positions according to different problem areas, so as to sufficiently expose and have access to the area to be investigated. The practitioner should be standing on the right hand-side of the patient, with fingers of the hand close together and gently moving along the skin with the palm.

For palpating the skin of the forearm, the patient may be in a sitting or in a supine position. When examining the skin of the left forearm, the practitioner should hold the patient's upper arm, near the elbow, with the right hand and hold the patient's palm with the left hand, in order to bring the medial surface of the arm to face upwards, be flat and expose the skin of the forearm sufficiently. The practitioner should just stroke the skin of the forearm with their fingers or palms. When examining the skin of the right forearm, the handing skill is the mirrored opposite of the above, i.e. with left and right hands swapping position.

In palpating the hands and feet, the patient may be in the sitting or lying position (either supine or side lying) and should sufficiently expose the hands and feet. The practitioner should gently stroke using one hand, or stroke and hold the patient's hands and feet using both hands, comparing the left and right or the centre and dorsum of the hands and feet. The emphasis of the palpation examination here is to distinguish whether there is warmth or coldness in the centre of the hands or feet because for example if the hand or foot is hot, one can diagnose yin deficiency, etc.

SECTION 2
ANALYSIS OF CASES

1. xx, male, 35 years old. He has red urine, and generally has dry stool and often feels thirsty and has a dry pharynx. After he caught a cold two days ago, he developed aversion to cold with fever, anhidrosis (lack of or very minimal sweat), headache and body pain, stuffy nose with a deep and hoarse voice, a red tongue with yellow coating, a floating and tight pulse.

Which pattern should be diagnosed in this disease? Please make a pattern analysis.

Differentiation: Pattern of cold in the exterior and interior heat.

Analysis: The constitution of the patient is a yin deficient one, so he presented with red urine, dry stool, thirst and a dry pharynx. Due to catching wind-cold again, the interior heat was held back by the cold exterior and the yang qi was stagnated and blocked, so the patient manifested the symptoms of cold exterior as aversion to cold with fever, body pain and anhidrosis, etc. The red tongue with yellow coating is the manifestation of the interior heat fumigating and steaming. The floating and tight pulse are the characteristics of wind-cold harassing the exteriors.

2. ××, female, 38 years old. She was troubled by pulmonary tuberculosis (TB) for two years. In these last two months, she often presented with coughing up blood, cough, steaming bone with tidal fever, night sweating, loss of voice, a thin body, panting and shortness of breath, a cold body, aversion to wind, spontaneous sweating, reduced eating, loose stool, oedema of the face and limbs, a mirror-like, light red and fissured tongue with scant liquid coating, a deep and faint thready pulse.
Which pattern should be diagnosed in this disease? Please make a pattern analysis.

Differentiation: Pattern of deficiency of both yin and yang (deficiency of lung yin and yang deficiency of the spleen and kidney).

Analysis: The disease was caused by yin deficiency involving yang, and the functional disorder of the lung, spleen and kidneys, due to the chronic pulmonary tuberculosis. Chronic coughing up of blood damaged lung yin and then the vocal chords lost their moisture, and the damaged lung would not function normally, so the loss of voice appeared. The lung qi was dissipated so that the qi could not be dominated by the lung, then insecurity of *wei* yang, and then the panting, shortness of breath, cold body, aversion to wind and spontaneous sweating appeared. Steaming bone with tidal fever is caused by yin deficiency. Night sweating impaired the fluid. Essence and blood insufficiency often lead to thinness of the body. The spleen and kidney yang damage could produce reduced eating, loose stool, oedema of the face and limbs, which is the reduction of the life function, and the deficiency is difficult to recover from. The mirror-like, light red and fissured tongue with the scant fluid coating is due to yang deficiency and yin having dried up. The deep and faint thready pulse is the manifestation of failure of both yin and yang.

3. ××, female, 29 years old. The patient regularly breaks out with fever, in the afternoon, over the last two months and this fever aggravates after exertion, the degree of fever is sometimes low and sometimes high, wavering between 37.3℃ to 38℃. She often feels tired and fatigued, short of breath and experiences laziness in speaking, and spontaneous sweating. In addition she easily catches cold, has poor appetite and digestion, and loose stool. This current fever has lasted three days. The tongue is pale with a thin white coating. The pulse is weak.
Please write the patient's complaints, eight principal patterns diagnosis and the pathogenesis analysis.

Patient's complaints: Recurrent fever over two months, three days' duration in this instance.

Differentiation: Interior pattern, deficiency pattern, heat pattern.

Analysis: Middle qi is insufficient, the interior produces yin fire and overexertion leads to qi consumption, which can lead to long-term recurrent fever and will aggravate when tired. Qi deficiency deprived of nourishment can induce lack of spirit and fatigue, shortness of breath and laziness of speaking. Qi deficiency and insecurity of the *wei* exterior can induce spontaneous sweating and make it easy to catch colds. The deficiency of spleen qi and the failure of transportation and transformation can result in reduced eating, loose stool, a pale tongue with a thin white coating, and a weak pulse.

Diagnostics in Chinese Medicine

4. ××, male, 48 years old. This patient developed hepatitis five years ago, even after the treatment, the symptoms were sometimes mild or sometimes severe, and he had a poor appetite and digestion, with hypochondriac pain. His abdomen was swollen, ascites (fluid accumulation) tight as a drum, has appeared over the last three months and his abdominal circumference is 90 cm now (the original was 81 cm). He has fever with dysphoria and a bitter taste in the mouth, thirst without a desire to drink, scanty dark urine, viscous stools, a red margins of the tongue with a yellow greasy coating, a stringy and rapid pulse.

Please write the patient's complaints, eight principal patterns diagnosis and the pathogenesis analysis.

Patient's complaints: Hypochondriac pain, poor appetite and digestion for five years, abdominal swelling for the last three months.

Differentiation: Interior pattern, heat pattern, excess pattern.

Analysis: Damp and heat are blocked in middle *jiao*, turbid water is stopped and gathering, so that abdominal swelling, tight as a drum appeared. The damp-heat was steaming in the upper *jiao* so that fever with dysphoria and the bitter taste in the mouth, and thirst without desire to drink appeared. There was damp-heat in the lower *jiao* so that scanty dark urine, and viscous stool appeared. Accumulated damp-heat is in the liver and spleen, so that poor appetite and digestion, and hypochondriac pain appeared. Both the red margin of the tongue with the yellow greasy coating and stringy and rapid pulse indicate that the damp-heat is severe, and the disease position is in the liver and spleen.

5. ××, male, 56 years old. The patient suddenly fainted and fell unconscious one year ago, and then regained consciousness after treatment. Now movement is difficult in his left upper and lower limbs. Constipation appeared and he passes a stool only every two or three days. Although there is awareness of wanting to pass stool, he feels too weak to pass it, moreover he experiences sweating and shortness of breath whenever he does defaecate. After passing stool, he feels tired, suffers agonising abdominal pains, becomes pale, spiritless and has qi deficiency, a pale and tender tongue with a thin and white coating, and a feeble pulse without strength.

Please write the patient's complaints, eight principal patterns diagnosis and the pathogenesis analysis.

Patient's complaints: Left hemiplegia and constipation for a year.

Differentiation: Interior pattern, deficiency pattern, yin pattern.

Analysis: The spleen is the acquired foundation, the lung governs qi. Qi deficiency of the spleen and lung, weakness of the blood movement, malnutrition of the channels, caused the hemiplegia to appear. The lung and the large intestine are interior-exteriorly related, qi deficiency of the lung can cause weakness to transfer to the large intestine, so that there is awareness of defaecation, but he feels too weak to pass stool. Lack of consolidation of the lung *wei* qi caused the sweating and shortness of breath after passing the stool. Deficiency of the spleen can cause insufficiency of transportation and transformation, so that the paleness, lack of spirit and qi deficiency appeared. The tongue and pulse both indicate the deficiency of qi.

6. ××, female, 38 years old. The patient experiences insomnia and many dreams, dizziness, palpitations and shortness of breath, limb numbness, soreness and weakness of

the waist and knees, tidal fever with night sweating, dysphoria with a feverish sensation in the chest, palms and soles, early menstruation with a normal red colour, a red tongue with reduced coating, a thready and rapid pulse.

Please write the eight principal patterns diagnosis and the pathogenesis analysis.

Differentiation: Yin deficiency (patterns of yin deficiency of the heart and kidney).

Analysis: The patient has tidal fever with night sweating, dysphoria (restlessness) with a feverish sensation in the chest, palms and soles, a red tongue with reduced coating, a thready and rapid pulse; these are all indicative of endogenous heat due to yin deficiency. Insomnia and excess dreams, dizziness, palpitations and shortness of breath, and limb numbness are all indicative of insufficiency of heart blood. Soreness and weakness of the lumbar region and knees, and dizziness are both indicative of deficiency of the kidney. Based on the above the patient belongs to patterns of yin deficiency of the heart and kidney.

7. ××, male, 40 years old. The patient complains of dizziness and has a fever in the head, left sided migraine, left face numbness, tinnitus in the night, distending pain of the eyes, disturbed sleep, palpitations, spasm and pain of the whole body, chest pain, feels like throwing up occasionally, is impatient and irritable, when he is angry his hand trembles, he has weakness of the legs and cold feet, a floating pulse without strength, a red dry tongue without coating.

Please make diagnosis and the pathogenesis analysis.

Differentiation: Patterns of intermingled deficiency and excess (upper excess and lower deficiency).

Analysis: The patient has disturbed sleep, palpitations, facial numbness, spasm and pain of the whole body, a red dry tongue without coating which are all indicative of insufficiency of yin blood. Dizziness and fever in the head, left sided migraine, distending pain of the eyes, impatience and irritability are all indicative of upper hyperactivity of liver yang. Hand-trembling when angry is indicative of hyperactive liver yang causing wind. Weakness of the legs and cold feet, a floating pulse without strength are all indicative of lower yin deficiency and upper yang excess, patterns of intermingled deficiency and excess, that is upper excess and lower deficiency.

8. ××, male, 9 years old. The patient had aversion to cold with fever at first, and then developed whooping cough due to retention of phlegm in the throat, that sounds like a see-saw, has a stuffy nose, and dry mouth, difficulty with urination and defaecation, red mouth and lips, a floating, slippery and rapid pulse on the right, a stringy and floating pulse on the left, a yellow and white mixed tongue coating.

Please make diagnosis and the pathogenesis analysis.

Differentiation: Simultaneous exterior and interior pattern, exterior pattern involving the interior (a pattern of asthma with wind-cold tightening the lung, and phlegm-fire interior stagnation).

Analysis: Aversion to cold with fever at first, and then cough is indicative of a exterior pattern with wind-cold tightening the lung. A floating pulse and white coating still remain which indicates that the exterior pathogens are not expelled. The red mouth and lips, whooping cough wheezing due to retention of phlegm in the throat, stuffy nose and dry mouth, difficulty in urination and defaecation, slippery and rapid pulse, and yellow coating are all indicative of heat due to exterior pathogens entering into the interior, burning fluid into phlegm, the lung is burned by fire and loses its function of dispersion and descending. An overview of the above clinical manifestations indicates that the patient belongs to the pattern of asthma with wind-cold tightening the lung, phlegm-fire interior stagnation, and the disease's nature is a simultaneous exterior and interior pattern, an exterior pattern involving the interior.

9. ××, male, 28 years old. He suddenly collapsed during a flood when fighting to rescue others, his fever and sweating cannot abate. The mind is clear after emergency treatment, but he feels thirsty, tired, has dark urine, a red tongue, a feeble and rapid pulse. Which pattern should be diagnosed in this disease? Please make a pattern analysis.

Differentiation: pattern of summer-heat.

Analysis: This pattern is due to prolonged labour in the summer time, summer heat steaming, invading upper orifices, burning the interior spirit, so that sudden collapse manifested. The summer-heat can injure the fluid and qi, so that fever and sweating can not abate. Although the mind is clear, the fluid was injured by heat, so that thirst and dark urine manifested. Excessive sweating is the condition of summer, the qi disappeared with the sweating, so that tiredness, feebleness and a rapid pulse manifested.

10. ××, female, 67 years old. She has dry skin and desquamation, which is very itchy at night, dizziness, sallow complexion, a pale tongue, and a weak pulse.
Which pattern should be diagnosed in this disease? Please make a pattern analysis.

Differentiation: Pattern of blood deficiency causing wind.

Analysis: The blood deficiency causes the malnutrition of the skin, so that a sallow complexion, dry skin and even desquamation manifest. Blood deficiency causes wind, so itchiness, which is the characteristic of wind being mobile, manifested. Blood deficiency can cause the malnutrition of the brain marrow, so that dizziness manifested. A pale tongue and weak pulse indicated that it is the pattern of blood deficiency.

11. ××, male, 25 years old. He had a pain in the lumbus and lower limb ankylosis for three years. Currently he feels pain in the chest, lumbus and lower limb joints, has swelling of the knee and ankle joints which are difficult to straighten, and needs to use crutches to walk. The pain becomes worse during the cold rainy weather. The leg muscle has atrophied, he is tired and fatigued, has a pale tongue with a thin coating, a thready and slippery pulse. Please make pattern differential diagnosis of pathogen and pathogenesis analysis.

Differentiation: Pattern of dampness (cold-dampness).

Analysis: The wind-cold dampness pathogen invaded the meridians and joints, the qi and blood were blocked, so that pain and swelling of the joints, and contorted joints manifested. The emphasis is on cold-dampness, so that the pain became worse during the cold rainy weather. The cold-dampness stagnated for a long time, causing malnutrition of qi and blood, so that tiredness, fatigue, and muscle atrophy manifested. The tongue and pulse also indicated cold-dampness and insufficiency of qi and blood.

12. ××, female, 37 years old. The last menstruation was five months ago; treatment was not effective. Now she experiences dizziness and forgetfulness, palpitations and shortness

of breath, fatigue and spontaneous sweating, the sleep is not good, with many dreams, she has body pain, leg soreness and cramps, and a reduction in vaginal discharge, a pale tongue with thin white coating, and a deep and thready pulse.

Please make pattern differential diagnosis of qi and blood, and pathogenesis analysis.

Differentiation: Pattern of deficiency of both qi and blood.

Analysis: The lack of *ying*-blood causes the lack of source of menses, so that the amenorrhoea manifested. The blood is malnourished, so that dizziness and forgetfulness manifested. The deficiency of blood causes malnutrition of the channels, so that leg soreness and cramps, and body pain manifested. The deficiency of heart blood can cause palpitations and insomnia. The deficiency of spleen qi can cause shortness of breath, fatigue and spontaneous sweating. The tongue and pulse also indicated deficiency of qi and blood.

13. ××, female, 37 years old. The patient has experienced pain of the left side of the chest in the last two weeks, has coughed for five days which produced white foamy phlegm, accompanied by headache, aversion to cold with fever, sweating, chest tightness and shortness of breath. In addition to these symptoms during visiting, the left chest and hypochondrium is distended with pain, she has poor appetite and digestion, the tongue coating is thin and greasy and the root coating is a little bit thick, she has a soft and rapid pulse that is also slippery.

Please make differential diagnosis of qi, blood and fluid, and pathogenesis analysis.

Differentiation: Pattern of fluid retention (exogenous disease due to wind pathogenic fluid retained in chest and hypochondrium).

Analysis: The patient had suffered from this condition for two weeks, felt pain in the left side of the chest in the beginning because of fluid retained in the chest and hypochondrium, the qi movement was blocked. Aversion to cold with fever, sweating with headache for five days occurred because of exogenous disease due to wind pathogens. The lung governs skin and hair. When the wind pathogen invades the exterior of skin and hair, it leads to failure of lung qi in dispersion, and adds fluid retained in the chest and hypochondrium, therefore chest tightness and shortness of breath, and chest and hypochondrium is distension with pain manifested. The pathogen invaded the spleen and stomach, so that poor appetite and digestion manifested. The thin and greasy coating and the root coating being a little bit thick, with the soft and rapid pulse with slipperiness all indicate fluid retention.

14. ××, female, 26 years old. She experiences dizziness, blurred vision, palpitations and insomnia, a fixed stabbing pain occurs in the abdomen due to postpartum excessive loss of blood one month ago. Dark and purple tongue with ecchymosis, thin and rough pulse.

Which pattern should be diagnosed? Please make a differentiation analysis of qi and blood.

Differentiation: Blood deficiency-stasis pattern.

Analysis: All the symptoms are caused by deficiency of blood, impeded flow of blood, and the blood stasis outside the vessels. The dizziness, blurred vision, palpitations and insomnia are due to blood deficiency, which leads to malnutrition of the brain and mind. When blood stasis accumulates in the abdomen, a fixed stabbing pain may manifest. Deficiency and stasis of blood result in a dark and purple tongue with ecchymosis, and a thin and rough pulse.

15. ××, female, 29 years old. Due to massive puerperal bleeding, the following suddenly occurred, a pale complexion, cold limbs, profuse sweating, syncope (transient unconsciousness), pale tongue, floating, large and scattered pulse.
Which pattern should be diagnosed? Please make a pattern analysis.
Differentiation: Collapse of qi due to haemorrhage.
Analysis: Blood and qi are interdependent, and qi has nothing to depend on due to the massive bleeding, since qi depletion leads to exhaustion of yang, qi and blood cannot nourish the upper part of the body. Cold limbs are due to failure of yang qi to warm the limbs; resulting in a pale complexion; the skin is no longer warm, which causes cold sweat. Mind scatters along with qi, and results in syncope. Blood vessels fail to be supported by qi and blood, so a pale tongue may occur.

16. ××, male, 28 years old, thin, he saw doctor on April 1st, he felt thirsty and had a dry pharynx, and cough, when he came back from Inner Mongolia, two days ago. Today his cough is worse, with a little sputum, which is difficult to expectorate, he is thirsty with a desire to drink, has a dry pharynx and lips, dry skin, a red tongue with a thin coating and a thready and rapid pulse.
Differentiation: Dryness pattern (pattern of dryness invading the lung *jīn*).
Analysis: The patient is very thin, and has experienced an invasion by a wind and dry pathogen during the windy spring, which results in consumption and deficiency of body fluids (*jīn*), especially in the lung. The dry pharynx and mouth, cough, a little sputum which is difficult to expectorate, thirst with a desire to drink, dry skin, red tongue with thin coating and thread and rapid pulse, are all symptoms of the pattern of injury to body fluid (*jīn*).

17. ××, male, 36 years old. Chronic spermatorrhoea, two to three times every week, with dizziness, tinnitus, restlessness, insomnia, palpitations, dream-disturbed sleep, a dry mouth and throat, night sweats, weakness in the lower back and knees, a red tongue with a scanty coating and a thready and rapid pulse.
Which pattern should be diagnosed? Please make a pathogenesis analysis.
Differentiation: Heart-kidney disharmony pattern.
Analysis: Insufficient kidney yin and heart yin, and then with hyperactive heart fire disturbs the mind, leading to restlessness, insomnia, palpitations, and dream-disturbed sleep. Weakness in the lower back and knees, with dizziness and tinnitus are due to reduced marrow due to insufficient kidney yin. Disturbance of the sperm chamber due to yin deficiency and fire blazing can lead to spermatorrhoea. The dry mouth and throat, night sweat, red tongue with scanty coating and thready and rapid pulse all indicate yin deficiency and fire blazing.

18. ××, male, 58 years old. He has a history of hepatitis. Over the last half a year, he has often experienced a scurrying and distending pain in the hypochondrium, depression and irritability, anorexia, fullness in the abdomen, borborygmus, flatulence or abdominal pain, tenesmus (alleviated after diarrhoea), a pale tongue with a white coating and a wiry moderate pulse.
Which pattern should be diagnosed? Please make a pathogenesis analysis.

Differentiation: Pattern of stagnation of liver qi with deficiency of the spleen.

Analysis: The scurrying and distending pain in the hypochondrium is due to failture in the smooth flow of liver qi. Depression and irritability results from unsmooth flow of liver qi. Anorexia and fullness in the abdomen are caused by failure of the spleen's transportation from the liver problem. Stagnant qi and retention of dampness can lead to borborygmus, tenesmus, and abdominal pain. Alleviation of pain after diarrhoea is due to the temporarily smooth flow of qi. Lassitude is a symptom of spleen deficiency. A pale tongue with white coating and a wiry pulse are symptoms of stagnation of liver qi with deficiency of spleen.

19. ××, female, 65 years old. The patient often has diarrhoea once every morning for the last six months; she has an urgent desire to defaecate and does with watery stools, and experiences dizziness, lassitude, and prolapse of the anus. This is accompanied by loss of appetite, weakness in the lower back and knees, aversion to cold and cold limbs, a pale tongue with a white coating and thready weak pulse.
Which pattern should be diagnosed? Please make a pathogenesis analysis.

Differentiation: Spleen-kidney yang deficiency pattern.

Analysis: Diarrhoea at dawn is caused by spleen-kidney yang deficiency, insufficient fire of the *mingmen* and sinking of clear yang. Dizziness, lassitude, and prolapse of the anus are symptoms of qi deficiency and qi sinking. The loss of appetite is due to spleen deficiency. Weakness in the lower back and knees, dizziness, aversion to cold and cold limbs, are caused by deficiency of kidney yang. A pale tongue with white coating and a thready weak pulse are the manifestation of a deficiency-cold pattern. The above pattern is diarrhoea before dawn due to deficiency of spleen-kidney yang and disturbance of transportation and transformation.

20. ××, female, 38 years old. She has insomnia and dream-disturbed sleep, dizziness, tinnitus, palpitations, shortness of breath, numbness in the hands and feet, weakness in the lower back and knees, tidal fever and night sweating, heat in the chest, palms and soles, early menstrual cycle, scanty and red menorrhoea, a red tongue with a scanty coating, and a thin and rapid pulse.
Which pattern should be diagnosed? Please make a pathogenesis analysis.

Differentiation: Heart-kidney yin deficiency pattern.

Analysis: The tidal fever and night sweating, heat in the chest, palms and soles, red tongue with scanty coating, thin and rapid pulse are all due to yin deficiency and internal heat. The insomnia and dream-disturbed sleep, dizziness, tinnitus, palpitations, numbness in the hands and feet are caused by the deficiency of heart blood. Weakness in the lower back and knees, dizziness, and tinnitus results from the deficiency of kidney. The early menstrual cycle is a symptom of yin deficiency of the heart and kidney.

21. ××, female, 14 years old. The patient has cough and fever for three days, headache, mild aversion to wind, little sweat, with expectoration of yellow sputum, dry mouth and painful throat, yellow urine, dry stools, a red tongue, a thin white with a little yellow coating, and a floating rapid pulse.
Which pattern should be diagnosed? Please make a pathogenesis analysis.

Differentiation: Wind-heat attacking the lung pattern.

Analysis: Fever, headache, mild aversion to wind, little sweat, red tongue, thin white with a little yellow coating, and floating rapid pulse are all the symptoms of wind-heat. The function of the skin and body hair has failed, cough is due to invasion of the lung by exogenous pathogens, leading to failure of the lung qi to disperse and descend. Thirst, a painful throat and yellow urine are due to impairment of body fluids by exuberant heat. The lung and the large intestine form a *zang-fu* pair, when the lung heat spreads to the large intestine there is dry stool. This pattern is caused by external contraction of wind-heat and failure of the dispersing functions of the lung.

22. ××, male, 40 years old. The patient said that she feels dizzy, has heat in the head, left sided migraine, numbness on the left side of the face, tinnitus at night, swollen and painful eyes, bad sleep, palpitations, pain in the chest, vomits regularly, depression and irritability, hand tremors, weakness of the legs and cold feet, a floating and weak pulse, a red and dry tongue and no coating.
Which pattern should be diagnosed? Please make a pathogenesis analysis.
Differentiation: Pattern of liver yang hyperactivity.
Analysis: Insomnia, palpitations, numbness of left side of the face, a red tongue and no coating are the manifestation of insufficiency of yin-blood. Dizziness, heat in the head, left sided migraine, swollen and painful eyes, depression and irritability, are symptoms of liver yang hyperactivity. Irritability, and hand tremor indicates liver yang transforming into wind. Weakness of the legs and cold feet, and a floating and weak pulse result from upper excess and lower deficiency due to yang hyperactivity and yin deficiency.

23. ××, male, 34 years old. He recently often experiences nausea on seeing food and vomits seriously once he has eaten a little, and has not been able to attend work due to this. He experiences belching, discomfort of the gastric cavity, oppression in the chest and pain in the hypochondrium, heat of the upper body and cold of the lower limbs, and disturbed sleep at night. He has a red tongue tip with a thin white coating, wiry pulse.
Which pattern should be diagnosed? Please make a pathogenesis analysis.
Differentiation: Liver-stomach disharmony pattern.
Analysis: Belching, discomfort of the gastric cavity, nausea, and vomiting after eating, all result from counterflowing rise of qi due to failure of stomach qi to descend. Oppression in the chest and pain in the hypochondrium, and a wiry pulse are due to qi stagnation in the liver. All the above symptoms are due to liver-qi attacking the stomach and disharmony of the liver and stomach. Heat of the upper body and cold of the lower limbs, a red tongue tip with white coating all result from upper heat and lower cold.

24. ××, female, 34 years old. She had an abortion three years ago, and since then she often experiences spontaneous sweating, aversion to wind, tingling in the abdomen, invasion of cold wind, poor appetite, wasting away and weakness, shortness of breath, scanty menstruation, a pale tongue with a white coating and a weak pulse.
Which pattern should be diagnosed? Please make a pattern analysis.
Differentiation: Spleen-lung qi deficiency pattern.
Analysis: Wasting away and weakness, shortness of breath, scanty menstruation, a pale tongue and weak pulse are due to injury of qi and blood after the abortion. Spontaneous

sweating is due to qi deficiency, which results in the interstitial spaces of the muscles becoming loose and releasing the body fluids. Aversion to wind, and often experiencing invasion of cold wind are due to feeble defensive power of external or *wei* qi. Poor appetite and shortness of breath are the symptoms of qi deficiency of the lung and spleen.

25. ××, male, 50 years old. He often experiences palpitations after a meal, which is often induced by fatigue and fevered emotion, accompanied by chest distress, shortness of breath, pale complexion, dizziness, and cold sweating. He also has mild oedema of the lower limbs, a little phlegm in the morning, loose stools, a deep and slippery pulse on the right side, weak on the left side, knotted and intermittent on both, a pale tongue with a thin white coating.
Please make differentiation diagnosis and pathogenesis analysis.
   Differentiation: Heart qi deficiency pattern accompanied by spleen deficiency and exuberance of dampness.
   Analysis: The heart is situated in the chest, *zōng* (gathering) qi fails to work well because of deficient heart qi, this causes chest distress, shortness of breath, and palpitations. The pale complexion is due to deficient qi not pushing blood to nourish. Deficient qi leads to spontaneous sweating due to hypofunction of the superficial portion. Qi is consumed when active, resulting in deterioration. Phlegm, oedema and loose stools are due to spleen deficiency and exuberance of dampness. The tongue and pulse are also manifestations of the above pattern.

26. ××, female, 35 years old. She experiences pain in the hypochondrium on both sides, which became more serious on the right side, eight days ago. Now she has alternating chills and fever, yellow skin and eyes; distension in the chest, nausea, loss of appetite, a bitter taste in the mouth, dark urine, dry stools, distending pain in the forehead, a red tongue tip and sides with a white and yellow greasy coating, and a soggy rapid pulse.
Please make differentiation diagnosis and pathogenesis analysis.
   Differentiation: Liver and gallbladder damp-heat pattern.
   Analysis: Alternating chills and fever, yellow skin and eyes, a bitter taste in the mouth, dark urine, and dry stools are caused by an accumulation of damp-heat in the liver and gallbladder. Pain in the hypochondrium is due to uneven qi flow of the liver and gallbladder. Damp-heat of the liver and gallbladder affects the stomach, leading to distension in the chest, nausea and loss of appetite, a red tongue with a white and yellow greasy coating, and a soggy rapid pulse.

27. ××, male, 44 years old. Swelling and prolapse of his right scrotum for three years. The symptoms change regularly becoming greater or lesser and moving up and down. The symptoms are in the scrotum when he stands up but are accompanied by swelling and pain of the lower abdomen as well as a sensation of cold. The pain becomes more serious when he gets cold and improves when he warms up. He has a white-slippery coating and a wiry pulse.
Please state the chief complaints and make the differentiation, diagnosis and analysis of pathogenesis.
   Chief complaints: Swelling and prolapse of his right scrotum, for three years.

Differentiation: Cold stagnating in the liver channel pattern.

Analysis: The liver channel surrounds the genitals, passing through the lower abdomen, when the cold invades the liver channel and accumulates in the genitals and the ensuing uneven flow results in swelling, prolapse and cold pain of the scrotum and contracture of the lower abdomen and thus improves when he warms up. The white slippery tongue coating is because of endogenous excessive cold, and the wiry pulse is due to cold accumulation in the liver channel.

28. ××, male, 62 years old. Over the past six months he often experiences more dribbling of urine after urination, frequent nocturia, but thin and clear urine, shortness of breath and lassitude, an ache in the lower abdomen, obvious decreased auditory function on one side, a pale tongue with a white coating and a weak pulse.
Please make an analysis for the diagnosis of this pattern.

Differentiation: Kidney qi insecurity pattern.

Analysis: Dribbling after urination, and frequent nocturia are due to insufficient kidney function from deficiency of kidney qi in the elderly, and disorder of the urinary bladder; the lower abdomen is the storage of the kidney, the ear is the window of the kidney, so there are aches in the lower abdomen, and decreased auditory function.

29. ××, female, 26 years old. Last September she experienced haemoptysis of about 500ml, and was diagnosed with bronchiectasis, with cough, phlegm with bright red blood again the following March, and has not improved at all, meanwhile she experiences burning pain in the chest and hypochondrium, irritability and bad temper, coughing, spitting blood, a red tongue with a thin and yellow coating, and a wiry thin and rapid pulse.
Please make the analysis of the diagnosis of pattern.

Differentiation: Pattern of liver fire invasion of the lung.

Analysis: The burning pain in the chest and hypochondrium, irritability and bad temper, and a wiry thin and rapid pulse are all due to liver fire flaming upward. When liver fire scorches the lung channel, vessels get injured and blood leaks out, leading to spitting of blood. The red tongue with thin and yellow coating, are heat symptoms.

30. ××, male, 24 years old. He experienced pain in the abdomen and diarrhoea one night due to eating too much raw or cold food, two months ago, and recovered after taking Western medicine, today he has serious diarrhoea, a sallow complexion, diarrhoea like water, seven or eight times everyday, distress in the abdomen and stomach, anorexia, nausea, lack of taste in the mouth, absence of thirst, heaviness in the head and body, a white greasy coating, and a soggy pulse.
Please make a pattern analysis.

Differentiation: Cold-dampness accumulating in the spleen pattern.

Analysis: Eating too much raw or cold food, causes cold-dampness to accumulate, causing dysfunction of the spleen and stomach in transporting and transforming, ascending and descending, marked by anorexia, and nausea. Heaviness in the head and body, lack of taste in the mouth, absence of thirst, and a white greasy coating are symptoms of cold-damp accumulating in the body, the soggy pulse is due to damp accumulating in the spleen.

31. ××, female, 45 years old. She experienced fullness in the stomach when eating larger portions or when cold, for several years. This week she has fullness and distending pain in the stomach, which dislikes palpation, fetid stools, twice everyday, and a sallow complexion, she is slim and weak, and has a thick and greasy tongue coating and slippery strong pulse.
Please make the analysis of the diagnosis of pattern.
   Differentiation: Food retention in the stomach and intestine pattern.
   Analysis: This refers to the pattern due to weakness of stomach qi, food retention in the stomach, failure of the function of the stomach and uneven flow of qi, which caused the fullness and distending pain in the stomach which cannot be palpated, the fetid stools, thick greasy tongue coating and slippery strong pulse.

32. ××, male, 25 years old. He experienced abdominal pain, and diarrhoea with foul smell and undigested food, two days ago and was diagnosed with acute enteritis. Currently he has abdominal pain, with yellow and fetid stools, accompanied by a burning feeling around the anus, dark urine, thirst, fever, a red tongue with a yellow greasy coating, a slippery and rapid pulse.
Please make a pattern analysis.
   Differentiation: Large intestine damp-heat pattern.
   Analysis: Damp-heat invasion of the large intestine obstructs qi movement causing yellow and fetid stools; the burning sensation around the anus is due to the invasion of heat into the large intestine. Scanty dark urine, thirst and fever are also symptoms of heat. The red tongue with yellow greasy coating, and the slippery and rapid pulse are symptoms of damp-heat.

33. Tong ××, female, 36 years old. For the past six months she often has ulcers in the mouth and tongue and feels depressed due to being laid off work. This week she has new ulcers in the mouth and tongue, which are large like soya beans and painful especially at night, even disturbing her sleep, she is thirsty with a sore-throat, hungry without a desire to eat, has dark and scanty urine, dry stools, a red tongue with a thin yellow coating, a rapid pulse.
Please make a pattern analysis.
   Differentiation: Heart fire hyperactivity pattern.
   Analysis: The depression, and the ensuing transformation from liver qi stagnation into fire that burned the tongue, results in ulcers in the mouth and tongue. Insomnia is due to heat harassing the mind and pain of the tongue. Hunger without a desire to eat is due to the pain of the tongue and the difficulty in eating. When heart fire moves into the small intestine, there is dark and scanty urine. Thirst and sore-throat, dry stools, a red tongue with thin yellow coating, and a rapid pulse are caused by injury to body fluids (jīn) invaded by heat.

34. ××, female, 18 years old. After she failed the university entrance exam half a year ago, she became restless, developed insomnia, and recently talks nonsense, experiences

irregular laughing and weeping. She is excited all day long, has a flushed face and bloodshot eyes, has much phlegm, dark and scanty urine, dry stools, a red tongue with a yellow greasy coating, and a slippery rapid pulse.

Which pattern should be diagnosed? Please make a pattern analysis.

Differentiation: Phlegm fire agitation pattern.

Analysis: The mind in disorder is due to qi stagnation or mental agitation is due to phlegm-fire. The flushed face and bloodshot eyes, constipation, yellow urine, red tongue with yellow greasy coating, and slippery rapid pulse are due to internal exuberance of phlegm and fire.

Index

A

abdominal colicky pain, 161
abdominal distending pain, 136
abdominal distension, 31, 78, 85, 87, 124, 149, 153, 186, 222, 223, 226, 228, 249, 250, 251, 262, 266, 267, 270, 272, 274, 300
abdominal dull pain, 226
abdominal fullness, 124, 284, 297
abdominal fullness with distension and pain, 281
abdominal masses, 175, 184, 238, 241
abdominal pain, 18, 26, 63, 84, 124, 131, 161, 217, 228, 229, 230, 231, 234, 270, 272, 333
abdominal pain with refusal for pressure, 220
abdominal sagging and distension, 166
abdominal swelling, 324
abnormal amount of menstrual flow, 97
abnormal behaviour, 201
abnormal breath, 65
abnormal colour and texture of menstrual flow, 98
abnormal form of the skin, 35
abnormal frequency of defaecation, 94
abnormal frequency of urine, 96
abnormal menstrual cycle, 97
abnormal menstruation, 238, 246
abnormal movements, 17
abnormal passage to the pericardium, 291
abnormal posture, 17
abnormal sensation of urination, 96
abnormal sensation on defaecation, 95
abnormal speech, 8
abnormal testis, 34
abnormal texture of stool, 95
abnormal volume of urine, 96
abnormality of the heart mind, 267
abnormality of *wei*, 130
abortion, 330
abscess, toxin or furuncle complicated by septicaemia, 64
absence of sweating, 159, 207
absence of taste, 132, 222
absence of taste with lack of thirst, 133
absence of thirst, 91, 228, 332
absent-mindedness, 255, 258
accompanying pus and blood, 160
accumulated heat, 39, 134
accumulated heat of the *zang-fu* and external pathogens, 29
accumulated toxin attacking upward, 28
accumulating and binding of damp and heat, 85
accumulation and gathering, 125
accumulation and stagnation in the stomach and intestines, 70
accumulation and stagnation of damp-heat, 95
accumulation and stagnation of damp-heat with wind-pathogen depressing damp in the muscles and skin, 37
accumulation and stagnation of liver qi, 86
accumulation and stagnation of qi and blood, 30
accumulation and stagnation of yin-cold, 38
accumulation of damp-heat, 38
accumulation of damp-heat in the middle *jiao*, 81
accumulation of damp-heat in the spleen, 223
accumulation of food, 53, 54, 63
accumulation of heat in the lung and stomach, 26, 37
accumulation of heat in the stomach, 39

accumulation of heat in the *yangming*, 64
accumulation of phlegm and food, 111
accumulation of phlegm-heat, 50
accumulation of the pathogenic qi, 56
accumulation of wind-dampness, 33
accumulations and gatherings, 31, 110
acerbic taste, 94
ache in the lower abdomen, 332
aching and weakness of the lumbar region and knees, 86
aching back and knee joints, 268
aching lumbus and knees, 83
aching of the lumbar region and knee joints, 20
aching pain, 82
acid and undigested food, 236
acid regurgitation, 87, 161, 222, 234, 235, 236, 269, 272, 312
acid-putrid odour, 71
acne, 199
acquired constitution deprived of nourishment, 30
acquired constitutional deprivation of nourishment, 32
acrid, spicy or hot foods, 233
acromphalus, 31
acute course, 211
acute enteritis, 333
acute gastritis, 312
acute infectious inflammation, 21
acute mastitis, 31

acute onset, 245
acute pain, 63
acute pain below the heart, 300
acute pain pattern, 25
acute throat disorder, 31
additional patterns differentiation, 275
adverse rising of the liver wind with phlegm, 63
afternoon fever, 191, 216, 217, 256
ageing process, 261
aggravated by cold, 157, 231, 236, 252
aggravated by pressure, 218, 220, 281
aggravated on exertion, 265
aggressive and violent behaviour, 192
agitation of liver wind, 158
allergic rhinitis, 39
alleviated by warmth, 231, 252
alleviation by sighing, 167
alliaceous (like garlic) odour, 71
alopaecia, 20, 256, 257
alternating chills and fever, 78, 249, 251, 283, 301, 331
alternating constipation and diarrhoea, 270
alternating loose and dry stool, 95
alternating vomiting and diarrhoea, 161
amenorrhoea, 98, 170, 239, 241, 255, 256, 257, 259, 266, 267, 327
amnesia, 266
an aversion to pressure, 122
anal abscesses, 34

anal fissure, 34, 40
anal fistula, 34
anal prolapse, 95
analysis of pattern differentiation, 312
analysis of pattern differentiation of diseases due to improper diet and activity, 161
analysis of the exterior patterns, 130
anger, 160, 242, 269
anger damage, 160
anhidrosis, 322
ankyloglossia, 52
anorexia, 92, 182, 222, 233, 234, 249, 250, 285, 312, 328, 332
anterior yin, 33
antrum auris, 243
anxiety, 8, 160, 198, 263, 266
anxiety damage, 160
anxiety injuring heart blood, 267
apathy, 143, 144, 201, 204
aphasia, 162
aphasia with a stiff tongue, 247, 250
aphonia, 62
aphtha, 27
apical pulse, 122
apoplexy, 238
appetite and quantity of food, 92
apprehension, 263
apprehensiveness and lack of peace, 161
arched-back rigidity, 24, 32
arrangement of the fingers, 321
arthritis, 63

ascendant hyperactivity of liver yang, 30, 190, 239
ascending counter-flow of damp-heat, 25
asthma, 31, 206, 211, 213, 265, 319
asymmetry of both sides of the bony thorax, 31
atrophy-flaccidity illnesses, 18
attack of cold, 131, 157
attack of dampness, 159
attack of exterior pathogens, 66
attack of wind, 131
attack of wind-heat, 34, 131
attack on the pericardium by heat, 295
aversion to cold, 76, 79, 129, 131, 132, 138, 140, 142, 146, 157, 159, 162, 180, 196, 207, 213, 215, 221, 255, 276, 277, 278, 285, 322, 325, 327, 329
aversion to cold and fever, 131
aversion to cold and preference for warmth, 135
aversion to cold with a preference for warmth, 132
aversion to cold with fever, 76, 299, 300
aversion to cold without fever, 131
aversion to food, 91
aversion to food smells, 236
aversion to heat, 244
aversion to heat and preference for cold, 135
aversion to pressure, 124
aversion to wind, 76, 77, 131, 146, 156, 206, 215, 262, 277, 323, 329, 330
aversion to wind and cold, 277
aversion to wind-cold, 208, 209

B

back and knee pain, 162
back pain, 262
backache, 84
back-*shu* points, 30
bad breath, 70
bad sleep, 330
bad temper, 332
barrel chest, 31
barrel-chested, 122
basic principles in diagnosis of CM, 3
Basic Questions: Discussion on Heat, 275
Basic Questions-Needling the Febrile Disease, 9
bean-rolling pulse, 116
bearing down sensation in the abdomen, 223
bearing down sensation of the anus, 223, 228
Bèi Jí Qiān Jīn Yào Fāng, 备急千金要方, 15
belching, 69, 168, 222, 242, 269, 270, 272, 300, 330
belching with acid and putrid odour, 69
běn, 59, 305
bending back and flagging shoulders, 32
benign colour, 10, 12
between the eyebrows, 9

bì, 85
bì pattern caused by cold-damp, 82
bì pattern caused by wind-damp, 82
bì patterns, 18
bì zhèng 痹症, 63
bì, 蔽, 9
biàn bìng, 305
biàn zhèng, 305
biāo, 58, 305
big head, 19
big toe, 300
binding constraint of liver qi, 69
binding constraint of pathogenic heat, 25
binding of phlegm and qi, 24
birthing pulse, 117
bitter taste, 87, 94, 238, 243, 245, 246, 249, 251, 252, 253, 269, 283, 301, 324, 331
BL 13, 127
BL 19, 127
BL 20, 127
BL 25, 127
black burnt coating, 282
black coating, 57
black jaundice, 35
black nose, 26
black rim around the eyes, 14
black stool with blood, 279
blackish complexion with scaly skin, 14
bladder channel, 276
bladder channel of the foot *taiyang*, 30, 300
bladder damp-heat, 190

bladder failing to ensure retention, 97
bland but slimy taste, 228
bland taste, 93, 140, 222, 226, 231
blazing of both qi and blood, 292
blazing of both qi and *ying*, 59
blazing of liver fire, 244
bleeding, 162, 222
bleeding after defaecation, 95
bleeding after delivery, 219
bleeding in the nose, 26
bleeding spots under the skin, 266
blepharoptosis, 25
bloating especially after meals, 223
bloating or pain, 222
blockage and blood stasis obstructing the brain vessels, 86
blockage in urination or defaecation, 153
blockage of an excessive pathogen, 82
blockage of phlegm-damp, 62, 97
blockage of the channels, 82
blockage of the channels and collaterals, 32
blockage of the channels by wind-phlegm, 22
blockage of the movement of qi, 63
blocked heat of the heart and spleen steaming upward, 27
blood accumulation pattern, 65
blood and essence exhaustion, 109
blood and water gathered in the

abdomen, 87
blood clots, 174
blood cold pattern, 174
blood collapse, 18
blood counterflow, 168
blood deficiency, 20, 23, 27, 28, 51, 83, 89, 97, 126, 135, 239, 326
blood deficiency causes wind, 326
blood deficiency pattern, 13, 170
blood deficiency unable to nourish tendons and channels, 33
blood deficiency-stasis pattern, 327
blood heat or blood stagnating around the anus, 34
blood heat pattern, 173, 178
blood in the stools, 228, 235
blood in the stools and urine, 222
blood in the urine, 192, 227, 261
blood level pattern, 173
blood *lín*, 40
blood loss pattern, 219, 266
blood not nourishing the skin, 35
blood seeps from the vessels, 238
blood spots under the skin, 228
blood level, 248
blood stasis, 14, 25, 35, 49, 53, 82, 83, 84, 92, 97, 110, 123, 126, 136, 165, 192, 193, 199, 201, 241
blood stasis and blockage of qi, 58
blood stasis and obstruction by dampness, 33
blood stasis blocking the *chong mai* and *ren mai*, 98
blood stasis due to stagnation of qi, 174

blood stasis in the channels, 32
blood stasis in the stomach, 39, 190, 235, 236
blood stasis in the uterus, 84
blood stasis not nourishing the skin, 35
blood stasis obstructing the brain collaterals, 204
blood stasis obstructing the brain networks, 190
blood stasis pattern, 27, 170
blood stasis with pathogenic fluid attacking the heart, 21
blood system, 289
blood tinged sputum, 216
blood vomiting, 199
blood wheel, 22
blood-flecked phlegm, 83
blood-retention pattern, 276
bloodshot eyes, 334
blood-tinged sputum, 159, 268
bloody phlegm, 70
blue and purple spots, 204
blue and purple tongue, 49
blue purplish lips and nails, 170
blue-black ear, 25
blue-green, 12, 14
blue-grey complexion, 83
blue-purple tongue, 58
blue-purple veins in the sides of the tongue, 170
blurred vision, 89, 239, 240, 257, 267, 327
body fluids discharging with qi, 167
body fluids intact, 133
body mass index (bmi), 15

Index

body odours, 70
body pain, 129, 131, 146, 322
body shape, 6
boils, 37
bone diseases, 122
borborygmus, 69, 142, 236, 300, 328
borderland, 9
both pupils become completely dilated, 24
both severe deficiency and severe excess, 147
bounding and rapid pulse, 160
bow legs, 32
(bow-string) pulse, 200, 242
bowel changes, 242
bow-string pulse, 244
branch, 58, 305
breath holding, 18
breath odours, 70
bright hall, 9
bright red and thick menses, 173
bright red spotted tongue, 50
bright white or dark complexion, 254
bright-white complexion, 274
bright-white tongue with a mirror-like coating, 55
broken metal failing to sound, 63
bronchial wheezing, 149
bronchiectasis, 332
brownish and thick menstrual flow, 98
brownish scanty urine, 96
brownish urine, 140
bruises, 192
bubble-rising pulse, 116

bulging of the eye, 24
burning feeling around the anus, 333
burning heat in the chest and abdomen, 152
burning pain, 82, 83
burning pain in the chest and hypochondrium, 269, 332
burning pain in the costal and hypochondriac regions, 243
burning pain in the costal regions, 241
burning pain in the soles, 301
burning pain in the stomach, 312
burning pain in the urethra, 192
burning pain on urination, 204, 205, 261, 262
burning sensation and pain in the epigastrium, 232, 236
burning sensation in the chest, palms and soles, 272
burning sensation of the anus on passing stool, 218
burns, 162
burnt dry mouth and lips, 297
bursts of anger, 162

C

cacosmia, 71
calculous stones, 167
cancer, 34, 71
canthus outcrop creeping over the eye, 24
carbuncles, 34, 37
cardiac pain, 300, 301
cardiac palpitations, 170

case analysis, 314
case history, 73, 312
case record, 302
Case Records (Zhěn Jí, 诊籍), 4
cellulitis, 37
Central Treasury Classic (Zhōng Zàng Jīng, 中藏经), 4
centre of the tongue, 45
cerebrospinal damage, 30
cháng mài 长脉, 112
changes in the quantity of food, 93
changes of the illness, 319
changes of the speech and breath, 62
channel pathway, 299
channel qi disturbance, 85
channel-bypassing transmission, 288
channels and joints, 157
chaotic mind, 161
chaperone, 315
chapped lips, 27
chattering jaws, 27
cheek swelling, 21, 300
chén mài 沉脉, 109
chen yan, 155
chest accumulation pattern, 124
chest *bì*, 83
chest distress, 86, 184, 187, 193, 194, 331
chest oppression, 196, 201
chest oppression and pain, 196
chest pain, 63, 83, 159, 192, 194, 206, 209, 210, 211, 214, 215, 217, 244, 262, 325
chest stuffiness, 159, 173, 211,

213, 214, 253
chest stuffiness or an oppressed feeling of the chest, 265
chest sweating, 81
chest tightness, 327
chǐ, 103
chickenpox, 37
chief complaint/concern, 318, 319
chief symptom, 318
childbearing, 223
childhood measles, 25
child's index finger, 315
child-organ affecting the mother-organ, 267
children's voices, 62
chills, 78
chills without fever, 76, 148
chilly feeling, 182
chilly with cold limbs, 194
chǐ-region, 321
cholera, 68
chōng yáng, 103
choppy pulse, 110, 114, 115, 235, 236, 240
chronic blood loss, 177
chronic cough, 173, 206, 211, 261, 267, 268
chronic course, 211
chronic diarrhoea, 95, 166, 259, 274
chronic diarrhoea with undigested food, 274
chronic disease, 133, 177, 220, 272
chronic disease damages yang, 133
chronic diseases of the nose, 63
chronic dysentery, 274

chronic illness, 265
chronic onset upper excess and lower deficiency, 245
chronic panting, 261, 262
cinnabar eye, 24
clear (清), 11
clear and abundant drool, 39
clear and dilute sputum, 265
clear and profuse urine, 132
clear and thin phlegm, 71
clear and thin vomitus, 71
clear and turbid (清浊), 10
clear drooling, 231
clear frequent urination, 254, 259
clear nasal discharge, 26
clear nasal mucus, 71
clear profuse leucorrhoea, 260, 262
clear sputum, 132
clear urine, 140
clear vomit, 157
clear watery leucorrhoea, 228
clear watery sputum, 207
clear-watery sputum, 215
clenched hands, 18
clenched jaw, 28
clinical manifestations, 129
clonic convulsions, 296
cloud or shelter, 9
clouded spirits, 169
clouding of consciousness, 204
clouding of the mind, 157
cloudy consciousness, 201
cloudy *lín*, 40
cloudy mind, 296
clubbing of the fingers, 33
coarse breathing, 136, 153, 203

coating, 154
coating texture, 53
coherent, 62
cold, 13, 14, 112, 121, 125, 128, 155
cold and dampness, 85
cold and heat, 132
cold and heat patterns, 300
cold attack, 18, 157
cold *bì*, 157
cold body, 196, 254
cold body and limbs, 174, 210, 221, 236, 252, 254, 264, 274
cold body and limbs without fever, 213
cold coagulation, 193, 199
cold congealing, 94, 97
cold congealing and blood stasis, 97, 98
cold congealing and obstruction of phlegm, 98
cold congealing in the liver channel, 33, 84
cold congealing in the muscles and vessels, 52
cold constrains *wei* qi, 157
cold damage, 27, 277
cold damages the spleen and stomach yang, 157
cold excess, 133
cold feeling at the auricle, 25
cold feet, 330
cold fluid-retention, 187
cold forearm skin, 126
cold hands and feet, 83
cold invades channels, 157
cold invades muscles, 157

Index

cold invading lung, 142
cold invading the exterior, 157
cold invading the stomach, 231
cold limbs, 86, 132, 138, 139, 140, 144, 162, 178, 194, 196, 200, 201, 226, 228, 231, 254, 260, 295, 328
cold limbs due to reverse flow of qi, 166, 285
cold obstruction, 201
cold of the hands and feet, 144
cold of the lower limbs, 330
cold of the spleen and abdominal pain, 63
cold of the spleen and stomach, 84
cold or heat patterns, 131, 151
cold pain, 82, 174
cold pain in the epigastrium, 147, 236
cold pain in the lower abdomen and pudendum, 252
cold pain of the lumbar region, 255
cold pain of the lumbar region and knee joints or the lower abdomen, 274
cold pathogen, 68, 131
cold pathogen assailing the lung, 206
cold pathogen congealing under the skin, 157
cold pathogen congesting the lung, 210
cold pathogen intruding into the lung, 86
cold pathogen settled in the stomach, 69

cold pattern, 42, 58, 59, 68, 69, 70, 71, 91, 93, 110, 124, 126, 132, 149, 275
cold pattern or phlegm-damp pattern, 53
cold phlegm, 38, 110
cold profuse sweating, 260
cold rainy weather, 326
cold soreness of the lumbar region and knees, 254, 259
cold stagnating in the liver channel, 252, 332
cold strike, 157
cold sweating, 194, 196, 331
cold patlerns, 232
cold uterus, 254, 255, 260
cold vomit, 39
cold-damage patterns, 118
cold-damp, 71, 85
cold-damp diarrhoea, 40
cold-damp due to an exterior invasion, 56
cold-damp encumbering the spleen, 223, 228
cold-damp obstructing internally, 54
cold-damp of the spleen and stomach, 35
cold-damp pouring down, 98
cold-dampness, 326
cold-dampness accumulating in the spleen pattern, 332
cold-dampness congestion, 51
cold-dampness encumbering the spleen, 229, 230
cold-dampness obstructing the middle *jiao*, 228

coldness in the perineal region in male, 254
cold-pathogen congesting the lung, 190, 211
cold-water flooding upward, 94
colicky pain, 82
collapse, 17
collapse of blood, 162
collapse of qi, 163, 328
collapse of qi and yang, 166
collapse of qi resulting from excessive haemorrhage, 174
collapse of qi resulting from haemorrhage, 178
collapse of qi with collapse of blood, 166
collapse of the nose, 26
collapse of yang, 144, 196, 292
collapse of yin, 144, 292
collection of phlegm-damp, 29
colour of the coating, 316
colour of the eye, 23
colour of the lips, 27
colour of the nose, 26
coma, 8, 9, 136, 158, 160, 168, 173, 192, 194, 196, 204, 218, 220, 244, 248, 250
combination of pathogenic wind with latent phlegm, 67
combination of patterns, 288
combined patterns, 146, 190
combined pressing, 106
combined pulses, 115
common contagious diseases in paediatrics, 37
comparison of exterior and interior patterns, 131

complexion, 315
complication, 288
compound pulse, 115
Comprehensive Treatise on Protecting Children's Lives, 15
concealed papulae, 35, 36
concrete location, 128
concretions, 110
concretions and conglomeration, 110
concretions or accumulation, 125
condition of summer, 326
condition of the hair, 19
confidentiality, 307
congealed cold, 82
congenital anomaly, 52
congenital cracked tongue, 51
congenital deficiency, 21
congenital heart disease, 49
congenital mental deficiency, 52
congenital syphilis, 20
congested varicose veins under the tongue, 170
conglomerate (括), 11
conglomerations, 110
conglomerations or gathering, 125
consciousness, 192
constant hunger, 222, 232, 233
constipation, 40, 70, 94, 132, 142, 146, 160, 169, 173, 203, 206, 211, 214, 218, 219, 221, 232, 233, 234, 235, 236, 243, 244, 245, 246, 297, 300, 324
constitution of patient, 154
constitutionally weak, 18
constraint of liver qi, 83, 123

constriction of the *wei* qi, 277
consumption of the body fluids, 54
contagious disease in children, 36
container of phlegm, 38
contention between wind and water, 88
contents of the inquiry examination, 74
continual and loud belching, 69
continual belching, 69
continuous hiccough in a long-term or severe illness, 68
continuous sweating, 149
contracted or stiff neck, 30
contraction and pain of the lumbar region, 32
contraction and pain of the scrotum and testes, 238
contraction of the external genitalia or scrotum, 252
contracture of the hands and feet, 33
contracture of the tendons and channels, 33
contradictory, 138
contusion, 32, 162
convulsions, 14, 17, 27, 42, 63, 127, 156, 158, 160, 201, 238, 246
convulsions in children, 14, 22
convulsions of the limbs, 238, 248, 250
convulsive disease, 28
convulsive spasms of the four limbs, 33
cool dryness, 159
cool-dryness patterns, 209

copious menstruation, 176
copious sweating, 158, 291
cord-like substances, 127
cornea is muddy with grey and white colouring, 23
cough, 129, 131, 149, 156, 157, 159, 162, 168, 184, 187, 206, 208, 210, 211, 213, 214, 215, 216, 217, 244, 257, 265, 268, 269, 295, 299, 319, 323, 325, 327, 329, 332
cough and asthma, 17
cough with scanty sputum, 268
cough with sticky yellow sputum, 208
cough with watery sputum, 262
coughing, 62, 332
coughing up blood, 323
counter flow rising of stomach qi, 39
courtyard, 9
cracked white coating, 57
cracks or creases on the dorsum of the tongue, 50
cramps, 267
crane's-knee wind, 32
craniocerebral trauma, 24
creeping of the limbs, 240
crimson tongue, 160, 291, 296
crimson-purple colour, 50
crimson-purple tongue, 49
critical disease, 25
critical illness, 24, 54
critical pattern of umbilical wind, 31
critical sign, 42
critical stage of chronic diseases, 21

critically ill, 15
cù mài, 111
cubit skin, 125
cùn, 103
cùn kǒu diagnostic method, 101
cùn kǒu pulse, 41
cùn kǒu area, 321
curd-like coating, 54
curled-up tongue, 192
curling up in bed, 133, 135
cyanosis, 260
cyanotic (blue) lips, 194
cyanotic spots and purple dots, 204

D

dà cháng shù, 127
dà líng, 127
dà mài, 112
dacryorrhoea, 89
dài mài, 111
dai mai, 30
damage of body fluid, 27, 28
damage of kidney-essence, 21
damage of the body fluid, 91
damage of the *dai mai* (带脉), 85
damage of the *du mai*, 84
damage of the *zang-fu* essence, 32
damage of yin fluids, 35
damage to the collaterals caused by the wind-pathogen, 22
damp accumulating in the spleen, 332
damp heat in the bladder, 261
damp heat in the liver and gallbladder, 86
damp pathogen, 82
damp pattern, 59, 110
damp phlegm, 38
damp warmth disease, 70, 78
damp warmth tidal fever, 78
damp-cold, 158
damp-heat, 23, 53, 54, 71, 84, 95, 158
damp-heat accumulated and obstructed in the intestines, 34
damp-heat accumulating in the spleen, 190, 251
damp-heat accumulation, 31
damp-heat blockage in the nose, 26
damp-heat brewing internally, 23
damp-heat burning and condensing impurities in the urine, 40
damp-heat diarrhoea, 40
damp-heat in the large intestine, 95, 231
damp-heat in the liver and gallbladder, 35, 39, 92, 190, 239, 251, 331
damp-heat in the middle *jiao*, 229, 297
damp-heat in the spleen and stomach, 229
damp-heat invasion, 333
damp-heat of the bladder, 71
damp-heat of the liver and gallbladder, 25
damp-heat of the spleen and stomach, 39, 50, 92
damp-heat of the spleen and stomach with gathering pathogenic qi attacking upward, 54
damp-heat overflowing onto the skin, 70
damp-heat pathogen, 59
damp-heat pattern, 91
damp-heat pouring down, 34, 35, 99
damp-heat pouring down via the liver channel, 33, 34
damp-heat pouring downward, 96
damp-heat spleen and stomach pathologies, 35
damp-heat sweltering, 23
dampness, 54, 111, 155, 158, 249, 284, 296, 331
dampness attacking, 87
dampness *bì*, 159
dampness blocking and stagnating qi movement, 82
dampness encumbering spleen yang, 228
dampness in the qi system, 59
dampness pathogen blocking the vessels, 109
dampness pattern, 91, 108, 158
dampness spreads under the skin, 159
dampness-heat in the lower *jiao*, 324
damp-phlegm and static blood obstructing the channels, 88
damp-phlegm confusing the upper orifices, 89
damp-turbidity, 54, 56

damp-warmth, 54
dǎn shù, 127
dàn zhōng, 126
dangerous sign, 69
dark and dusky complexion, 170, 204
dark and gloomy face, 8
dark and greasy coating, 316
dark and purple tongue with ecchymosis, 327
dark and scanty urine, 204, 333
dark black without lustre, 14
dark eyelids, 23
dark purple maculopapular eruptions, 160, 291
dark purple tongue, 170, 235, 236
dark tongue, 201
dark tongue with blue and purple spots, 199
dark urine, 257, 331, 333
dark-purple tongue, 204
dark-yellow urine, 151
dead pulses, 116
deafness, 88, 238, 243, 255, 258, 259, 296, 300, 301
debilitation of heart qi and heart yang with blood stasis, 14
debilitation of qi and blood, 21
debilitation of stomach qi, 68
debilitation of the kidney, 71
debilitation of yang, 97
debilitation of *zang-fu*'s essential qi, 32
debilitation of *zheng* qi, 55
decline in the *mingmen* fire, 95
declining kidney essence in old age or with excessive sexual activity, 254
decreased auditory function, 332
deep (沉), 11, 107
deep and choppy pulse, 279
deep and faint pulse, 285
deep and faint thready pulse, 323
deep and gruff cough, 68
deep and hacking cough, 68
deep and hoarse voice, 322
deep and knotted pulse, 279
deep and slippery or deep and choppy pulse, 200
deep and slippery pulse, 201, 331
deep and slow or deep and tense pulse, 200, 201
deep and slow pulse, 139, 221
deep and tense pulse, 151
deep and thready pulse, 327
deep and tight or taut pulse, 157
deep and tight pulse, 252
deep and weak pulse, 265
deep breathing, 122
deep in winter, 108
deep palpation, 121
deep pulse, 109, 114, 131, 182
deep weak and slow pulse, 194
deep yellow coating, 56
deep, 226, 229, 254, 259, 264, 274
deep, slow, and forceless pulse, 182
defaecation once every several days, 219
defensive qi, 79
deficiency, 13, 64, 128
deficiency and cold of the lower *jiao*, 96
deficiency and damage of the spleen and stomach, 85
deficiency and failure of the kidney essence qi, 88
deficiency and failure of the spleen and kidney, 95
deficiency and failure of yang, 109
deficiency and sinking of middle *jiao* qi, 34
deficiency and sinking of the *zheng* qi, 37
deficiency and weakness of the spleen and stomach, 92, 95
deficiency and weakness of the spleen qi, 88
deficiency cold of the spleen and stomach, 39
deficiency fire flaming upward, 25
deficiency heat, 12
deficiency in the root and excess in the branches, 213, 246, 247
deficiency of blood, 110, 327
deficiency of blood generating wind, 52
deficiency of body fluids, 126
deficiency of both heart and spleen pattern, 266
deficiency of both qi and blood, 85, 174, 176
deficiency of both qi and yin, 59
deficiency of essence and marrow, 136
deficiency of essence qi, 8
deficiency of fluid, 94
deficiency of heart and spleen, 64
deficiency of heart blood, 193

Index

deficiency of heart qi, 86, 193, 194, 196
deficiency of heart yang, 193, 196
deficiency of heart yin, 193
deficiency of heart-blood, 329
deficiency of kidney, 329
deficiency of kidney essence, 30
deficiency of kidney qi, 32, 97, 332
deficiency of kidney yang, 96, 254, 329
deficiency of kidney yin, 29, 254
deficiency of lung qi and kidney qi, 66, 260
deficiency of lung yin, 67
deficiency of the spleen and kidney, 323
deficiency of prolonged disease, 64
deficiency of qi, 26, 48, 57, 161
deficiency of qi and blood, 20, 23, 25, 32, 48, 50, 51, 86, 88, 98, 111
deficiency of qi and yin, 55
deficiency of qi, blood and essence, 82
deficiency of the spleen, 39
deficiency of spleen and kidney, 31
deficiency of spleen qi, 323, 326
deficiency of stomach qi, 56
deficiency of the body fluids, qi and blood, 48
deficiency of the heart, 18
deficiency of the heart and spleen, 81
deficiency of the kidney, 324
deficiency of the kidney qi, 31
deficiency of the kidney yang and fluid retention in the brain, 19
deficiency of the liver and kidney, 89
deficiency of the qi and blood, 38, 51, 52
deficiency of the spleen, 54, 324
deficiency of the spleen and accumulation of dampness, 14
deficiency of the spleen and dampness patterns, 13
deficiency of the spleen and kidney associated with damp-heat, 40
deficiency of the spleen and stomach unable to perform transportation and transformation, 87
deficiency of the spleen or qi and blood, 42
deficiency of the spleen qi, 25
deficiency of the stomach qi, 26
deficiency of the *yuan* qi (元气), 66
deficiency of the *zang* essence, 23
deficiency of the *zong* qi, 123
deficiency of *wei* qi, 136
deficiency of yang, 91, 125
deficiency of yang and blood, 35
deficiency of yang in the middle *jiao*, 284
deficiency of yang qi, 77
deficiency of *ying* blood not nourishing the skin, 35
deficiency of *ying* qi, 136
deficiency of *ying*-blood, 13, 90
deficiency of *zheng* qi and damp-turbidity unable to transform, 55
deficiency of *zong* (gathering) qi (宗气), 64
deficiency or cold patterns, 68
deficiency or excess patterns, 152
deficiency or exhaustion of lung qi and kidney qi, 66
deficiency or weakness of the spleen and stomach, 87
deficiency panting, 66
deficiency pattern, 8, 17, 27, 29, 42, 50, 82, 84, 88, 89, 108, 124, 135, 229, 275, 319, 323, 324
deficiency pattern transforming into an excess pattern, 151
deficiency pattern with pseudo-excess pattern, 153
deficiency pulse, 113
deficiency resulting in vigourous fire, 49
deficiency-cold pattern, 17, 40
deficiency-cold pattern of the spleen, 226
deficiency-consumption of the kidney, 40
deficiency-fire harassing the interior, 93
deficient and cold patterns, 65
deficient and exhausted posture, 17
deficient and weak pulse, 66
deficient blood causing liver wind, 239, 250
deficient cold, 58

deficient cold body invaded by damp-heat, 58
deficient cold of the spleen and stomach, 71, 95
deficient cold pattern, 58, 96
deficient fire flaming upward, 28, 29
deficient fire flaring, 30
deficient fire scorching the lung, 63
deficient heart qi, 331
deficient heat pattern, 49
deficient pain, 82
deficient pattern, 60, 68, 69, 88, 150
deficient pattern accompanied by an excessive pattern, 147
deficient pulse, 111, 115, 262, 296
deficient qi, 15
deficient rapid pulse, 158
deficient spleen and exuberant dampness in infants, 27
deficient yang and exuberant yin, 49, 90
deficient yin causing liver wind, 239, 250
deficient *zang-fu* organs, 109
deficient-cold of the spleen and stomach, 95
deficient-cold pattern, 31
deficient-fire harassing, 241
deficient-heat harassing internally, 241
deficient-heat pattern, 240, 296
deficient-heat rises upward, 241
deformity of the fingers, 33
degree of urgency, 319

dehydration, 179
delayed closure of the fontanel, 258
delayed menstruation, 97, 170
delayed menstruation with purple menstrual blood, 174
delirious speech, 64
delirium, 8, 136, 160, 173, 199, 203, 204, 218, 220, 244, 282, 295, 296
dementia, 8, 201, 204
deplete kidney essence and primary qi, 136
depletion of lung qi functions of dispersing and descending, 26
depressed, 333
depressed and stagnated, 130
depressed emotions, 247, 270
depressed eyeballs, 179
depressed gallbladder with phlegm harassing, 190, 239, 253
depressed gallbladder with phlegm harassing pattern, 252
depressed qi transforming into fire, 239
depression, 8, 160, 201, 204, 238, 241, 269, 270, 272, 328, 329
depression of qi, 232, 233
depressive-psychosis, 201
depth of the disease, 128
dermal burning pain, 199
desertion of blood, 13
desertion of *yuan* (original) qi, 81
desire for cold drinks, 233
desire for drinking, 68
desire for drinking in small sips, 229

desire to be covered, 152
desire to drink, 328
desire to drink in small sips, 230
desire to drink water, 91
desire to gargle, 92
desire to see family members, 8
desires to be covered with clothes and quilt, 152
despondency, 246
desquamation, 326
desquamation on the scalp, 20
deterioration of the spirit, 48
deterioration of the *zang-fu* organs, 71
development, 319
development of the disease, 319, 320
developmental retardation, 257, 258, 259
deviation inward, 32
deviation of the eyes and mouth, 18, 247, 248
deviation of the face and mouth, 21
deviation of the mouth, 300
deviation outward, 32
devitalised heart yang, 86
devitalised spleen yang or water-dampness collecting internally, 56
diabrosis, 34
diagnosing bladder diseases, 127
diagnosing gallbladder diseases, 127
diagnosing heart diseases, 127
diagnosing kidney diseases, 127

diagnosing large intestine
  diseases, 127
diagnosing liver diseases, 127
diagnosing lung diseases, 127
diagnosing small intestine
  diseases, 127
diagnosing spleen diseases, 127
diagnosing stomach diseases, 127
diagnostic indicators, 304
diān 癫, 9
diarrhoea, 70, 84, 95, 126, 131,
  136, 149, 157, 161, 206, 218, 219,
  220, 221, 222, 223, 228, 233, 234,
  255, 270, 284, 332
diarrhoea at dawn, 254, 259, 260,
  274, 329
diarrhoea due to deficiency of
  the spleen or kidney, 40
diarrhoea due to heat, 95
diarrhoea due to indigestion, 95
diarrhoea like water, 332
diarrhoea with blood and mucus,
  217
diarrhoea with foul smell, 236,
  332
diarrhoea with undigested food,
  285
dietary irregularities, 92
differentiation of patterns
  according to pathogenic
  factors, 155
difficult and painful urination,
  96, 136
difficult defaecation, 219, 234
difficult digestion, 146
difficult to observe, 138
difficulty in inhaling, 260, 261,
  262
difficulty in lying down, 65
difficulty in micturition, 182
difficulty in movement, 8
difficulty in speaking, 192
difficulty in urination and
  defaecation, 325
difficulty in walking, 161
difficulty with urination, 300
diffuse swelling, 32
digestive problems, 241
dilute and white leucorrhoea,
  226
dilute cold sweat, 143
dilute sweating, 144
dim and purple face, 192
diminished coating, 256, 257, 259,
  263, 268, 296
diminished or no coating, 233,
  234
diminished yellow coating, 269
diphtheria, 29, 31
diplopia, 89
direct attack of a pathogen on a
  certain channel, 288
direct invasion of pathogens on
  the zang-fu organs, 131
direct tapping, 121
dirty greasy coating, 54
discharge of fetid pus, 28
discontinuous breath, 66
disease, 2
disease subsiding, 55
disequilibrium, 89
disharmony between the heart
  and kidney, 190, 263
disharmony between the liver
  and spleen, 95, 270
disharmony between the liver
  and stomach pattern, 269
disharmony between the *ying*
  and *wei*, 276
disharmony between yin and
  yang, 128
disharmony of qi and blood
  impairing the *chong mai* and
  ren mai, 242
disharmony of yin and yang, 111
disharmony of *zang-fu* organs,
  137
dislike being pressed, 124
dislike of flexing or stretching, 17
dislike of pressure, 232, 236
dislike of speaking, 222
dislikes palpation, 333
disorder of closing eyes, 24
disorder of qi and blood, 111
dispiritedness, 66
distal bleeding, 40, 95
distending and burning pain in
  the right hypochondrium, 251,
  249
distending and wandering pain,
  242
distending headache, 159, 245,
  246, 269
distending pain, 81, 83, 200, 201,
  270, 272
distending pain in the chest, 238
distending pain in the chest and
  hypochondrium, 238
distending pain in the forehead,
  331
distending pain in the head and

eyes, 244, 245, 248, 273
hypochondriac burning pain, 244
distending pain in the legs, 170
distending pain in the lower abdomen, 261
distending pain in the right hypochondrium, 250
distending pain in the epigastrium and abdomen, 242
distending pain in the head, 238
distending pain or wandering pain in the chest, epigastrium and hypochondrium, 269
distension, 175, 187, 218, 219, 233
distension and bearing down sensation in the pudendal area, 252
distension and distending pain, 167
distension and fullness of the chest and epigastrium, 299
distension and fullness of the chest, 299
distension and fullness of the lesser abdomen, 278
distension and pain in the epigastrium, 236
distension and pain in the breasts, 242
distension and pain in the lumbar region, 261
distension of the epigastrium, 222
distension in the epigastrium and abdomen, 228
distension of the breast, 238
distinguishing cold and heat patterns, 132
distinguishing exterior and interior patterns, 131
disturbance in joint movements, 157, 238
disturbance of channel qi, 30
disturbance of *fu* qi, 54
disturbance of opening and closing, 96
disturbance of qi transformation, 96
disturbances in digestion, 238
disturbances of the lung, spleen, kidney, 31
disturbances of the spleen, 87
disturbed sleep, 325, 329
disturbing the mind, 142
disturbs the mind, 134
dizziness, 20, 66, 146, 162, 165, 166, 168, 170, 176, 186, 187, 191, 192, 197, 198, 204, 219, 220, 238, 240, 243, 244, 245, 246, 247, 248, 252, 253, 256, 257, 262, 263, 265, 266, 267, 269, 272, 273, 283, 324, 325, 326, 328, 329, 330
dizziness that upsets balance, 246
dizzy, 330
dizzy vision, 89
dòng mài, 111
dorsal curvature, 17
dorsally located radial artery, 108
dream-disturbed sleep, 192, 197, 198, 246, 248, 252, 263, 266, 267, 272, 273, 328, 329
dream-disturbed sleep with vivid dreams, 243
dribbling after urination, 255, 259, 260, 262, 332
dribbling urinary block, 96, 301
drool, 39, 45
drooling, 201
drooped shoulders, 17
drooping of the upper eyelid, 25
drowsiness, 161, 182
drum distension, 31
drumskin pulse, 109, 113, 114
dry and black complexion, 14
dry and chapped auricle, 25
dry and pale tongue, 159
dry and rough skin, 126
dry and yellow coating, 248
dry and yellow coating or prickly coating, 146
dry coating, 53
dry cough, 67, 68, 159, 209, 216, 257
dry cough with scanty sputum, 209
dry eyes, 246, 257, 267
dry faeces, 95
dry fissured coating, 282
dry greasy coating, 54
dry hair, 206
dry lips, 215
dry lips and tongue, 144
dry mouth, 91, 92, 140, 209, 215, 217, 219, 234, 236, 243, 246
dry mouth and pharynx, 216
dry mouth and throat, 240, 248, 250, 256, 263, 268, 272, 273, 296, 328
dry mouth and tongue, 160
dry nose, 159

dry or splitting lips, 179
dry pharynx, 146, 322, 328
dry pharynx and lips, 328
dry phlegm, 38
dry red tongue, 257
dry skin, 35, 126, 179, 326, 328
dry sores on the lips, 300
dry stool, 135, 136, 140, 179, 199, 209, 217, 219, 220, 233, 234, 236, 257, 312, 322, 329, 330, 331, 333
dry teeth, 28
dry throat, 159, 257, 283, 301
dry throat and lips, 159, 179
dry tongue coating, 317
dry tongue with yellow coating, 159
dry white tongue, 48
dry yellowish coating, 132
dry, scaly skin, 35
dry, thin, grey-yellow or white hair, 20
dry-heat, 268
dry-heat damaging the fluid, 57, 94
dry-heat pattern, 204
dryness, 155, 281
dryness accumulation and bowel excess, 57
dryness and swelling of the tongue and throat, 301
dryness invading the lung, 67, 206, 209
dryness of the eyes, 238, 240
dryness of the large intestine, 234
dryness of the mouth, 236, 300
dryness of the mouth and throat, 233, 234, 285

dryness of the throat, 300
dryness pattern, 91, 159, 327
dry-yellow coating, 142
du mai, 19, 30
dual deficiency of the heart and spleen, 190
duǎn mài, 111
dull abdominal pain, 221
dull burning pain in the costal and hypochondriac regions, 240
dull eyes, 8
dull pain, 82
dull pain in the epigastrium, 233, 234, 236
dull pale complexion, 267
dull purplish complexion, 196
duodenobulbar ulcer, 312
duration of these ailments, 318
dusty complexion, 301
dwarfism, 258
dwarfism in children, 259
dysentery, 40, 68, 95, 136, 218, 223, 231, 274
dysentery due to damp-heat, 95
dysfunction of digestion, 283
dysfunction of the internal organs, 136
dysmenorrhoea, 98, 241
dyspepsia, 70
dyspepsia of the spleen and stomach, 94
dyspeptic retention, 54
dysphasia, 173, 246, 250
dysphoria, 36, 324, 325
dysplasia, 32, 34
dysplasis, 30

dyspnoea, 8, 66, 149, 187, 210, 211, 213, 214, 215

E

early menstrual cycle, 329
early menstruation, 97, 173
early onset of exogenous disease, 48
early senility, 258, 259
earth, 13
earth insulting wood, 249
easily observed, 138
eating too late, 233
ecchymosis, 170
eczema, 37, 159, 249
eczema on the anterior yin, 33
Effective Formulas from Generations of Physicians (*Shì Yī Dé Xiào Fāng*, 世医得效方), 4
eight principles, 128
eliminated centre, 93
eliminated centre pattern of the spleen and stomach qi, 93
emaciated face with high cheek bones, 21
emaciated muscles, 8
emaciation, 8, 91, 92, 140, 153, 179, 216, 217, 223, 235, 236
emissions, 268, 273
emotional factors, 131, 201
emotional frustration, 232, 233, 240, 243, 270
emotional irritation, 203
emotional problems, 272
emotional upsets and stagnation of liver, 87

emotions, 35
empathic, 318
empty pain, 82
endogenous heat, 325
enlarged, 51
enlarged pale tongue, 138, 139
enlarged tongue, 228, 229, 230
enuresis, 96, 255, 259, 262, 301
epidemic infection, 21
epidemic pestilence, 155
epigastric burning pain, 244
epigastric discomfort, 269, 272
epigastric distension, 222, 272
epigastric fullness, 159, 234, 236
epigastric pain, 84, 222, 231, 232, 300
epigastric stabbing pain, 235, 236
epigastric stuffiness, 159
epigastric upset, 312
epilepsy, 8, 9, 18, 64, 201
epistaxis, 26, 132, 199, 209, 222, 227, 228, 243, 246, 291, 300
ěr mén, 103
erratic behaviour, 160, 161
erysipelas, 34
essence damage, 110
essence not nourishing upward, 28
essence qi, 7
essential qi exhaustion, 21
Essentials from the Golden Cabinet, 186, 187
evening vomiting, 68
examination method at st 9 (*rén yíng*) and *cùn kǒu*, 101
examinations of inspection, palpation, listening and

smelling, 312
excess, 64, 128
excess and deficiency, 135
excess and heat patterns, 68
excess conditions of damp obstruction, 80
excess fire, 160
excess gallbladder fire, 83
excess heat, 12, 214
excess heat in the small intestine, 204
excess heat in the *yangming*, 295
excess heat pattern, 17, 23, 49
excess of cold, 14
excess panting, 66
excess pattern, 17, 42, 49, 60, 64, 68, 69, 83, 85, 88, 89, 96, 97, 124, 136, 150, 229, 245, 275, 324
excess pattern transforming into a deficiency pattern, 150
excess pattern with pseudo-deficiency pattern, 153
excess pulse, 111, 112, 113, 115
excess qi and blood, 112
excess salivation, 231
excess-deficiency, 128
excess-heat pattern, 14, 40, 250
excessive bleeding, 178
excessive cold, 27
excessive consumption of raw and cold foods, 133
excessive drinking, 23
excessive drinking of alcohol and contracted warm disease, 50
excessive fire of liver and gallbladder attacking upward, 23

excessive fire of the liver and gallbladder, 50
excessive heart-fire, 23
excessive heat, 27, 110, 111
excessive heat causing cold, 151
excessive heat damaging fluids, 49, 51
excessive heat generating wind, 52
excessive heat in the liver channel, 49
excessive heat in the lung, 66
excessive heat of the heart and spleen, 50
excessive heat of the stomach or intestines, 40
excessive heat of the *zang-fu* organs or blood, 50
excessive heat pattern, 31, 80, 125
excessive heat transforming into wind, 52
excessive intake of alcohol, 33
excessive intake of raw or cold foods, 228
excessive internal heat, 91
excessive menstrual flow, 222
excessive pain, 82
excessive pathogens blocking, 111
excessive pattern accompanied by a deficient pattern, 147
excessive phlegm, 17, 201
excessive phlegm and dampness, 15
excessive rising of liver yang, 273
excessive seven emotions, 134
excessive sexual activities, 136,

254, 263, 268, 272
excessive shortage of qi and fluid, 15
excessive speaking, 64
excessive sweating, 326
excessive tears, 89
excessive thirst, 92
excessive urination, 286
excessive yang keeping yin externally, 151
excessive yin rejecting yang, 151
excited behaviour, 184
exertion of standing for a long time, 33
exhausted bone, 28
exhausted pulses, 116
exhausted *yuan* qi, 116
exhaustion of blood and essence, 21
exhaustion of bones, 17
exhaustion of essence and spirit, 17
exhaustion of essential qi, 31
exhaustion of kidney essence, 25
exhaustion of kidney yin, 25
exhaustion of stomach yin, 55
exhaustion of the heart and lung, 17
exhaustion of the heart and lung qi, 123
exhaustion of the kidney essence, 17
exhaustion of the kidney essential qi, 24
exhaustion of the kidney yin, 28
exhaustion of the tendons, 17
exhaustion of the *zang-fu*

essential qi, 24
exhaustion of the *zang-fu's* essence, 23, 30
exhaustion of yang, 328
exhaustion of yang on the outside, 116
ex-hn5, 102
exogenous disease, 327
exogenous factors, 127
exogenous heat disease, 51
expectoration, 214
expectoration of yellow sputum, 329
expectoration with foul smelling pus sputum with blood, 215
expiratory dyspnoea, 31
expiring of yang qi, 55
expiry of heart qi, 52
expiry of the spleen and stomach qi and kidney yang qi, 116
exposure to a cold and damp, 228
expression of the eyes, 7, 314
exterior, 128
exterior and interior and moving out or entering in of the pattern, 148
exterior cold patterns, 115
exterior deficient heat, 115
exterior heat patterns, 115, 127
exterior pathogen, 125
exterior pathogen entering the interior and transforming into heat, 57
exterior pathogens, 35
exterior pattern, 42, 49, 60, 108, 129

exterior pattern involving the interior, 325
exterior wind, 156
exterior wind-cold, 77, 207
exterior wind pattern, 77
exterior wind-heat pathogen, 36
exterior wind-heat pattern, 57, 77, 208
external attack of wind-cold, 69
external attacking of a wind pathogen, 34
external blockage of wind-cold, 37
external cold patterns, 69
external contraction, 121
external contraction of wind-cold, 71
external deficiency and internal excess, 146
external excess and internal deficiency, 146
external heat disease, 8
external heat pathogen, 58
external injury, 32
external invasion of a wind pathogen, 38
external invasion of a wind-pathogen and fire toxin with accumulation of pathogen, 38
external invasion of wind-heat, 37
external pathogen blocked around the anus, 34
external pathogens, 31
external pathogens attacking the lung, 67
external pattern, 79

external wind-cold, 62, 276
externally contracted diseases, 275
externally contracted fever, 127
externally contracted heat diseases, 289
externally contracted pathogenic qi, 65
externally contracted pestilence, 28
Externally-Contracted Warm-Heat Diseases (Wài Gǎn Wēn Rè Piān, 外感温热篇), 5
externally-contracted wind, 77
externally-contracted wind-cold, 62
externally-contracted wind-heat, 26, 39, 77
extreme (甚), 11
extreme cold in the three yin, 116
extreme damage of the body fluid, 91
extreme deficiency of qi and blood, 17
extreme deficiency of *zheng* qi, 64
extreme heat, 27, 29, 116, 125
extreme heat damaging fluids, 54
extreme heat damaging yin, 292
extreme heat disturbing mental activity, 64
extreme heat generating wind, 28, 239, 250, 292
extreme heat in the *yangming*, 81
extreme heat of the forearm skin, 126
extreme heat of the lung and stomach, 29
extreme heat of the stomach and kidney, 28
extreme heat of the *yangming*, 28
extreme heat pattern, 58, 109
extreme heat stirring the blood, 292
extreme loss of kidney essence, 25
extreme pain, 27
extreme pain in the spinal column and lumbus, 300
extreme weak pulse, 178
extreme yin-cold, 26
exuberance and debility of the yin and yang, 132
exuberance of blood heat, 21
exuberance of dampness, 51
exuberance of internal heat, 33
exuberance of lung heat, 70
exuberance of pathogens and decline of the *zheng* qi, 77
exuberance of the pathogens and the *zheng* qi, 77
exuberance of stomach fire, 28
exuberance of the pathogenic qi, 54
exuberance of yang qi, 81
exuberant, 111
exuberant dampness encumbering the spleen, 92
exuberant heart fire, 205
exuberant heat, 112
exuberant heat in the blood, 98
exuberant heat of the liver and gallbladder, 24
exuberant internal yin-cold, 13
exuberant summer-heat injures *ying* qi, 158
exuberant *yang*, 111
exuberant yang and heat of the *zang-fu* organs, 94
exuberant yang causing heat, 134
exuberant yang-heat, 134
exuberant *yin*, 110
exuberant yin and reduced yang in a deficient body, 69
eye discharge, 89
eye diseases, 238
eye pain, 89
eye spirit, 314
eyes and body all yellow, 14

F

fã, 305
face, 13
facial complexion, 314
facial erysipelas, 21
facial expression, 7, 315, 318
facial oedema, 13, 156
facial paralysis, 156
facial swelling, 21
facial swelling with hot pain, 21
facing upwards and out towards the room, 17
fading or faint pulse, 178
faecal impaction, 220
faecal incontinence, 95, 221, 255
faeces mixed with blood, 95
failing to control discharge of stool and urine, 254
failure and weakness of *zang* qi, 111
failure of both yin and yang, 323
failure of clear yang to rise, 90

failure of kidney qi to control water, 96
failure of middle qi, 123
failure of nourishment of the eyes, 267
failure of the body fluid to flow and spread, 91
failure of the heart and kidney to interact, 81
failure of the kidney in receiving qi, 261
failure of the spirit to keep to its abode, 65
failure of the spleen in controlling blood, 223
failure of the spleen to transform and transport, 90
failure of the spleen to transport, 92
failure of the stomach qi, 26
failure of the stomach qi with damp-turbidity floating upward, 54
failure of transportation and transformation, 222
failure of warmth, 133, 162
failure to control the blood, 222
failure to nourish the bones, 255
failure to nourish the heart-mind, 64
failure to nourish the mind, 64
failure to produce enough marrow to fill the brain, 255
failure to recognise people, 18
failure to warm the body, 133
failure to warm water and fluids, 133

faint (微), 11
faint and expiring pulse, 169
faint and extreme (微甚), 10
faint pulse, 80, 111, 113, 144, 166
faint, 194
fainting, 201, 246
falling asleep, 90
false coating, 56
false cold pattern, 151
"false" deficiency, 153
false deficient pattern, 65
"false" excess, 153
"false" heat, 151
false spirit, 8
false symptoms, 152
"false" cold, 151
false-cold pattern, 152
false-heat pattern, 152
family history, 74
fān, 藩, 9
fat but eats only small amounts, 15
fat pigmentation, 23
fatigue, 138, 158, 159, 161, 182, 221, 222, 223, 226, 227, 236, 260, 326, 331
fatigue of limbs and body, 159
fatigued, 323
fatigued limbs, 88
fatness, 15
fear, 160
fear damage, 161
fear of cold, 76
fear of touch, 18
febrile disease, 216, 233, 286
feeble and rapid pulse, 326
feeble pulse without strength, 324

feeble voice, 189, 206
feeling, 121
feeling of body heaviness, 222
feeling of heat in the mouth, 301
feeling of heaviness, 230
feeling of hunger, 301
fèi shù, 127
fell unconscious, 324
fēng guān, 41
fēng lóng, 313
fetid stools, 333
fever, 78, 129, 146, 149, 156, 157, 158, 159, 173, 203, 204, 207, 208, 209, 211, 213, 214, 215, 217, 218, 230, 231, 233, 261, 263, 276, 277, 278, 289, 295, 322, 325, 326, 330, 333
fever at night, 160
fever that is worse at night, 292
fever with malar flush, 296
fever without aversion to cold, 131
fever without chills, 77, 148
feverish, 121
feverish dysphoria, 152
feverish sensation, 124
feverish sensation in the chest, 240, 296, 325
feverish sensation in the chest, palms and soles, 191, 216, 250
feverish sensation in the five centres, 140
feverishness, 269, 272
feverishness in the chest, 140
feverishness in the chest, palms and soles, 246, 263, 273

fine and rapid pulse, 179
fine and weak pulse, 176
fingers and toes, 17
fingers become submerged on palpation, 182
fire, 12, 155
fire and heat attacking the head and eyes, 86
fire blazing, 328
fire disturbance, 193
fire pathogen attacking the throat, 67
fire pathogen of warm disease attacking upward, 30
fire pattern, 159
fire tends to flame, 134
fire toxin, 70, 160
fire-heat scorching upwards, 142
firm pulse, 110, 113, 114
first visit record, 312
fish and turbid nasal discharge, 26
fish-swimming pulse, 116
fishy smell, 70, 71
fishy smell menstruation, 71
five colours, 12
five human forms, 15
five kinds of flaccidity, 20, 99
five kinds of flaccidity in childhood, 255
five kinds of retardation, 20
five kinds of tardy growth in childhood, 255
five phases, 12
five retardations, 99
five *zang*-organs, 12
fixed pain, 82, 83

flaccid hands, 18
flaccid muscles and tendons, 18
flaccid tongue, 51, 154
flaccid type, 18
flaccidity, 32
flaccidity disease, 33
flaccidity of muscles, 222
flaccidity of the bones, 258
flaccidity of the lower limbs, 301
flaccidity of the pores, 277
flank pain, 149
flaring nares, 26, 65, 244
flaring nostrils, 83, 86
flaring up of liver wind, 201
flat chest, 31
flat philtrum, 27
flatulence, 270, 272, 328
flicking stone pulse, 116
floating and large pulse without root, 166, 169
floating and moderate pulse, 156
floating and rapid or tense pulse, 215
floating and rapid pulse, 131, 159, 208, 215, 217, 289, 295
floating and tense pulse, 131
floating and tight pulse, 157, 207, 209, 217
floating and weak pulse, 329
floating feeling of the feet, 244
floating feet sensations, 247
floating in autumn, 108
floating of deficient yang, 116
floating or deep pulse, 153
floating or rapid pulse, 278
floating pulse, 106, 108, 114, 129, 131, 159

floating pulse without strength, 325
floating rapid pulse, 330
floating yang pattern, 12, 14
floccillation, 281
flooding and spotting, 98
flourishing of stomach fire, 232, 244
fluent pulse, 114
fluid following yang, 81
fluid forming the superficial nodules, 30
fluid retention, 222, 327
fluid retention in the chest and hypochondrium, 87
fluid retention oedema, 206
fluid-retention in the chest and hypochondria, 187
fluid-retention stagnating in the lung, 187
fluid-retention stagnating in the stomach and intestines, 186
fluids, 136
fluorescent lamp, 316
flushed cheeks, 140
flushed complexion and eyes, 245, 248
flushed face, 142, 160, 243, 296, 301, 333
flushed red complexion and eyes, 245
foaming at the mouth, 18
foetal distress, 259, 262
foetus interfering with the collaterals, 63
fontanel, 19, 20
food accumulation, 56, 71, 112,

137
food damage, 39
food poisoning, 68
food predilection, 93
food retention, 39, 69, 112, 332
food retention in the stomach
   and intestine pattern, 333
food stagnation, 94, 234
food stagnation becoming putrid,
   57
food stagnation in the stomach
   and intestines, 95
food stagnation stomach
   disharmony leading to restless
   sleep, 90
foods stagnate in the stomach
   and intestinal tract, 224
foot *taiyang* channel, 275
forceful or forceless pulse, 153
forceful pulse, 136
forceful, deep and rapid pulse,
   233
forceless pulse, 165
forehead, 9
foreign body sensation in throat,
   184
forerunner of macular eruption,
   49
forerunner of stroke, 52
forewarning of stirring wind, 33
forgetfulness, 20, 21, 161, 192,
   263, 266, 267, 272, 273, 279, 327
form of the constitution, 16
form of the eye, 23
form of the mouth and lips, 27
forms cold-dampness interiorly,
   133

foul belching, 235, 236
foul blood smell, 71
foul breath, 70, 233
foul breath odour, 232, 234
foul breath with rotten gingiva,
   70
foul odour menstruation, 71
foul smell of sweat, 70
foul smelling breath, 219
foul smelling diarrhoea, 71
foul smelling stools, 218
foul turbid qi steaming upward
   to the mouth, 27
foul turbidity gathering in the
   middle *jiao*, 54
four aspect pattern identification,
   288
four diagnostic methods, 1
four level pattern differentiation,
   288
four limbs and joint migratory
   pain, 319
four limbs oedema, 32
fox *shàn*, 33
foxy mounting, 301
fractures, 162
frequency and urgency of
   defaecation, 228
frequent and urgent defaecation,
   223
frequent and urgent urination,
   261, 262
frequent sighing, 200
frequent urination, 96, 260, 262
frequent urine, 147
fresh yellow skin and yellow
   sclera, 230

fright, 111, 123, 160
fright damage, 161
fright palpitations, 252
frightened, 63
frightened and fearful face, 22
front of the tongue is red, 208
frostbite, 162
fŭ fēi mài, 116
fú mài, 108, 109
fu organs, 129
fú tù, 300
full coating, 55
fullness, 218, 219, 220, 234, 235
fullness and distending pain, 332
fullness and distending pain in
   the epigastrium and abdomen,
   228
fullness and distension, 161
fullness and distension of the
   chest and hypochondrium, 253
fullness and distension of the
   epigastrium, 222
fullness and pain in the chest
   and hypochondria, 187, 301
fullness in the abdomen, 229, 328
fullness in the chest, 136, 184, 252
fullness in the chest and
   hypochondrium, 187, 283
fullness in the epigastrium, 182,
   201, 233
fullness or pain in the
   epigastrium and abdomen,
   230, 231
functional failure of the spleen
   and stomach, 93
funnel chest, 31
furuncles, 37

G

ga, 312
gallbladder channel, 237
gallbladder channel of the foot shaoyang, 301
gallbladder heat, 65
gallbladder qi deficiency, 238
gān shù, 127
gangrene, 71
gas poisoning, 27
gastrelosis, 312
gastric antrum, 312
gastric fullness, 124
gate tower, 9
gb 24, 127
gé mài, 109
general aching, 146
general examination method, 102
general information, 74
general pain, 85
generalised oedema, 21
genitals and anus, 33
genu valgum, 32
genu varum, 32
geographic tongue, 55
gingival bleeding, 227, 238
gingival haemorrhage, 232
glaucoma, 24
globus hystericus, 241, 242
glomus lumps, 170
glossolalia, 201
goatish smell of sweat, 70
goitre, 22, 24, 30, 184, 241, 242
goitre tumour, 24
governing colour, 10, 11
gradual exuberance of the pathogenic qi, 53
gradual tinnitus, 88
greasy coating, 54, 59, 78, 154
greasy hair with pruritus, 20
greasy taste, 94
greasy tongue coating, 182, 201, 230
great anger, 18, 123
greater yang, 275
greater yin, 275
green-blue nose, 26
grey black coating, 57
grey coating, 57, 317
grey-white turbid circle around the cornea, 23
grief, 160
grinding of the teeth, 28
grinding of the teeth in sleep, 28
groaning, 63
guān, 104
guān yuán, 127
guān-region, 321
guest colour, 10, 11
guidelines for inquiry, 317
guidelines for the inspection examination, 314
gum bleeding, 233
gums, 28
gums are inflamed, 28
gunshots, 162
gurgling sound in the throat, 201, 214

H

habitual intolerance to cold, 139
haemafaecia, 173, 227, 228, 235
haematemesis, 132, 168, 173, 192, 199, 235, 243, 246, 292
haematuria, 40, 173, 192, 204, 227, 228, 261, 292
haemoptysis, 39, 162, 173, 209, 210, 217, 257, 269, 301, 332
haemorrhage, 71, 136, 198, 227, 266, 328
haemorrhage into the skin, 227
haemorrhoids, 34, 40, 166
hair, 20
hair loss, 256
half coating, 56
half-exterior and half-interior pattern, 79
halitosis, 151, 232, 244
hand trembles, 325
hands are clasped firmly, 169
hardness and pain of the abdomen or around the umbilicus, 218, 233
harmonious tone, 62
harmony of qi and blood of a healthy person, 48
hasty panting, 158
hasty pulse, 111, 114, 118
having eaten excessive cold or uncooked food, 63
hé gǔ, 103
head and body pain, 207
head bent down, 17
head circumference, 19
head erysipelas, 35
head is wrapped in a cloth, 86
head sweating, 81
headache, 18, 63, 82, 129, 131,

Index

146, 156, 157, 168, 173, 204, 246, 250, 293, 301, 327, 329
headache and neck pain, 277
heart, 12, 83
heart and kidney yang deficiency, 21, 190, 263
heart and liver blood deficiency, 190, 267
heart and lung diseases, 83
heart and lung qi deficiency, 190, 265
heart and lung qi exhaustion, 122
heart and small intestine patterns, 190
heart blood deficiency, 190, 197, 198, 266
heart channel of the hand *shaoyin*, 44, 191, 300
heart disease, 118
heart fire, 65, 333
heart fire flaming upward, 49, 198
heart fire hyperactivity, 198, 244, 333
heart fire moving downward, 262
heart orifice being obstructed by phlegm-damp, 64
heart pain, 194
heart qi deficiency, 165, 193, 262
heart qi deficiency pattern accompanied by spleen deficiency and exuberance of dampness, 331
heart vessel obstruction, 190
heart vexation, 146, 160, 199, 203, 204, 262, 263, 286, 291, 300, 301

heart yang deficiency, 190, 194
heart yin deficiency, 190, 197, 198, 257, 263
heart-kidney disharmony pattern, 328
heart-kidney yin deficiency pattern, 329
heart-mind and *zang-fu's* vital essence, 315
heart-qi deficiency, 190
heat, 23, 76, 125, 128, 159, 281
heat agitates blood, 134
heat *bì*, 32
heat congesting the lung, 206
heat damaging the *chong mai* and *ren mai*, 98
heat declining and fluid recovering, 54
heat disease, 70
heat disease damaging the fluid, 52
heat disturbing the mind, 68
heat driving into the *ying* (nutritive) and blood levels, 36
heat dysentery and prolapsed sensation, 151
heat entering the pericardium, 64, 65
heat entering the *ying* and blood levels, 49, 59
heat harassing the heart spirit, 33, 64
heat in the blood, 20, 26
heat in the blood and dry intestines, 34
heat in the chest, 329
heat in the exterior, 125

heat in the head, 330
heat in the heart disturbing the mind, 192
heat in the interior, 125
heat in the lung and spleen channels, 26
heat in the stomach, 222
heat in the *ying* level, 59
heat in the *ying* level and dampness in the qi level, 59
heat injures yin-fluid, 142
heat invading the blood chamber, 64
heat is attacking the pericardium, 63
heat obstructing the large intestine, 218, 233
heat of the upper body, 330
heat on the exterior-cold in the interior, 146
heat on the lateral side of the feet, 301
heat or poisoning, 50
heat pathogen combined with alcohol obstructing upward, 50
heat pathogen congesting the lung pattern, 211, 214
heat pathogen damaging the body fluids, 57
heat pathogen damaging yin, 51
heat pathogen invading the stomach, 69
heat pathogen or phlegm-heat obstructing the lung, 86
heat pattern, 14, 42, 48, 58, 59, 68, 71, 91, 96, 124, 126, 132, 149, 275, 286, 323

heat phlegm, 38
heat sensation in the palms, 300, 301
heat stagnates in the intestines, 142
heat stagnation in the intestines, 71
heat steaming upward, 81
heat symptoms, 331
heat toxin, 23
heat toxin obstructing upward, 50
heat toxin of the lung and stomach has damaged yin, 29
heat toxin settling in the throat, 29
heat transports into the pericardium and disturbs the mind, 249
heat vomit, 39
heat-dryness injures the lung, 217
heat-stroke, 157
heavily sagging in lower abdomen, 166
heavily sagging in the right rib-side, 166
heaviness in the head and body, 332
heaviness of the body, 85, 87, 91, 156, 199, 201, 300
heaviness of the body and limbs, 228, 229
heaviness of the head, 244, 245, 246, 248, 273
heaviness of the head and body, 228, 251
heaviness of the limbs, 297
heavy and gruff voice, 62
heavy cold feeling, 149
heavy dampness, 54
heavy head, 83
heavy limbs, 182
heavy pain, 82
hemi-lateral sweating, 81
hemi-paralysis, 18, 32
hemiplegia, 247, 250
herbal prescription, 306
hereditary weakness, 136, 223
hereditary weakness of *yuan* (original) qi, 261
hernia, 33, 238
hesitation, 238
hiccough, 68, 168, 222, 233, 234, 242, 269, 270, 272, 312
hidden pulse, 109, 169
high fever, 77, 83, 86, 142, 158, 160, 215, 220, 248, 250, 291, 295
high fever with mild aversion to cold, 77
high fever without aversion to cold, 291
high or low pitch, 62
histories of prophylactic immunisation and infectious diseases, 99
history of present illness (hpi), 319
hoarse voice, 268
hoarseness, 62, 206, 216, 257
hollow pulse, 109, 113
hóng mài, 109
hot limbs, 144
hot or burning sensation of the tongue body, 316
hot sensation in the chest, 198, 199
hot skin, 144
hot-cold, 128
house the mind, 192
howling, 63
HT 7, 104
hú shàn, 301
huá mài, 112
huǎn mài, 110
Huáng Dì Nèi Jīng, 黄帝内经, 4
huddled up when lying in the bed, 17
humpback, 31
hunger, 236
hunger but no appetite, 234
hunger with no desire to eat, 286
hungry without a desire to eat, 333
hydrocele, 33
hyperactive heart fire, 328
hyperactive liver qi, 95
hyperactive liver qi attacking the spleen, 95
hyperactive liver yang causing wind, 325
hyperactivity of fire, 51
hyperactivity of fire due to yin deficiency, 59
hyperactivity of heart fire, 34, 192, 193
hyperactivity of heart fire disturbs the mind, 264
hyperactivity of liver yang, 245, 246, 248
hyperactivity of liver yang

causing wind, 246, 248, 250
hyperactivity of the body mechanisms, 132
hyperfunction, 137
hypermenorrhoea, 98, 238
hypersensitiveness, 36
hypertonicity or contracture of the arms and elbows, 301
hypochondriac burning pain, 245, 246
hypochondriac distension, 86, 312
hypochondriac lumps, 123
hypochondriac pain, 84, 246, 257, 272, 273, 300, 324
hypochondrium and abdomen, 167
hypofunction, 138
hypofunction of respiration, 205
hypofunctional reproduction, 255, 258, 259, 260
hypofunctional sexual activity and reproduction, 254
hypomenorrhoea, 97, 255, 256, 257
hysteria, 8

I

ill at ease, 198, 199
illnesses due to block or obstruction, 18
imminent death, 116
impaired harmonious down-bearing of the stomach, 94
impaired movement of the little finger, 301
impaired movement of the small toe, 300, 301
Important Formulas Worth a Thousand Gold Pieces for Emergency, 15
impotence, 162, 255, 260
improper diet, 131, 134, 155, 223, 228
improper posture during sleep, 63
improvement of *zheng* qi, 55
inability to bend, 84
inability to move, 17
inability to rotats, 301
inability to speak, 295
inability to swallow food, 284
inability to turn the head, 300
inability to walk, 63
inappropriate eating, 35
incisions, 162
incoherent speech, 160, 203
incomplete defaecation, 296
incomplete perspiration, 37
incontinent diarrhoea, 95
increase or decrease of the qi and blood, 126
indigestion, 90, 167
indirect tapping, 121
indistinct pulse, 194, 196
individual life history, 74
individual-finger palpation, 321
infant (one month to three years), 99
infant's malnutrition with accumulation, 42
infant's slobbering, 39
infertility, 254, 255, 259, 260
infestation or injury by parasites, insects, snakes and other animals, 155
inflammation, 232
inflammation of the throat, 300
influence of food, 316
informed consent, 303
inherent deficiency, 25, 30, 31
inhibited lactation, 31
inhibited urination, 136, 279
injures fluids, 158, 216
injures body fluids, 134
injury includes falls, 162
injury to the heart and kidney, 285
innate colour, 11
innate deficiency, 19
innate yin deficiency, 220
inner disharmony, 276
inner heat, 21
inner invasion, 148
inner-transmission of a superficial pattern, 288
inquiring into diet and partiality, 90
inquiring into sleep, 90
inquiring of children, 99
inquiry examination, 72, 312
inquiring into cold and heat, 76
inquiring into menstruation and vaginal discharge, 97
inquiring into pain, 81
inquiring into sweating, 79
inquiring into the ears, 88
inquiring into the head, body, chest and abdomen, 85

inquiring into the nature of pain, 81
inquiring into the position of pain, 82
inquiring into the urine and stool, 93
insect and animal bites, 162
insect bites, 162
insecurity of the *wei*, 323
insecurity of *wei* (defensive) qi, 206
insomnia, 21, 90, 132, 161, 170, 192, 197, 198, 199, 203, 204, 238, 243, 246, 248, 252, 253, 256, 257, 262, 263, 266, 272, 273, 286, 291, 327, 328, 329, 333
insomnia and many dreams, 324
inspecting the spirit and the stomach qi of the tongue, 58
inspection examination, 6
inspection of colour, 9
inspection of drool, 39
inspection of excreta, 38
inspection of maculopapular eruptions or rashes, 35
inspection of nasal discharge, 39
inspection of phlegm or sputum, 38
inspection of posture and movement, 16
inspection of saliva, 39
inspection of skin blisters, 37
inspection of sores and ulcers, 37
inspection of the anterior and posterior yin, 33
inspection of the body, 29
inspection of the ears, 25

inspection of the face, 21
inspection of the five sense organs, 22
inspection of the form of the body, 14
inspection of the four limbs, 32
inspection of the head and face, 19
inspection of the mouth and lips, 26
inspection of the nose, 25
inspection of the *shen*, 7
inspection of the skin, 34
inspection of the skin and lower orifices, 315
inspection of the stool, 40
inspection of the superficial vein of the index finger, 41, 315
inspection of the teeth and gums, 27
inspection of the throat, 28
inspection of the tongue, 44
inspection of the tongue body, 48
inspection of the tongue coating, 53
inspection of vomit, 39
insufficiency of body fluids pattern, 179
insufficiency of earlier congenital constitution, 32
insufficiency of fluid and impairment of the lung in producing a normal voice, 63
insufficiency of fluids, 126
insufficiency of heart blood, 324
insufficiency of heart yang, 123
insufficiency of kidney essence and mal-development of the skull, 19
insufficiency of kidney essence and qi in childhood with hereditary insufficiency, 254
insufficiency of kidney qi, 31
insufficiency of kidney yin, 98
insufficiency of liver and kidney, 98
insufficiency of qi and blood, 31, 53, 109, 326
insufficiency of stomach yin, 28
insufficiency of stomach-spleen qi, 90
insufficiency of the spinal marrow, 88
insufficiency of yin-blood, 94, 330
insufficiency of *yuan* qi, 165
insufficiency of *zang-fu* essence, 15
insufficient body fluids, 136
insufficient essence-blood, 126
insufficient heart qi, 64
insufficient kidney essence, 255
insufficient kidney yin, 240, 328
insufficient production of qi and blood, 239
insufficient qi and blood, 81, 109
insufficient sources of *ying* qi and blood, 136
insufficient ying and blood, 109
insufficient *zheng* qi, 8, 65
insufficient *zong* qi and *wei* qi, 261
intense heart fire, 190
intense heat pathogen, 51

intense liver fire, 190
intense lung heat, 190
intense pain, 14, 63
intense stomach fire, 84
intense stomach heat with consequent excessive decomposition of the food, 92
intense summer-heat, 70
intentions, 305
inter-costal fullness, 87
interior, 128
interior accumulation of damp phlegm, 54
interior blockage of dampness and fluids unable to go upward, 54
interior cold, 226
interior cold patterns, 57
interior damage disease, 51
interior deficient cold pattern, 77
interior excessive cold pattern, 77
interior excessive heat pattern, 78, 218, 233
interior heat, 322
interior heat patterns, 42, 57, 127
interior pattern, 42, 60, 109, 131, 323, 324
interior pattern mixed with an exterior pattern, 57
interior phlegm fire, 203
interior stagnation of pathogens, 109
interior wind, 156
interior-exterior, 128
intermingled phlegm and qi, 242
intermittent and rapid pulse, 192
intermittent constipation and diarrhoea, 272
intermittent pulse, 111, 114, 118
internal accumulation of damp-heat, 57, 70
internal accumulation of damp-heat due to upward reverse flow of gallbladder qi, 94
internal accumulation of the kidney fire, 35
internal accumulation of yin-cold, 110
internal damage, 65, 121
internal damage disease, 78
internal damage fever, 127
internal damage of the essential qi, 63
internal damage of the lung or other *zang-fu* organs, 67
internal deficiency fire, 15
internal disturbance of liver wind, 17, 88
internal dryness pattern, 179
internal excess of heat pathogen, 37
internal exuberance of phlegm-heat, 90
internal exuberance of yin-cold, 81
internal eye disease, 23
internal food retention, 59
internal harassment of heart spirit, 90
internal heat, 216, 329
internal injury disease, 319
internal invasion of cold-dampness, 32
internal obstruction of phlegm-dampness, 86
internal or external conditions, 126
internal retention of damp-heat, 37
internal retention of excessive heat, 87
internal retention of phlegm-rheum, 66, 91
internal sinking of measles toxin, 37
internal stirring of liver wind, 20, 24, 32, 33
internal ulcer, 71
internal ulcer or abscess, 70
internal-external cold, 146
internal-external deficiency, 146
internal-external excess, 146
internal-external heat, 146
intestinal abscess, 125
intestinal damp-heat, 190
intestinal dryness, 179
intestinal dryness and liquid depletion, 40, 190
intestinal flatus, 234
intestinal heat and bowel excess, 190
intestinal rumbling, 157
intestinal wind, 40
intestines, 87
invasion by exterior pathogens, 206
invasion by external warm-heat, 91
invasion by toxin in the black (pupil) part of the eyes, 23
invasion of a cold pathogen,

132
invasion of an external warm-heat pathogen, 36
invasion of cold wind, 330
invasion of cold-damp, 32, 33
invasion of exterior pathogenic factors, 129, 188
invasion of external wind-cold, 67
invasion of pathogen, 276
invasion of pathogenic wind, 87
invasion of the lung, 330
invasion of the lung by liver fire, 269
invasion of the stomach by liver, 269
invasion of wind combined with cold and dampness in the joints and channels, 156
invasion of wind-damp, 35
invasion of wind-heat, 49
investigating moistness or dryness, 125
investigating the existence or depletion of yang, 127
investigating the pain, 126
invisible phlegm, 185
involuntary shaking of the head, 246, 248, 250
involuntary wriggling of hands and feet, 257
inward, 138
inward invasion of a carbuncle, 64
inward invasion of toxin, 21
irregular alternating chills and fever, 78

irregular and rapid pulse, 122
irregular bowel habits, 221
irregular defaecations, 249
irregular diet, 223, 235
irregular inter-menstrual cycle bleeding, 256
irregular menstrual cycle, 97
irregular menstruation, 255, 257, 268
irregular respiration, 65
irregular rhythm of breath, 31
irregular thrashing and waving of the limbs, 18
irritability, 8, 78, 175, 204, 242, 243, 244, 245, 248, 269, 270, 272, 273, 286, 328, 329, 330
irritation, 238
irritation of the mind, 291
itching, 230
itching of the skin, 230
itchy eyes, 89
itchy skin, 156
itchy throat, 206

J

jaundice, 13, 23, 35, 40, 83, 173, 238, 249, 250, 251, 300
jaundice due to sexual intemperance, 35
jaundice of the skin and sclera, 230
jí mài, 110
jī mén, 104
jié mài, 110
jiě suǒ mài, 117
jǐn mài, 112

jǐng yuè quán shū, 景岳全书, 5
joint pain or swelling, 18
joy damage, 160
jù liáo, 102
jù quē, 127
jueyin, 275
jueyin channel headache, 83
jueyin liver channel, 84
jueyin pattern, 286

K

K 3, 127
ké, 67
ké sòu, 67
KI 3, 104
kidney and bladder patterns, 190
kidney and liver yin deficiency, 197, 198, 296
kidney and lung yin deficiency, 190, 268
kidney and spleen yang deficiency, 190, 274
kidney channel of the foot *shaoyin*, 44, 301
kidney deficiency, 14, 20, 21, 23, 26, 28, 83, 85, 91, 94, 95
kidney deficiency and water flooding, 190
kidney diseases, 122
kidney essence deficiency, 88, 190, 255, 257, 259
kidney failing to absorb qi, 255
kidney failing to grasp qi, 190
kidney failing to receive qi, 255, 260, 262
kidney prolapse, 166

Index

kidney qi deficiency, 165, 259, 260, 262
kidney qi insecurity, 96, 190, 331
kidney qi not firm pattern, 255
kidney yang deficiency, 13, 14, 190, 254, 255, 259, 260
kidney yin deficiency, 13, 14, 25, 190, 191, 244, 255, 257, 259, 263, 296
kidney yin deficiency with heart fire flaring-up, 24
kinds of bleeding, 160
knees swelling, 32
knife wounds, 162
knock knees, 32
knotted and intermittent pulse, 170, 192, 194, 265
knotted or intermittent pulse, 193, 199
knotted pulse, 110, 114, 118
kōu mài, 109
kuáng 狂, 8

L

laboured breathing, 86, 168, 173, 265
lack of ability to taste foods, 223
lack of appetite, 8, 189
lack of aversion to cold, 285
lack of coating, 86
lack of courage, 238, 252, 253
lack of distribution of wei qi, 205
lack of movement, 138
lack of nourishment of the skin, 35
lack of qi transformation, 138

lack of spirit, 8
lack of strength, 87, 88, 139, 158, 159, 161, 165, 176, 221, 222, 223, 226, 227, 236, 262, 264, 265, 266, 267
lack of strength to move blood, 133
lack of sweating, 277
lack of taste in the mouth, 332
lack of the sense of taste, 186
lack of thirst, 132, 138, 186, 231
lack of transformation of the accumulated damp-turbidity or food, 54
lack of vitality in the activity of the eyeballs, 314
lack of warmth, 138
language, 318
láo mài, 110
large and moderate pulse, 161
large but forceless pulse, 260
large intestine channel of the hand yangming, 280, 300
large intestine damp-heat pattern, 217, 333
large intestine deficient-cold, 190, 221
large intestine dryness pattern, 219
large pulse, 112
laryngopharynx, 28
lassitude, 66, 153, 160, 161, 189, 193, 194, 222, 254, 259, 265, 301, 329, 332
lassitude of the body and limbs, 223
lassitude of the limbs, 228

late afternoon fever, 218, 220
late afternoon tidal fever, 78
laughing and weeping, 334
laziness in speaking, 139, 161, 165, 176, 223, 227, 228, 267, 323
leaning on objects, 17
left face numbness, 325
left sided migraine, 325
leg erysipelas, 35
leonine (lion-like) face, 22
leprosy, 22, 26
lesser yang, 275
lesser yin, 275
lethargic sensation, 87
lethargy, 8
lethargy in speaking, 260
leucorrhoea due to cold-dampness, 14
lǐ, 305
LI 11, 313
LI 4, 103, 313
[Li] Bin-Hu's Teachings on Pulse Diagnosis (Bīn Hú Mài Xué, 濒湖脉学), 4
life gate, 226
life pass, 41, 42
lifting, 105
less pathogens and failure of the zheng qi, 77
light-purple lips and tongue, 265
light red and fissured tongue, 323
light swollen and bleeding gums without redness and pain, 28
light yellow and moist appearance on the tip of the nose, 26

light yellow coating, 57
light-dark or purple tongue, 264
light-white tongue with cracks, 51
limb numbness, 324
limbs paralysis, 33
Líng Shū-Wǔ Sè, 灵枢·五色, 9
lips, 17, 196, 209, 217
listening and smelling examination, 61
listening to sounds, 61
listening to the respiration, 65
listening to the sound of the cough, 67
listening to the sound of vomiting, 67
listening to the speech, 63
listening to the voice, 62
listlessness, 8, 265, 285, 296
little coating, 272
liù jīng 六经, 218
liver, 12
liver abscess, 123
liver and gallbladder damp-heat pattern, 331
liver and gallbladder diseases, 83
liver and gallbladder fire disturbing the upper orifices, 88
liver and gallbladder fire flaring up and congesting the ears, 88
liver and gallbladder patterns, 190
liver and gallbladder qi deficiency, 165
liver and kidney deficiency, 23
liver and kidney yin deficiency, 88, 190, 272, 273
liver and stomach disharmony, 94
liver and stomach qi stagnation, 168
liver blood deficiency, 190, 239
liver blood deficiency leading to liver wind, 246
liver cancer, 123
liver channel, 237
liver channel of the foot *jueyin*, 19, 44, 301
liver cold pattern, 252
liver constraint, 246
liver constraint and qi stagnation, 190
liver constraint and spleen deficiency, 190, 270
liver constraint pattern, 242
liver deficiency, 123
liver disease, 82, 238
liver fire, 23
liver fire blazing upward, 238, 243, 245, 246
liver fire flaming upward, 86, 89, 332
liver fire invading the lung, 190, 268
liver fire invading the stomach, 39
liver invading the spleen, 40, 270, 272
liver prolapse, 166
liver qi attacking the stomach, 69
liver qi counterflow, 168
liver qi stagnation, 97, 168, 333
liver stagnation and deficiency of the spleen, 14
liver wind agitating within, 190
liver wind pattern, 158, 248
liver wind stirring internally pattern, 246
liver wind with phlegm, 52
liver yang hyperactivity, 330
liver yang rising, 238
liver yang rising and troubling the upper orifices, 86
liver yang stirring causing wind, 239
liver yang transforming into wind, 52, 330
liver yin deficiency, 190, 239, 246, 257
liver yin deficiency leading to liver wind, 246
liver-gallbladder damp-heat fuming and steaming, 25
liver-kidney yin deficiency, 30
liver-stomach disharmony, 190, 330
living in a cold environment, 138
local sweating, 81
locked jaw, 18, 169
long course, 131, 229, 245
long pulse, 112, 113, 115
long-standing phlegm turns into heat, 206
looking examination, 6
loose bones, 255
loose coating, 54
loose stool, 132, 135, 138, 146, 158, 159, 182, 222, 223, 225, 226, 227, 231, 236, 262, 266, 267, 268, 270, 272, 297, 300, 323, 330

loose stools with a foul odour, 229, 230
loose stools with an offensive odour, 251
loose teeth, 255, 256, 257, 258
loss of appetite, 284, 329, 330
loss of blood, 27, 28, 162
loss of blood due to deficiency of qi, 174, 176
loss of consciousness, 17, 201, 296, 297
loss of essence, 136
loss of excessive blood, 143
loss of hair, 20, 255, 258
loss of speech, 18
loss of vitality, 33
loss of voice, 62, 323
loss of voice during pregnancy, 63
loss of yang qi, 194
loud breathing with phlegm gurgling in the throat, 169
loud voice, 153
low and weak speech, 64
low libido, 254, 258
low lumbar region pain, 255
low pitched sound, 66
low tension pulses, 114
low voice, 215
low, weak and slow borborygmus, 69
lower *jiao*, 261, 294
lower limb ankylosis, 326
lower yin deficiency, 325
LU 1, 127
LU 9, 127
lubricated skin, 126

lumbago, 63, 85, 121
lumbar cold and heavy pain, 85
lumbar pain, 18
lumbus and lower limb joints, 326
lumps in the abdomen, 125
lumps in the nares, 26
lumps in the neck, 301
lung abscess, 38, 83
lung and large intestine patterns, 190
lung and stomach brewing into heat and then burning the nasal vessels, 26
lung channel of the hand *taiyin*, 41, 295, 299
lung deficiency, 17
lung distension, 17, 24, 31, 122, 187
lung dryness, 179, 209, 210, 214, 216
lung excess and qi counter-flow, 17
lung fails to disperse and descend, 157
lung fire, 23, 211
lung governs qi, 61
lung heat pattern, 211
lung is obstructed by phlegm-dampness, 86
lung is the master of qi, 205
lung qi counterflow, 168
lung qi deficiency, 31, 86, 165, 189, 190, 206, 215, 262
lung qi failing to diffuse and purify, 63
lung qi failing to disperse, 130

lung qi rises counter flow, 130
lung *wei qi*, 324
lung yin deficiency, 83, 190, 206, 216, 257
lung-dryness, 190
lung-kidney qi deficiency, 31
lustre, 9
lustreless skin, 206, 227, 301
lustrous, 315
lustrous tongue, 60
LV 10, 104
LV 13, 127
LV 14, 127, 313
LV 3, 104, 127, 313
lying in a supine position with extension of the limbs and refusal to cover, 17
lying on the bed, 17
lying on the bed facing downwards or facing the wall, 17
lying on the bed with inability to sit up, 17

M

maculae, 36, 149
maculopapular eruptions, 35, 36
main complaint, 304
main symptoms, 74, 319
major blood loss, 18
major chest accumulation pattern, 124
malar flush, 14, 191
malaria, 18, 27, 79, 123
mal-development, 31
malformation of the lower limbs,

32
malfunction of the liver, 87
malignant colour, 10, 12
malnutrition, 21, 82
malnutrition of the channels, 17, 85, 327
malnutrition of the ear orifices, 88
malnutrition of the eyes, 89
malnutrition of the heart spirit, 90
malnutrition of the skin, 326
malnutrition of tissues and organs, 82
malnutrition of *ying*-blood, 86
mammary pain, 18
mania, 8, 65, 160, 173, 192, 199, 203, 204, 218, 220, 248, 250, 253, 300
manic disease, 8
manic raving, 64
manifestation of the tongue spirit, 57
manifestations of the spirit, 7
margins of the tongue, 45
marked symptoms from *zang-fu* organs, 131
Mài Jīng, 脉经, 4
measles, 35, 36, 149
medical encounter, 302
medical history, 304
medical record, 302
medical terms, 318
membranous screen, 23
men's voices, 62
meningitis, 36
menorrhagia, 227, 228
menorrhoea, 258

menstrual and vaginal discharge odours, 71
menstrual or essence incontinence, 167
menstrual pulse, 117
menstruation, 97
mental activity, 192
mental confusion, 8, 192, 201
mental confusion due to phlegm, 193
mental depression, 246
mental derangement, 64
mental disorders, 8, 201, 203, 204, 301
mental fatigue, 139, 160, 165, 215, 254, 259, 262, 264, 265, 266
mental restlessness, 203, 244, 248, 253
mental restlessness and sadness, 192
mental retardation, 258
mental status, 7, 314
messenger of the heart, 314
metal, 13
method and guidelines of pulse examination, 320
method and guidelines of the tongue examination, 315
method of the inquiry examination, 73
method of the tongue examination, 45
metrorrhagia, 109, 222, 227, 256, 259, 260, 262
metrorrhagia and metrostaxis, 228, 238
metrostaxis, 109, 256

middle *jiao*, 205, 218, 221, 249, 294
migraine, 330
migratory pain, 82
mild aversion to wind and cold, 295
mild damage of the body fluid, 91
mild disease and with good prognosis, 92
mild fever, 77, 78, 156, 159
mild pressing, 106
miliaria alba, 37
mìng guān, 41
mingmen fire, 40, 276
mingmen fire deficiency, 254
míng táng, 明堂, 9
mingmen, 226, 329
minor chest accumulation pattern, 124
miosis, 24
mirror-like, 323
miserable expression, 161
mixed cold and heat pattern, 147
mobility of the head, 19, 20
moderate and weak pulse, 223
moderate pulse, 110, 115
moderate, 284
moist, 121
moist and slippery whitish coating, 138
moist coating, 53
moist facial colour, 11
moist slippery and white coating, 135
morbid colour, 10, 12
mouldy and curdy coating, 316

mouldy bean curd-like coating, 54
mounting qi pain, 301
mouth and lips ulcers, 27
mouth breathing, 317
mouth opening and eyes closing, 166, 169
movement of the body, 314
movement of the mouth and lips, 27
movement of the *wei* qi, 90
movements of the eyes, 24
mucky damp-heat pathogen overflowing, 55
muffled metal failing to sound, 63
muscle dystrophy, 32
muscle has atrophied, 326
muscle wheel, 22
muscular spasms, 162
muscular twitching, 246, 248
muttering and mumbling to oneself, 64
mutual transmission and transformation, 288
mydriasis, 24

N

nails, 177, 196
nasal bleeding, 228
nasal discharge, 132
nasal obstruction, 277, 300
nasal polyps, 26
nasopharynx, 28
natural light, 314

nature of the disease, 128, 132
nausea, 158, 159, 161, 168, 182, 184, 201, 222, 228, 229, 230, 231, 242, 249, 251, 252, 253, 272, 297, 330, 332
nausea on seeing food, 330
nebula, 23
neck rigidity, 30
neck swelling, 300
nèi guān, 313
nèi tíng, 313
neonates (birth to one month), 99
new disease, 119
night blindness, 89, 238
night sweat, 78, 80, 83, 140, 162, 191, 197, 198, 216, 217, 240, 246, 255, 256, 257, 259, 263, 268, 272, 273, 323, 328, 329
nine orifices being obstructed, 169
no appetite, 236
no aversion to cold, 295
no coating, 330
no desire to eat or drink, 8
no desire to speak, 8, 153
no evident pulse, 170
no hair for a long time after birth, 21
no pain on pressure, 87
no past history, 211
no strength for raising the head, 30
no sweat, 126, 129, 157, 180
no thirst, 159, 226, 236
no treatment or incorrect treatment, 136

nocturia, 254, 332
nocturnal emissions, 162, 255, 259, 260, 263, 268, 272
nocturnal emissions without dreams, 262
nodules, 30, 127
non-ascending of clear yang, 86
non-floating pulse, 148
non-meaningful speech, 201
non-pitting oedema, 126
non-productive cough, 67
non-traumatic haemorrhage, 192
normal breath, 65
normal colour, 10
normal mental status, 312
normal pulse, 107
normal sounds, 62
normal tongue body or slightly red in the tip and sides, 131
normal tongue coating, 56
normal tongue manifestation, 47
normal tongue with slight red on the sides and tip, 208
normal urine, 40
nose, 9, 209, 215, 217
nose bleeding, 132, 199, 209, 217, 227, 243, 246, 292, 300
nostrils flaring, 211, 214, 215
numbness, 87, 149, 156, 173, 238, 246, 316, 329
numbness in the hands and feet, 329
numbness of the limbs, 170, 184, 239, 246, 248, 249, 250, 267
nutation, 30

O

obese build, 15
obesity, 123, 161
objective focus, 318
oblique flying pulse, 108
obstruct the circulation of qi, 87
obstructed defaecation, 95
obstructing middle yang, 142
obstructing qi movement of the middle *jiao*, 69
obstructing the channels, 142
obstruction and accumulation of the phlegm-turbidity, 62
obstruction and stagnation of static blood, 86
obstruction and stagnation of the channels and collaterals, 85
obstruction and stagnation of wind, 85
obstruction by dampness and blood stasis, 31
obstruction of the blood vessels suggesting a severe case, 42
obstruction of the collaterals by wind-phlegm, 65
obstruction of the heart vessel, 193, 199, 201
obstruction of the lung by heat or asthma, 26
occurrence of the disease, 319
odours of the vomitus, 67
oedema, 23, 31, 33, 71, 87, 96, 126, 138, 180, 213, 222, 226, 228, 230, 254, 255, 260, 262, 264, 267, 274, 331
oedema of the face and limbs, 323
oedematous disease, 32
old circle, 23
oliguria, 180, 192
one pupil is dilated, 24
one-sided paralysis, 17
onset, 319
onset of measles, 127
opacity of the eye (nebula), 23
opisthotonos, 162, 238, 248
opposite pulses, 114
oppressed feeling, 269
oppression in the chest, 196
oppression of emotions, 83
ordinary transmission, 292, 298
organ patterns, 189
organo-phosphate poisoning, 71
oropharynx, 28
otopyorrhoea, 25
outburst of *zong* qi, 123
outbursts of anger, 238, 242, 243, 245, 248, 269, 270, 272, 273
outcome measures, 306
outward, 138
outward overflow of bile, 251
over consumption of raw and cold foods, 221
over intake of warm and dry medicines, 141
over thinking, 223
over worrying, 223
over-controlling of yang, 133
overexertion damaging the kidney, 35
overflowing of water-damp, 21
overstrain, 131, 155, 186, 223

P

PC 6, 313
PC 7, 127
pain, 14, 109, 111, 112, 125, 157, 162, 173, 222, 231, 277, 286, 330
pain aggravated by pressure, 235
pain alleviated by pressure, 153
pain and dyskinesia, 301
pain and dyskinesia along the lateral aspect of the chest and hypochondrium, 301
pain and fullness of the chest and hypochondrium, 301
pain and heavy sensation of the joints and limbs, 159
pain and stiffness in the head and neck, 276, 277
pain and ulcers in the gums, 244
pain around the breasts, 300
pain caused by deficiency, 81
pain caused by excess, 81
pain during breathing, 187
pain in the abdomen, 219, 332
pain in the chest, 199, 200, 201, 326, 330
pain in the ear, 246
pain in the hypochondrium, 329
pain in the lumbus, 326
pain in the nape of the neck, 300
pain in the posteriomedial aspect of the thigh, 301
pain in the posterior border of the medial aspect of the upper limbs, 300

pain in the retroauricular region, 301
pain of the chest and hypochondrium, 301
pain of the heels, 85
pain of the joints and limbs, 157
pain of the limbs, 85
pain of the lower abdomen, 331
pain of the lumbus that inhibits stretching, 301
pain of the mandible, 301
pain of the outer canthus, 301
pain of the supraclavicular fossa, 299
pain on pressure, 87
pain or dysfunction of the knee, 300
pain or dysfunction of the shoulders, 300
pain or dyskinesia of the thigh, 300
pain patterns, 42, 111, 118
painful, 255
painful and bleeding gums, 232
painful body, 157
painful eyes, 89
painful throat, 329
painful urine, 147
pair of principles, 128
pale and enlarged tongue, 196
pale and lustreless complexion, 239
pale and moist tongue body, 194
pale and plump tongue, 182, 226
pale and receding gums, 28
pale and tender tongue, 58, 164, 176, 262, 266, 324

pale and thin menstrual flow, 98
pale and white lips, 177
pale auricle, 25
pale canthus, 23
pale complexion, 8, 18, 132, 138, 142, 161, 166, 176, 189, 193, 194, 196, 198, 215, 227, 262, 265, 267, 328, 331
pale cyanosis of the lips and nails, 264
pale enlarged tongue, 229, 274
pale face, 249, 250
pale face with occasional migratory bright-red, 14
pale gums, 28
pale lips, 262
pale lips and nails, 170, 197, 198, 266
pale menstrual flow, 239
pale or blue complexion, 231
pale or light pale face, 192
pale or pallid complexion, 196
pale red tongue, 200, 201
pale tongue, 58, 86, 92, 132, 135, 151, 166, 193, 196, 197, 198, 201, 210, 211, 213, 215, 221, 227, 228, 231, 236, 239, 249, 250, 252, 254, 258, 259, 260, 267, 326, 327, 328, 330, 331
pale tongue coating, 270, 272
pale tongue with a peeled coating, 55
pale tongue with a thin coating, 326
pale tongue with a white coating, 170, 223
pale tongue with slippery

coating, 182
pale tongue with thin white coating, 326
pale without lustre, 13
pallid or gloomy complexion, 196
pallor, 178
pallor or sallow complexion, 170, 176
palms and soles, 140, 197, 198, 217, 240, 256, 257, 259, 324, 329
palpating, 106
palpating sores and ulcers, 126
palpating the area below heart, 123
palpating the chest, 122
palpating the chest and hypochondrium, 122
palpating the hands and feet, 126, 127
palpating the hypochondrium, 123
palpating the skin, 125
palpating the swelling, 126
palpating the transport points, 127
palpating to discern the coldness or heat of the skin, 125
palpation, 121
palpating examination, 120
palpation of BL 59 (*fū yáng*) pulse, 105
palpation of KI 3 (*tài xī*) pulse, 105
palpation of the *cùn kǒu* pulse, 105
palpation of the forearm skin,

126
palpitations, 18, 21, 87, 131, 146, 161, 187, 192, 193, 194, 196, 197, 200, 201, 204, 213, 240, 246, 253, 257, 262, 263, 264, 265, 266, 296, 301, 319, 324, 326, 328, 329, 330
palpitations due to fright, 87, 238, 252
panic, 8, 161, 238
panting, 65, 66, 131, 142, 146, 157, 184, 187, 260, 265, 267, 268, 277, 296, 299, 301, 323
panting breath, 24
panting cough, 301
papulae, 35, 36
papulovesicular, 249
paralysis, 156, 173, 246
paraphasia, 64
paraplegia, 33
parasite accumulation, 28
parasites, 63
parched teeth with no sordes, 28
parched teeth with sordes, 28
paroxysmal howl in infants, 63
parturition pulse, 117
past medical history, 74
pathogen is moving from the exterior into the interior, 59
pathogen is transforming into heat, 59
pathogen stagnating, 109
pathogenic changes of the spleen and stomach, 87
pathogenic cold invading the stomach, 84
pathogenic factor, 275
pathogenic heat entering the *ying*, 91
pathogenic invasions, 80
pathogenic qi, 135
pathogenic qi in superabundance, 54
pathogenic qi invading the channels, 42
pathogenic qi invading the *zang-fu* organs, 42
pathogenic qi of damp-turbidity is being dispelled, 54
pathogens harassing the interior and results in a restless spirit, 90
pathogens invade the *zang-fu* organs, qi-blood and marrow, 131
pathogens obstruction, 137
pathogens prevailing over *zheng* (healthy) qi and internal sinking of pathogenic qi, 36
pathological changes in the ears, 25
pathological changes in the nose, 26
pathological manifestations of the twelve channels, 299
pathological products cause obstruction, 137
pathological sounds, 62
pathological sweating, 79
patient care, 302
patient record, 302
pattern differentiation, 2
pattern differentiation according to qi, blood and body fluids, 163
pattern differentiation according to the eight principles, 128
pattern differentiation according to the twelve channels, 299
pattern differentiation according to the *wei*, qi, *ying*, and blood, 288
pattern identification, 2, 128
pattern of blood deficiency causing wind, 326
pattern of blood loss, 13
pattern of cold in the exterior and interior heat, 322
pattern of dampness, 326
pattern of deficiency of both qi and blood, 326
pattern of deficiency of both yin and yang, 323
pattern of dryness invading the lung *jin*, 327
pattern of excess heat in the lung, 83
pattern of extreme cold appearing with heat signs, 151
pattern of fluid retention, 327
pattern of liver fire invasion of the lung, 332
pattern of liver yang hyperactivity, 330
pattern of liver-stomach disharmony, 312
pattern of stagnation of liver qi with deficiency of the spleen, 329
pattern of summer-heat, 326
pattern of the *ying* (nutrient)

stage of warm disease, 92
pattern of upper cold and lower heat, 147
pattern of upper heat and lower cold, 147
pattern of yang deficiency, 13
patterns of intermingled deficiency and excess, 325
patterns of yin deficiency of the heart and kidney, 325
peeled coating, 55, 236
penetration of the heat pathogen, 291
percussion, 121
pericardium channel of the hand *jueyin*, 295, 301
peripheral coldness, 151, 152
perishing (夭), 11
persistent cold-damp, 32
persistent thirst, 286
personal profile, 303
pes valgus, 32
pes varus, 32
pestilence, 70, 71
pestilent diseases, 57
petechiae, 170, 227, 228
pharynx, 209, 215, 217
phlegm, 38, 136, 331, 332, 334
phlegm and nasal mucus odours, 70
phlegm and qi stagnation, 168
phlegm damp obstructing the lung, 206
phlegm fire agitation pattern, 334
phlegm fire harassing, 203
phlegm fluids obstructing the lung, 211

phlegm heat obstructing the lung, 206
phlegm in the throat, 325
phlegm misting the heart orifices, 201, 203, 204
phlegm misting the heart spirit, 190
phlegm nodes, 301
phlegm obstructing the heart, 143
phlegm or fluid retention, 66
phlegm patterns, 201
phlegm retention, 112, 201
phlegm rheum, 54
phlegmatic turbidity, 88
phlegm-damp, 53
phlegm-damp obstructing the lung, 190, 211
phlegm-dampness disturbing the spleen, 90
phlegm-dampness obstructing in the interior, 58
phlegm-dampness obstructing the middle *jiao*, 56
phlegm-fire, 25, 112, 334
phlegm-fire disturbing the heart, 64
phlegm-fire disturbing the mind, 193
phlegm-fire harassing the heart, 190, 204, 253
phlegm-fluid retention, 184
phlegm-fluids, 180
phlegm-fluids obstructing the lung, 211
phlegm-fluids or blood stasis, 167

phlegm-heat, 23, 54, 57
phlegm-heat brewing internally, 39
phlegm-heat disturbing the heart, 64
phlegm-heat harassing the heart spirit upward, 90
phlegm-heat obstructing the lung, 122, 190, 214
phlegm-retention, 123
phlegm-rheum, 56, 66, 94, 126
phlegm-rheum accumulating and transforming into heat, 57
phlegm-rheum disease, 23
phlegm-rheum obstructing in the middle *jiao* with fluids not nourishing upward, 56
phlegm-rheum retention and malaria, 112
phlegm-turbidity, 51
photophobia, 89
physically weak body, 153
physiological differences of the tongue manifestation, 47
physiological sweating, 79
pǐ, 78
pí shù, 127
pigeon breast, 31
pitting oedema, 126, 182
Pivot for Diagnosis (*Zhěn Jiā Shū Yào*, 诊家枢要), 4
pǐ-with fullness and distension, 124
pleural effusion, 187
pleural rheum, 31, 84
plum-stone throat, 241
pneumothorax, 31, 122

point prescription, 306
polydipsia, 92
polyorexia, 244
polyphagia, 91
polyuria, 93
poor appetite, 90, 146, 158, 159, 160, 161, 222, 223, 226, 227, 228, 229, 230, 231, 235, 236, 251, 262, 266, 267, 268, 270, 272, 323, 327, 330
poor appetite and digestion, 323
poor memory, 192, 197, 204, 255, 256, 257, 258, 259
popliteal fossa, 300
position for tongue observation, 315
posterior yin, 34
postnatal deficiency, 255
postpartum excessive loss of blood, 327
posture, 6, 315
posture of tongue extending, 315
powder-like coating, 56
powerful and rapid pulse, 160, 173, 199, 244, 290
powerful and smooth pulse, 161
powerful and wiry pulse, 246
powerful deep and rapid pulse, 218, 220
powerful pulse, 153
powerful wiry and rapid pulse, 169, 250
precordial pain, 83
predilection for lying down, 301
preference for cold, 124, 142, 244
preference for cold drinks, 91, 232, 236

preference for hot drinks, 91
preference for lying in a curled-up posture, 285
preference for pressure, 124
preference for warmth, 124, 147, 221, 229, 230, 236
preference for warmth and pressure, 221
prefers to drink warm liquids, 152
pregnancy reaction, 92
pregnant women, 112
premature ejaculation, 162, 254, 256, 259, 260
premature senility in adults, 255
presence of stomach qi, 56
present illness history, 74, 75, 304
present symptoms, 304, 319, 320
pressing, 121, 321
pressing and searching, 321
prickly tongue, 50, 192
principles, 305
principles of the tongue examination, 44
principles of treatment, 128
procedure of the diagnosis and treatment, 319, 320
proctoptosis, 34
production of phlegm, 64
productive cough, 67
profuse and clear urine, 221, 285
profuse clear dilute sputum, 267
profuse clear leucorrhoea, 259
profuse clear urine, 135, 142, 274
profuse cold, 144
profuse cold sweating, 178
profuse leucorrhoea, 228, 230
profuse nocturia, 259

profuse sputum, 86, 136, 162
profuse sweating, 80, 158, 166
profuse urine, 96
profuse urine and loose stool, 139
profuse watery frothy sputum, 211
profuse white sticky sputum, 211
prognosis, 149
prolapse of internal organs, 222
prolapse of organs, 222
prolapse of the anus, 328
prolapse of the rectum, 166
prolapse of the rectum or uterus, 222, 223, 228
prolapse of internal organs, 166
prolonged anxiety, 197
prolonged blood stasis, 14
prolonged cough, 267
prolonged disease, 119
prolonged dysentery, 95
prolonged expiratory phase, 31
prolonged illness, 51, 263
prolonged inspiratory phase, 31
propensity to catch colds, 262
propensity to fright, 301
prosperity of qi and blood, 126
protruding tongue, 52
protrusion of the female yin, 34
protrusion of the fontanel, 20
proximal bleeding, 40, 95
pruritus, 33
pruritus vulvae, 249
pseudo-cold manifestations, 151
pseudo-deficiency pattern, 153
pseudo-excess pattern, 152
pseudo-heat manifestations, 151

pseudomembrane, 29
psycho-social factors, 305
psychotic diseases, 64
pterygium, 24
ptosis, 25
pudendal eczema, 34
pudendal sores, 34
puerperal bleeding, 328
puffiness, 187
puffiness of the head and face, 180
puffy face and eyes, 156
puffy swelling, 300
pulling pain, 82
pulmonary abscess, 70
pulmonary tuberculosis, 323
pulsation of the neck artery, 30
pulse, 153, 242
pulse examination, 101
pulse of a child, 117
pulse of pregnancy, 117
pulse of the four seasons, 108
pulse reading and palpation, 1
pulse taking, 105, 320
pungent foods, 313
purgatives, 284
purple maculae under the skin, 170
purple tongue, 174, 192, 235
purple-black skin, 35
purple-red tongue, 49, 178
purplish menstrual flow, 98
purulent stool with blood, 95
purulent throat, 29
pus, 192
pus and blood in the vomitus, 71
pus and swelling, 199

pus and swelling pain in the ear, 243
pus or curd-like coating, 54
pushing, 106
pus-like sputum, 214
putrefactive odour, 71
putrid belching, 87
pyodermal, 192
pyodermic, 199
pyretic sores, 37

Q

qi and blood deficiency, 111, 266
qi and blood deficiency unable to nourish tendons and channels, 33
qi and blood desertion, 48
qi and blood disharmony, 35
qi and blood exhaustion, 17
qi and blood failing to move freely, 130
qi and blood obstruction and stagnation, 85
qi and blood rushing, 86
qi and blood stagnation, 25, 162
qi and yang deficiency with retention of body fluids, 50
qi and yin deficiency, 31
qi blocking pattern, 158, 163
qì chōng, 300
qi collapse, 18
qi constraint transforming into fire, 64
qi counterflow, 163
qi deficiency, 13, 51, 83, 94, 96, 97, 135, 163, 165, 189, 323, 328, 330
qi deficiency and blood stasis, 176
qi deficiency and fever, 78
qi deficiency and weakness, 94
qi deficiency of the heart and gallbladder, 90
qi deficiency of the heart and lung, 33
qi deficiency of the lung and kidney, 86
qi deficiency of the spleen and kidney, 98
qi deficiency of the spleen and lung, 324
qi deficiency of the spleen and stomach, 13, 33, 93
qi deficiency of the stomach and intestines, 70
qi deficiency pattern, 80, 196
qi disorder, 126
qi drum distension, 125
qi failing to control blood, 176
qi failing to hold blood, 179
qì guān, 41
qì hǎi, 127
qi level pattern, 211, 218
qī mén, 127, 313
qi movement being obstructed, 54
qi pass, 41, 42
qi prolapse of the anus, 95
qi rising counterflow, 301
qi sinking, 163, 328
qi stage of warm disease, 78
qi stagnated by blood, 111
qi stagnation, 14, 64, 83, 84, 97, 110, 111, 137, 163, 165, 200, 201,

269, 333
qi stagnation and blood stasis, 97, 168, 175, 238
qi stagnation and dampness blocking, 168
qi stagnation and obstruction due to stasis, 66
qi stagnation and poor function of the stomach and intestines, 70
qi stagnation and water retention, 168
qi stagnation due to depressed liver, 239
qi stagnation in the intestines, 84
qi stagnation misting the heart orifice, 64
qi stagnation of the stomach, 84
qi syncope, 18
qi system, 288
qi wheel, 22
qi-constraint fever, 78
qing dynasty, 288, 294
qīng qi (clear yang qi), 222
qū chí, 313
quality of the breath sounds, 65
què zhuó mài, 116
què, 阙, 9

R

rabies, 22, 162
racing pulse, 110
radial pulse, 104
ragged throat, 29
rales in throat, 137
rampant heat toxin, 59

rancid breath, 70
rapid and deficient pulse, 296
rapid and forceless pulse, 144
rapid and frequent hungering, 300
rapid and powerful pulse, 152
rapid hungering, 92
rapid pulse, 110, 114, 132, 160, 204, 211, 215, 251, 295, 296, 332
rapid weak pulse, 193
rapid wiry pulse, 86
rash behaviours, 253
rattling sound in the throat, 201
rattling sound of phlegm in the throat, 187
reactions, 306
recovery of the stomach qi, 55
rectal or anal prolapse, 221
recurrent flatus, 236
red, 12, 14, 28, 58
red and dry tongue, 140, 330
red and painful eyes, 238
red and swollen eyelids with ulceration, 23
red and swollen throat, 29
red canthus, 23
red cheeks, 78, 140, 197, 198, 216, 217, 240, 246, 248, 257, 268, 272, 273
red cheeks in the afternoon, 256, 259
red colour on the tip of the nose, 26
red complexion, 83, 199, 238
red complexion and eyes, 132, 244, 269, 273
red dry tongue, 256, 259, 325

red eyes, 160, 203, 243
red face, 18
red face and red eyes, 160
red margins of the tongue, 324
red margins of the tongue with a thin yellow coating, 312
red nose with acne-like pustules on the tip of the nose, 26
red on the sides and tip of the tongue, 289
red or dark tongue, 196
red skin, 34
red swelling and pain of the nose, 26
red swelling of the surrounding skin, 160
red swollen auricle, 25
red tip and sides of the tongue, 295
red tip of the tongue, 208, 215, 286
red tongue, 59, 78, 86, 132, 135, 142, 149, 160, 180, 192, 198, 199, 203, 204, 211, 214, 215, 217, 218, 220, 230, 231, 232, 233, 234, 236, 243, 246, 248, 250, 251, 252, 253, 262, 263, 268, 269, 272, 273, 291, 316, 322, 325, 327, 328, 329, 331, 332, 333
red tongue body, 58
red tongue tip, 329
red tongue tip and sides, 330
red tongue with a mirror-like coating, 55
red tongue with a peeled coating, 55
red tongue with diminished

Index

fluids, 197
red tongue with yellow coating, 244
red tongue with little fluid, 179, 240, 246
red tongue with red-crimson tip, 199
red tongue with scanty fluid, 216, 219, 220, 244
red tongue with scanty fluids and a thready pulse, 241
red tongue with yellow coating, 158, 215, 244
red urine, 291, 322
red-crimson tip of the tongue, 199, 244
red-crimson tongue, 173, 248
red-crimson tongue with cracks, 51
reddish complexion, 203, 204
redness, 149
redness and swelling in the entire eye, 23
redness of the eyes, 89
redness of the whole face, 14
reduced coating, 325
reduction in vaginal discharge, 327
red-white leucorrhoea, 99
refusal of abdominal pressure, 234
refusal of pressure, 142, 146, 233
region anterior to the ear and below the cheekbone, 9
regular alternating chills and fever, 78
regurgitation, 168

relative concepts, 128
relative property of exterior and interior, 129
relative yang excess, 134
relieved by warmth or pressure, 226, 229
reluctance for pressure, 229
reluctance to speak, 64
ren, 13, 313
ren mai, 19
rén yíng, 105
repeated onset, 211
respiratory rhythm, 65
restless, 138, 199, 333
restless heart spirit, 90
restlessness, 132, 136, 142, 144, 149, 160, 198, 214, 244, 249, 252, 291, 328
restlessness of emotions, 312
restlessness of the hands and feet, 33
restrain, 138
resuming work immediately after delivery, 34
resurgence of yang qi, 69
retained disease, 66
retarded closure of the fontanel, 20
retching, 67, 233, 234, 283
retention, 39
retention and collection of cold-phlegm and damp-turbidity, 67
retention and stagnation of damp-turbidity, 94
retention of body fluids pattern, 180

retention of cold in the liver channel, 239
retention of cold-damp, 284
retention of damp-heat in the spleen, 229, 230, 231
retention of dampness, 328
retention of fluid due to kidney deficiency, 14
retention of fluid in the chest, 17, 122
retention of food, 71, 222
retention of food in the stomach, 92, 190, 234, 236
retention of food in the stomach and intestines, 87
retention of heat, 159
retention of heat in the intestines, 94
retention of heat in the lung, 244, 295
retention of phlegm, 199
retention of secondary pathological products, 136
retention of water in the stomach, 92
retracted genitals, 33
reverse flow of qi, 144
reverse transmission, 298
reverting yin, 275
rheum, 38
rì yuè, 127
rib-side distension, 200
rickets, 20
right hypochondriac lumps, 123
rigid tongue, 153, 154, 233
rigidity of hands, 8
rigidity of the neck, 246, 248, 250

rising of hidden phlegm, 201
RN 14, 127
RN 17, 127
RN 3, 127
RN 4, 127
RN 6, 127
roof-leaking pulse, 116
root, 59, 305
root coating is a little bit thick, 326
root of phlegm, 38
root of the tongue, 45
rooted coating, 58
rootless coating, 58, 191
rosacea, 26
rotten apple odour, 71
rotten belching, 161
rotten or foul belching, 234
rotten smell, 71
rotten sore, 71
rough coating, 54
rough forearm skin, 126
rough tongue, 60
roundworms, 167
rú mài, 109
ruddy complexion, 8
rumbling intestines, 221
rumbling or gurgling, 69
running of purulent fluid from the ear, 25
runny nose, 129, 156, 206
ruò mài, 109

S

saddle nose deformity, 26
saliva, 45, 132
salivation from the corners of the mouth, 39
salivation in sleeping, 39
sallow complexion, 182, 201, 223, 228, 301, 326, 331, 332
sallow or pale complexion, 266
salty taste, 94
sanjiao channel of the hand shaoyang, 301
sanjiao pattern differentiation, 294
Sān Yīn Jí Yī Bìng Zhèng Fāng Lùn, 三因极一病证方论, 4
săn mài, 109
sanjiao, 283
sardonic smile, 22
scaly dry skin, 170
scaly skin, 126
scant liquid coating, 322
scanty and red menorrhoea, 329
scanty coating, 328, 329
scanty dark urine, 214, 218, 232, 249, 323
scanty dark-yellow urine, 261
scanty deep-red urine, 211
scanty deep-yellow urine, 132, 134
scanty fluids, 217, 273
scanty light menstruation, 267
scanty menstruation, 272, 273, 330
scanty or no sweat, 169
scanty pale menstruation, 266
scanty semen, 255, 258, 259
scanty sputum, 209, 210, 211, 215, 216, 217, 257, 268
scanty sticky sputum, 216

scanty sweating, 209, 217
scanty urine, 96, 138, 140, 144, 156, 158, 179, 209, 217, 226, 228, 230, 233, 254, 260, 274
scanty yellowish urine, 243, 256, 259
scanty-dark urine, 147, 244
scattered (散), 11
scattered and conglomerate (散 抟), 10
scattered heart-mind, 64
scattered pathogenic qi, 56
scattered pulse, 109, 113, 114
sclerotic skin, 35
scorched dry and withered ear, 25
scorched yellow and dry coating, 58
scorched yellow coating, 57
scorching dry-black ear, 25
scorching exuberance of stomach heat, 232
scorching sensation at the anus, 95
scraping, 316
scraping or wiping the tongue, 315
scraping the tongue, 46
scrofula, 30
scrotum hernia, 301
scurrying and distending pain in the hypochondrium, 329
scurrying pain in the chest and hypochondrium, 242
sè mài, 110
sea of blood, 240
sea of water and food, 222

searching, 321
seasonal wind-heat pathogen, 36
seeking, 106
sensation of cold, 331
sensation of heat in the heart, 286
sensation of incomplete defaecation, 95, 159, 270, 272
sequellae of lung atrophy, 31
sequellae of mumps, 34
sequellae of wind stroke, 18
seven emotional factors, 155
seven emotions, 111, 253
seven-emotion internal damage, 23
severe attack of a cold pathogen, 77
severe aversion to cold with low fever, 77
severe burn, 145
severe conditions, 131
severe distending pain in the head, 243
severe expiration of the *zheng qi* and extreme invasion of pathogenic qi, 55
severe fever at night, 291
severe inguinal hernia, 33
severe pain, 201
severe pain of the shoulder and arm, 300
severe palpitations, 18, 86
severe panting on exercise, 260
severe struggle of pathogenic qi and *zheng* qi, 27
severe trauma, 143
Shāng Hán Lùn, 伤寒论, 275
shàng wǎn, 313

shaoyang, 275
shaoyang channel, 25
shaoyang channel headache, 83
shaoyang disease, 281
shaoyang disease of cold damage, 78
shaoyin, 275
shaoyin channel headache, 83
shaoyin cold pattern, 285
shaoyin heat pattern, 285
shaoyin pattern, 285
shape of the head, 19
sheen (泽), 11
sheen and perishing (泽夭), 10
shen, 6, 7
shén mén, 103
shí mài, 111
shiver sweating, 80
shivering, 18, 76, 79
short and fat, 16
short and quick breathing, 187
short breath, 228
short course, 229, 245
short of breath, 323
short pulse, 111, 113, 115
shortage of congenital kidney essence, 25
shortage of essence and blood, 89
shortage of liver and kidney, 23
shortage of lung yin, 55
shortage of qi, 139, 161, 166, 206, 215, 222, 223, 226, 267, 299
shortage of qi and blood, 17, 126
shortage of stomach qi and yin, 55
shortage of the essence, 20

shortage of the essence and blood, 89
shortage of the lung qi, 66, 67
shortage of the qi and blood, 15
shortage of the *ying*-blood, 97
shortage of yang qi, 15
shortage of yin-blood, 15
shortened tongue, 52
shortness of breath, 8, 31, 65, 66, 86, 138, 153, 176, 187, 189, 192, 193, 194, 215, 227, 261, 262, 265, 266, 267, 268, 301, 322, 324, 326, 329, 330, 331
shortness of breath on exertion, 260
shoulders, 300
shrimp-darting pulse, 116
shù mài, 110
shū points, 127
shuttle shape of the finger joints, 33
sì zhěn 四诊, 1, 304
sickroom odours, 71
sighing, 69, 86, 238, 241, 246, 252, 253, 270
simultaneous disease in the middle and lower *jiao*, 298
simultaneous exterior and interior pattern, 147, 325
simultaneous palpation with three fingers, 321
single pressing, 106
single pulse shape, 118
sinking of spleen qi, 223, 228
sinking of the middle qi and non-ascending of the clear yang, 89
sinking pulse, 106

sinusitis, 26, 71
sitting position, 321
sitting up with inability to lie flat on the bed, 17
sitting with the head bent down, 17
sitting with the head raised, 17
six exogenous pathogenic factors, 129, 155
six pathogenic factors, 23
sj 21, 103
skin of the forearm, 322
skin rashes which are of sudden onset and migratory, 156
skin ulceration, 199
skin ulcers, 160
sleeping with eyes open, 24
sleeplessness, 160
slight aversion to wind or cold, 289
slight aversion to wind-cold, 217
slight borborygmus, 70
slight fever, 297
slight headache, 159
slight heat of the lung and stomach, 29
slightly deep pulse, 108
slightly superficial pulse, 108
slightly surging pulse, 108
slightly wiry pulse, 108
slim body, 140
slippery and rapid pulse, 169, 203, 214, 215, 218, 236, 253, 262
slippery coating, 53
slippery greasy coating, 54
slippery pulse, 112, 114, 115, 201, 211, 235, 236

slippery rapid pulse, 334
slippery strong pulse, 333
sloppy and fishy odour of the stool, 71
sloppy diarrhoea, 300
sloppy stools, 295
slow and moderate pulse, 210
slow and tight pulse, 231
slow and weak pulse, 138, 226, 229, 274
slow eye movements, 8
slow movements, 8
slow or tense pulse, 132
slow or wiry and tight pulse, 236
slow pulse, 106, 110, 114
sluggish response, 8
sluggish speech, 65
small head, 19
small intestine channel, 276
small intestine channel of the hand *taiyang*, 300
small intestine excess-heat, 190
small pulse pillow, 320
small red spots at the back of the ear, 25
smell of urine, 71
smelling odours, 61
smoky yellow skin, 228
smoky yellow skin and eyes, 229
smoky yellow skin and sclera, 230
smooth and rapid pulse, 232, 233
smooth breathing, 8
sneezing, 69, 129, 148, 206, 213
snoring, 63
soft and rapid pulse, 230, 231
soft and rapid pulse that is also

slippery, 327
soft foods diet, 313
soft or deep and thready pulse, 228, 229
soft pulse, 230
soft rapid pulse, 182
softness of the neck, 30
soggy or soft and moderate pulse, 159
soggy pulse, 107, 109, 113, 251, 332
soggy rapid pulse, 331
soles, 296
soliloquy, 64, 201
sombre and withered nose, 26
somniloquy, 65
somnolence, 90
sonorous voice, 153
sore throat, 129, 131, 206, 208, 211, 215, 300, 301
sore throat with redness and swelling, 215
soreness and pain of the lumbar region, 17
soreness and weakness of the lumbar region, 191
soreness and weakness of the lumbar region and knees, 255, 256, 257, 259, 268, 272
soreness and weakness of the waist and knees, 325
soreness of the lumbar region, 260, 261, 262, 263
soreness of the lumbar region and lower limbs, 260
sores on the anterior yin, 34
sore-throat, 333

Index

sorrow, 160
sorrow damage, 161
sòu, 67
sound production, 61
sour and turbid smell of vomitus, 71
sour breath, 70
sour odour of the stool, 71
sour taste, 93
sour vomiting, 235
source of phlegm, 38
SP 11, 104
SP 3, 127
sparkling eyes, 8
sparrow vision, 89
sparrow-pecking pulse, 116
spasm, 157
spasm and pain of the whole body, 325
spasm of the limbs, 17
spasm of the sinews and tendons, 249
spasm of the sinews due to retention of cold, 238
spasms and contraction, 33
spasms of the sinews and vessels, 33
spastic type, 18
special sweating, 80
spermatorrhoea, 255, 256, 257, 259, 328
spinal malnutrition, 32
spirit of the eye, 22
spirited, 8
spirit-lassitude, 90
spiritless, 8
spiritual lassitude, 88

spitting blood, 332
splashing sounds in the chest, 213
splashing sounds in the stomach and intestines, 186
spleen and kidney deficiency, 25
spleen and kidney yang deficiency, 21, 98
spleen and kidney depletion, 97
spleen and lung qi deficiency, 190, 267
spleen and stomach deficiency, 31
spleen and stomach deficiency-detriment, 85
spleen and stomach patterns, 190
spleen channel of the foot *taiyin*, 44, 300
spleen deficiency, 23, 28, 51, 93, 95, 110, 166, 197, 198, 329
spleen deficiency and sinking of the middle *jiao* qi, 34
spleen deficiency failing to govern blood, 36
spleen deficiency leading to damp encumbrance, 51
spleen failing to control blood, 40, 190, 227, 228
spleen fire, 23
spleen heat, 52
spleen not controlling blood, 266
spleen qi deficiency, 165, 189, 190, 206, 211, 223, 266
spleen qi deficiency and sinking, 190
spleen qi exhausted, 27
spleen qi sinking, 223

spleen yang deficiency, 190, 223, 226, 228, 229
spleen-kidney yang deficiency pattern, 329
spleen-lung qi deficiency pattern, 330
splenomegaly, 123
spontaneous sweating, 80, 138, 146, 165, 176, 193, 194, 196, 206, 215, 260, 262, 265, 323, 327, 330
spots and prickles on the margins of the tongue, 50
spotted tongue, 50
spouting diarrhoea, 218
spring, 211, 215
sprout of the heart, 44
sputum, 38
sputum with blood, 209
square-formed head, 20
ST 25, 127
ST 3, 102
ST 30, 300
ST 32, 300
ST 36, 127
ST 40, 313
ST 42, 104
ST 44, 313
ST 9, 105
stabbing intense pains, 241
stabbing pain, 82, 86, 175, 199
stabbing pain fixed in one place, 204
stabbing pain in a fixed location usually aggravated at night, 170
stagnated heat, 134
stagnated heat in the liver

channels, 99
stagnated qi, 193, 283
stagnating the movement of qi, 124
stagnation and stasis of qi and blood, 38, 49
stagnation in the limbs and joints, 159
stagnation of blood due to deficiency of qi, 174
stagnation of calculus (stones), 85
stagnation of channels and collaterals qi, 30
stagnation of damp-heat, 51
stagnation of excessive pathogens, 96
stagnation of food and drink, 92
stagnation of liver qi, 329
stagnation of liver qi and retention of phlegm, 30
stagnation of liver qi and stomach heat, 31
stagnation of lung qi, 66
stagnation of phlegm, 193
stagnation of qi, 81, 82, 111, 199
stagnation of qi and blood, 49, 98, 161
stagnation of qi movement by a cold pathogen, 82
stagnation of stomach qi, 56
stagnation of the cold-pathogen, 33
stagnation of the liver, 118
stagnation of the liver qi, 31, 33
stagnation of the liver qi and blood stasis, 31
stagnation of the seven emotions, 23
stagnation of the *ying* yin, 277
stagnation of water and dampness, 50
stagnation of yang qi, 77
stained coating, 317
staring of the eyes, 160
staring straight ahead, 24
stasis and blockage of heart blood, 86
stasis maculae tongue, 49
stasis of blood, 81
stasis of blood and channels, 49
stasis of channels or collaterals, 24
stasis spotted tongue, 49
static blood, 64, 84, 110
static blood accumulation and stagnation, 97
static blood blocking the channels, 52
static blood in the body, 49
steaming bone, 140, 323
steaming bone fever, 78
steaming by fire toxin, 29
steaming of accumulated heat in the spleen and stomach, 27
steaming of damp-heat, 24
steaming *ying*-yin bearing upward, 91
stench, 71
sterility, 255, 259
sticky drool, 39
sticky greasy coating, 54
sticky or oily sweating, 144
sticky sputum, 209, 217
stiff and red-crimson tongue, 295
stiff tongue, 51, 192
stiffness, 156
stiffness and pain in the root of the tongue, 300
stiffness in the head and neck, 277
stirring of the foetus, 259, 260
stirring of the heart, 296
stirring-up of the blood, 292
stirring-up of the wind, 296
stomach and intestine qi stagnation, 168
stomach being damaged by eating, 87
stomach cancer, 84
stomach cavity *pǐ*, 87
stomach channel of the foot *yangming*, 280, 300
stomach cold, 71, 231, 236
stomach deficiency and counterflow of qi, 69
stomach dryness, 179
stomach fire flaming upward, 28
stomach heat, 26, 28, 39, 70, 71, 233, 236
stomach heat and worm accumulation, 39
stomach pain, 312
stomach prolapse, 166
stomach qi counterflow, 168, 222
stomach qi deficiency, 165
stomach qi failure, 26
stomach qi returning again, 26
stomach yang deficiency, 84
stomach yin deficiency, 84, 190, 234

stomach yin defficiency, 93
stomachache, 161
stomach-cold, 190
stomach-heat, 190
stomach-qi weakness, 27
stone *lín*, 40
stones in the urine, 261
stones or blood in the urine, 262
stool is dark, 170
stool with blood, 236, 292
strabismus, 24
straining of the testes, 252
straining with difficulty, 218
strange diseases, 184
stranguria, 169
strategies and methods, 305
stretching pain in the nape of the neck, 300
string-like and rapid pulse, 178
stringy and floating pulse on the left, 325
stringy and rapid pulse, 324
strong constitution, 15
strong physique and body, 312
strong speech, 64
strong stomach and weak spleen, 93
struggle of pathogenic qi and *zheng* (healthy) qi, 27, 78, 276
stuffiness, 167, 215
stuffiness and fullness in the chest and hypochondrium, 246
stuffiness and suffocating feeling in the chest and hypochondrium or lower abdomen, 241
stuffiness below the heart, 124

stuffiness in the chest, 157
stuffiness in the epigastrium and abdomen, 158
stuffiness or pain of the epigastrium and abdomen, 251
stuffy nose, 26, 39, 129, 131, 156, 157, 159, 206, 208, 213, 322
stuffy nose with clear watery mucus, 207
stuffy nose with yellow thick discharge, 215
sty and cinnabar (red) eye, 24
Sù Wèn - Cì Rè, 素问·刺热, 9
Sù Wèn - Rè Lùn, 素问·热论, 275
subcutaneous ecchymosis, 176
subjective assumptions, 318
sublingual veins, 52, 317
sudden cloudiness, 17
sudden collapse of heart yang, 193, 196
sudden collapse of yang qi, 13
sudden coma, 8
sudden desertion of heart yang, 190
sudden desire to eat, 8
sudden emotional irritation, 69
sudden faint, 158, 166, 169, 201, 247
sudden falling down, 248
sudden fever, 158
sudden illness, 119
sudden loss of heart yang, 194
sudden loss of yang qi, 13
sudden mental improvement, 8
sudden onset, 158, 169, 211, 229
sudden onset of wheals, 156
sudden patchy or elliptical loss

of hair, 20
sudden severe cold pain in the epigastrium and abdomen, 157
sudden sneezing, 69
sudden sparkling of eyes, 8
sudden syncope, 160
sudden unconsciousness, 201, 247
suddenly fainted, 324
suffocating feeling, 199, 200, 201
suffocating feeling in the chest, 192, 203
suffocating pain, 199, 201
suggestive hints, 318
suitable environment, 317
summer febrile disease, 54
summer fever in children, 78
summer-heat, 155, 158
summer-heat damages qi, 158
summer-heat disturbs the mind, 158
summer-heat injures fluids and damages qi, 158
summer-heat invades the pericardium, 158
summer-heat pattern, 157
summer-heat stroke, 18, 158
summer-heat-dampness, 158
sunken eye socket, 23
sunken fontanel, 20
superficial (浮), 11
superficial and deep (浮沉), 10
superficial and rapid pulse, 180
superficial and tight pulse, 180
superficial gastritis, 312
superficial palpation, 121
superficial portion of the body,

129
superficial swelling of anterior yin, 33
superficial vein, 315
supine position, 321
suppurative parotitis, 21
surgery on the lung, 31
surging and rapid pulse, 158
surging headache, 300
surging in summer, 108
surging pulse, 108, 114, 113, 115
surging, bounding and powerful pulse, 152
sweat, 329
sweat and/or urine with apple odour, 71
sweat odours, 70
sweating, 18, 79, 126, 129, 131, 146, 156, 158, 159, 160, 217, 218, 220, 230, 233, 262, 277, 295, 296, 299, 301, 327
sweating in the armpits, 70
sweating of the palms and soles, 81, 281
sweating of yang exhaustion, 80
sweating of yin exhaustion, 80
sweating with no resolution of the fever, 159
sweet or greasy sensation in the mouth, 222
sweet taste, 93
swelling, 122, 125, 162
swelling and burning pain of the involved area, 149
swelling and burning pain of the testes, 249
swelling and pain in the gums, 233, 236
swelling and pain in the supraclavicular fossa, 301
swelling and pain of the axillary fossa, 301
swelling and pain of the cheeks, 301
swelling and pain of the throat, 91, 301
swelling and prolapse of his right scrotum, 331
swelling below the axilla, 301
swelling in the eye and eyelid, 23
swelling of the jaw, 300
swelling of the knee and ankle joints, 326
swelling of the lesser abdomen in women, 301
swelling of the neck, 24
swelling of the scrotum, 33
swelling of the throat, 180
swelling of vulva, 33
swellings, 125
swift digestion, 300
swift digestion with rapid hungering, 92
swill diarrhoea, 301
swollen and painful eyes, 330
swollen purple blue-green face and lips, 21
swollen-head infection, 21
symptoms, 2
syncope, 109, 162, 168, 201, 328
syphilis, 26, 34
Systematic Differentiation of Warm Diseases (*Wēn Bìng Tiáo Biàn*, 温病条辨), 5

T

tài bái, 127
tài chōng, 103, 127, 313
tài xī, 103, 127
tài yáng, 102
tài yuān, 127
taiyang, 275
taiyang blood-retention pattern, 276
taiyang channel headache, 83
taiyang channel disease, 24
taiyang pattern, 275
taiyang water accumulation pattern, 68
taiyang water-retention pattern, 278
taiyin, 275
taiyin spleen channel headache, 83
taiyin stage, 228
taking infested foods, 137
talkative without much sense, 8
talks nonsense, 333
tán, 38
tán shí mài, 116
tapping, 121
tasteless mouth, 236
tastelessness, 142
tastelessness in the mouth, 35
taut and rapid pulse, 269, 270, 272
taut or weak pulse, 270, 272
taut pulse, 167
taut, 240, 273
tearing pain of the calf, 300

teeth are bright and dry like stone, 28
teeth are dry, 28
teeth are like withered bone, 28
teeth are sparse, loosening, exposure of the roots of the teeth, 28
teeth marks on the tongue, 317
teeth-marked, 51
telangiectasia, 170
ten methods for observing colour, 10
Ten Question Song, 76
tendency to catch cold, 206, 215
tendency to sigh, 301
tender, 51
tender tongue, 59
tenderness of the stomach, 312
tenesmus, 95, 136, 217, 221, 328
tense pulses, 114
tension and spasm, 162
tension of the sinews, 32
testicular disorders, 238
testing abdominal tension, 322
tetanus, 22, 27, 32, 156, 162
The Assemble of Knack in Sphygmology (Mài Jué Huì Biàn, 脉诀汇辨), 5
the body posture of palpation examination, 321
The Classic to Obey for Inspection Diagnosis, 10
The Complete Works of [Zhang] Jing-yue, 5
the contents of the inspection of spirit, 314
the guidelines for tongue examination, 316
the heat entering the ying and blood levels, 54
the methods of the inspection examination, 314
The Orthodox Tradition of Medicine, 66
the pattern of extreme heat appearing with cold signs, 151
The Pulse Classic, 4
the relationship among the eight principles patterns, 146
The Spiritual Pivot-Treatise on Reversal, 灵枢·厥论, 15
The Spiritual Pivot-Yin and Yang Twenty-five People Types, 灵枢·阴阳二十五人, 15
The Spiritual Pivot-Five Colours, 9
the uterus or another internal organ, 166
theory of the five wheels (rings), 22
theory of the six channels, 275
therapeutic principles, 135
thick, 154, 269
thick and foul smelling leucorrhoea, 71
thick and greasy coating, 92, 136, 153, 213, 333
thick and sticky tongue coating, 161, 235
thick and yellow coating, 218, 220
thick coating, 53, 60
thick sticky coating, 236
thick tongue coating, 146, 317
thick-white coating, 56, 157
thick whitish and greasy coating on the tongue, 142
thick yellow coating, 233
thick-yellowish sputum, 132, 149
thickening of the skin, 22
thigh, 300
thin and clear urine, 332
thin and fishy smelling leucorrhoea, 71
thin and rapid pulse, 329
thin and rough pulse, 327
thin and slightly yellow coating, 131
thin and soft pulse, 107
thin and tall, 16
thin and white coating, 324
thin and white tongue coating, 129, 180, 200
thin and yellow coating, 332
thin body, 161, 222, 248, 250, 256, 257, 259, 262, 268, 323
thin coating, 53, 60, 273
thin dry tongue coating with little fluids, 209
thin hair, 21
thin hair in young people, 20
thin or no coating, 154
thin white and moist coating, 131
thin white coating, 56, 323, 330, 331
thin white or yellow coating, 270, 272
thin white with a little yellow coating, 329
thin yellow coating, 208, 215, 333
thin, dry and withered auricle,

25
thin, light yellow coating, 57
thin, white and dry coating, 56
thin, white and moist coating, 56
thin, white and slippery coating, 56
thinking, 192
thinness, 15
thin-pale coating, 159
thin-white and dry coating, 131, 208
thin-white coating, 156, 157, 207
thin-whitish sputum, 149
thin-yellow coating, 208
thirst, 90, 131, 158, 159, 160, 173, 199, 203, 208, 211, 214, 215, 218, 229, 230, 232, 233, 236, 245, 278, 295, 332
thirst and drinking, 91
thirst and preference for warm drinks, 140
thirst with a desire for cold drink, 132, 135, 160, 204, 244, 291, 295
thirst with a desire for hot drinks, 138, 139
thirst with a desire to drink, 158, 160
thirst with a desire to take sips of water, 251
thirst with much drinking, 91
thirst with parched mouth but disinclination to drink, 218
thirst without a desire to drink, 91
thirst, 262
thirsty, 328, 333

thirsty but has no desire to drink, 152
thorny tongue, 218
thought, 160
thought damage, 161
thready, 244, 246, 254
thready and choppy pulse, 170, 201, 204, 219, 220
thready and faint pulse, 264
thready and feeble pulse, 153
thready and rapid pulse, 80, 140, 191, 197, 198, 216, 217, 233, 234, 236, 240, 244, 246, 248, 250, 256, 257, 259, 263, 268, 272, 273, 292, 325, 328
thready and rough or choppy pulse, 234
thready and slippery pulse, 326
thready and weak pulse, 197, 198, 227, 249, 258, 259, 266, 267
thready pulse, 86, 111, 115, 161, 196, 239, 250, 267
thready weak pulse, 329
thready wiry but powerful pulse, 248
thready wiry pulse, 86
thready and choppy pulse, 199
three passes of the child's finger, 315
three portions, 117
three positions and nine pulse-takings, 101
three yang channels, 129
three yin channels, 129
three-section examination method of zhang zhong-jing, 101

throat pain, 244
throbbing pulse, 111, 113, 114
thrush, 27
tiān shū, 127
tic, 246
tidal fever, 78, 83, 140, 162, 198, 240, 246, 248, 250, 255, 256, 257, 259, 263, 268, 296, 323, 329
tidal fever in the afternoon, 197, 281
tidal redness only in the cheeks, 14
tight and oppressed, 68
tight pulse, 112, 114, 115
tightly closed jaw, 162
time for pulse examination, 320
time in bed, 90
timidity, 253
tíng, 庭, 9
tingling in the abdomen, 330
tinnitus, 86, 88, 191, 238, 240, 243, 244, 245, 248, 252, 256, 257, 258, 259, 260, 262, 263, 272, 273, 301, 328, 329
tinnitus in the night, 325
tip of the nose is dark and dry, 26
tip of the tongue, 45
tired and weak body, 8
tiredness, 166, 176, 215
tongue, 154, 215
tongue and mouth ulcers, 204
tongue body, 58
tongue changes, 316
tongue coating, 46, 58, 316
tongue coating changes from thick to thin, 53
tongue coating changes from

thin to thick, 53
tongue coating is thin and greasy, 327
tongue coating turns from dry to moist, 54
tongue coating turns from moist to dry, 54
tongue coating with root, 56
tongue coating without root, 56
tongue colour, 48
tongue contraction, 238
tongue depressor, 46
tongue diagnosis, 43
tongue examination, 43
tongue inspection, 153
tongue is extended, 52
tongue is pale, 323
tongue manifestation, 44, 316
tongue manifestation changes, 59
tongue motility, 51
tongue observation, 315
tongue shape, 49
tongue spirit, 48
tongue ulcers, 192, 199, 244
tongue with ecchymosis, 175
tongue-depressor, 316
tongue-tied, 52
tonify the deficiency, 135
tonsillitis, 29
toothache, 63, 300
tortoise back, 31
touching, 321
tough tongue, 136
toxicities from medicines or food, 49
tragus of the ear, 9
transformation, 146

transformation between cold and heat, 149
transformation between deficiency and excess, 150
transformation of patterns, 147
transmission of disease along the order of the channels, 288
transmission of diseases from one channel to another channel, 288
transmission of pathogens from exterior to interior, 129
transmission of pathogens from interior to exterior, 129
transmission of the four systems patterns, 292
transmission of the six channel pattern, 287
transverse invasion of hyperactive liver qi, 241
trauma, 155
Treatise on Cold Damage, 275
Treatise on Cold Damage And Miscellaneous Diseases (Shāng Hán Zá Bìng Lùn, 伤寒杂病论), 4
Treatise on Diseases, Patterns, and Formulas Related to the Unification of the Three Aetiologies, 4
Treatise on the Origins and Manifestations of Various Diseases, 4
treatment plan, 305
treatment progress, 319
trembling of the hands and feet, 33

trembling tongue, 52
tremor, 238, 246, 267
tremor of the eyelids, 17
tremor of the limbs, 238, 246, 248, 249, 250
tremor of the limbs and muscular twitching, 239
tremors, 156, 330
triggers, 319
"true" cold, 151
"true" deficiency, 153
"true" excess, 153
"true" heat, 151
true and false patterns, 152
true coating, 56
true heat with false cold, 125
true pulse, 320
true symptoms, 152
tuberculosis, 216, 217, 268
tuberculosis infection, 206
tumbling down and sudden sprain, 32
tumour, 22, 184
tumour in the lower *jiao*, 40
turbid (cloudy) urine, 261
turbid (浊), 11
turbid-dampness with heat pathogen, 57
turbid nasal discharge, 26
turbid nasal mucus, 71
turbid phlegm obstructing the lung, 24
turbid urine, 223, 228
turbid vomit, 39
turbid, purulent phlegm, 70
turbidity, 184
tympanites, 31, 87

U

ulceration and pain of the tongue, 199
ulcerative gingivitis, 28, 70
ulcerative perforation, 34
ulcers, 125, 192, 333
ulcers in the mouth, 262
umbilical sore, 31
umbilical wind, 22, 27
unable to stand for a long time, 17
unbearable itching of the scrotum, 249
unconsciousness, 160, 194, 247, 250
uncontrollable talking nonsense, 161
uncontrolled weeping and laughing, 203
under-nourishment of the spirit-essence, 20
undigested food in the stool, 95, 151
undigested food in the vomitus, 71
unhappiness, 241
unnourished tendons and channels, 33
unsteadiness, 89
unsurfaced fever, 91, 251
untwining rope pulse, 117
unusual facial, 22
unusual pulses, 116
up floating of yang, 151
upper abdominal pain, 84
upper excess and lower deficiency, 244, 248, 250, 273, 325, 330
upper fire toxin, 21
upper heat and lower cold, 330
upper *jiao*, 191, 205, 294
upper yang excess, 325
upturned knife pulse, 116
upward and outward movement of deficient yang, 81
upward attack in the *yangming* by a heat pathogen, 21
upward attack of a stagnated gallbladder channel, 26
upward attack of a heat-pathogen, 25
upward counterflow of qi and fire, 94
upward staring, 24, 201
upward turning of the eyes, 248
uraemia, 71
urgency, 192
urgent, 255
urinary and bowel incontinence, 166
urinary disturbances, 260
urinary incontinence, 18, 96, 161, 255, 259
urinary problems, 264
urine, 96
urine and stool odours, 70
urine with blood, 292
uterine prolapse, 166

V

vaccinations, 99
vaginal discharge, 97
vaginal eczema with severe itching, 249
vaginal itching, 250, 251
vaginal protrusion, 34
vanquished pulses, 116
vertebral illness, 32
vertex cold headache, 252
vertex headache, 252
vertigo, 83, 85, 184
very thin hair in children, 21
vesicles, 37
vexation, 214, 215
vexing heat, 252
vexing heat in the chest, 197, 198, 217, 256, 257, 259
vexing heat in the five centres, 78
vigourous empty fire, 89
vigourous fire, 50
vigourous flaring of liver-gallbladder fire, 94
violent and aggressive behaviour, 203
violent behaviour, 204
violent thoughts, 123
virulent poison, 143
viscous stools, 324
visible phlegm, 184
vital essences, 314
vitality, 6
vitiligo, 35
voice, 154
volume, 62
vomit, 39
vomiting, 67, 132, 136, 149, 158, 161, 168, 201, 219, 220, 222, 223, 228, 231, 233, 242, 249, 251, 252,

253, 272, 284, 285, 286, 297, 300, 301
vomiting after eating, 232
vomiting blood, 192, 236
vomiting of blood, 132, 160, 168, 173, 238, 243, 292
vomiting of clear fluid, 186
vomiting of sour and undigested food, 234
vomiting which contains blood, 235
vomiting with blood, 246
vomits, 330
vomitus odours, 71

W

waggling tongue, 52, 192
wandering itchy skin, 156
wandering pain, 246, 270
wandering pain in joints and limbs, 156
wandering pain in the chest, 167, 242
wandering pain in the chest and hypochondria, 175
wandering pain in the joints and limbs, 156
Wàng Zhěn Zūn Jīng, 望诊遵经, 10
waning or waxing of the tongue coating, 56
wanting to vomit, 147
warm disease pattern identification, 288
warm diseases, 294
warm dryness, 159
warm febrile disease, 49, 78

warm heat (*wēn bìng*) diseases, 173
warm patterns, 57
warm toxin, 21
warm-dampness, 159
warm-dryness, 209
warm-heat disease, 65, 126, 291
warm-heat pathogen accumulated in the upper *jiao* and confusing the orifices, 88
wasting away, 330
wasting-thirst, 91, 93, 96, 286
water, 13
water and dampness flowing over the skin, 31
water counterflow pattern, 91
water drum distension, 125
water floating oedema, 13
water in the stomach, 124
water not generating wood, 244
water not nourishing wood, 273
water pathogen begins to transform, 54
water retention, 51, 137
water *shàn*, 33
water wheel, 22
water-damp obstructing the spleen, 182
water-retention pattern, 276
water-rheum, 13, 14
water-swelling illnesses, 21
watery diarrhoea, 151, 274
watery stools, 329
weak, 15
weak and deep pulse, 261
weak and deficient pulse, 165
weak heart-beats, 195

weak body, 17
weak bones, 258
weak breath, 8, 18, 194, 196
weak breathing, 31, 66, 126, 166, 260
weak constitution, 164, 265
weak function of the *zang-fu*, 15
weak pulse, 92, 109, 113, 193, 196, 215, 254, 259, 284, 326, 330, 332
weak resistance against pathogenic invasion, 15
weak voice, 265, 267
weakness, 330
weakness and aching of the back and knees, 244, 245, 246, 248, 263, 273
weakness and pain of the back and knee joints, 272
weakness in the lower back and knees, 328
weakness of stomach qi, 333
weakness of the feet, 258
weakness of the legs, 330
weakness of the limbs, 161, 222
weakness of the spleen and kidney, 239
weakness of the spleen and stomach and mal-development of the skull, 20
wei (defensive) qi, 89
wēi mài, 111
wěi patterns, 18
wei qi, 79, 217
wèi shù, 127
wei system, 289
wei yang, 77
wet and white coating, 252

wheezing, 66, 211, 213, 244
wheezing asthma, 17
wheezy phlegm in the throat, 247
white, 13, 71
white and greasy coating, 58, 86, 201
white and grey complexion, 182
white and moist coating, 58
white and slippery coating, 196, 226, 264
white and thick coating, 317
white and watery sputum, 210
white and yellow greasy coating, 331
white coating, 56, 60, 149, 151, 196, 201, 210, 213, 215, 228, 250, 254, 259, 328, 330, 331
white colour on the tip of the nose, 26
white complexion, 226, 260
white dull complexion, 13
white foamy phlegm, 327
white greasy coating, 35, 201, 211, 332
white hair, 255
white hair in young people, 21
white leucorrhoea, 98
white moist and slippery coating, 132
white or greasy coating, 248, 250
white or thin yellow coating, 215
white sticky coating, 231
white sticky sputum, 211
white tongue coating, 193, 194, 227, 246, 284
white watery sputum, 210, 213
white, slippery, greasy coating, 59
white, thick, greasy and dry coating, 56
white-greasy, 228
white-moist and slippery coating, 231
white-slippery coating, 213, 221, 228, 229, 236, 267, 274, 331
white-sticky phlegm, 213
whitish slippery coating, 228
whooping cough, 325
wind, 155
wind attack, 20
wind *bì*, 156
wind cold invading the lung, 206, 207, 210
wind heat invading the lung, 206, 210
wind interferes with the circulation of qi and blood under the skin, 156
wind interferes with the circulation of *wei* qi, 156
wind invading the lung, 156
wind papulae, 35, 36
wind pass, 41, 42
wind pathogen, 131
wind pathogen attacking upward and obstructing the ears, 88
wind pathogen invading the channels and networks and obstructing the channels, 156
wind pathogen invading the exterior, 156
wind pathogen striking, 36
wind pathogenic fluid retained in chest and hypochondrium, 327
wind patterns, 111, 156
wind stirring, 140
wind stroke, 33, 277
wind stroke block pattern, 18
wind stroke desertion pattern, 18
wind stroke in the channels, 18
wind stroke in the *zang*, 17
wind wheel, 22
wind, cold and damp attacking the stomach and intestines, 70
wind, damp and heat interactive steaming, 80
wind-cold, 26
wind-cold attacking the lung, 66
wind-cold attacking the *taiyang* channel, 30
wind-cold dampness, 326
wind-cold harassing the exteriors, 322
wind-cold harassing the lung, 39
wind-cold headache, 83
wind-cold intruding, 85
wind-cold invading the lung, 190, 207, 211
wind-cold invading the *taiyang* channel, 276
wind-cold pattern, 127
wind-cold tightening the lung, 325
wind-cold transforming into heat, 57
wind-damp, 70
wind-damp disease, 70
wind-damp headache, 83
wind-damp transforming into heat, 32

wind-fire attacking the upper orifices, 89
wind-fire of the liver channel harassing the upper body, 89
wind-heat, 26, 329
wind-heat attacking the lung pattern, 329
wind-heat attacking upward, 89
wind-heat exterior pattern, 56
wind-heat headache, 83
wind-heat in the liver channel, 23
wind-heat invading the lung, 190, 208
wind-heat invading the lung pattern, 214
wind-heat obstructing the lung and heart channels, 24
wind-heat pathogen, 131
wind-phlegm blocked collaterals, 28
wind-phlegm blocking the channels, 51, 52
wind-phlegm obstructing the collaterals, 27
wind-phlegm transforming into heat, 59
wind-strike, 27, 65
wind-strike entering the *zang* organs, 63
wind-strike in adults, 27
wind-strike involving the collaterals, 24
wind-stroke, 24, 32, 157
wind-stroke due to ascendant hyperactivity of liver yang, 22

wind-stroke in the networks, 156
wind-warm, 62
wind-water, 156
wind-water fighting the lung pattern, 180
windy spring, 328
winter, 211, 215
wiping the tongue, 46
wiry, 200, 242, 244, 248, 250
wiry (taut) in spring, 108
wiry and rapid or slippery and rapid pulse, 249
wiry and rapid pulse, 241, 246, 248, 252, 253
wiry and thready pulse, 312
wiry and tight pulse, 252
wiry but powerful pulse, 247
wiry moderate pulse, 328
wiry or deep, 231
wiry pulse, 112, 113, 114, 201, 244, 246, 250, 251, 283, 329, 331
wiry pulse in left *guān*, 118
wiry thin and rapid pulse, 332
with qi counterflow, 168
withered, 315
withered and brittle nails, 238, 249, 267
withered skin, 144
withered tongue, 48
withered yellow complexion, 13
withered yellow facial colour, 161
withered-yellowish or pale complexion, 197
without an acid-putrid odour, 69
without coating, 256, 259, 263,

325
without sweating, 79
women's voices, 62
wood, 12
wood constraint transforming into fire, 24
wood not controlling earth, 241
wood overacting on the earth, 270
worm accumulation, 84, 137
worm accumulation in intestine, 190
worm accumulation pattern, 93
worry, 161, 198, 266
worry consuming the blood, 197
worrying, 223
wriggling of the hands and feet, 33, 296
wrist pulse, 104
wu ju-tong, 294
wŭ lĭ, 104
wū lòu mài, 116

X

xì mài, 111
xiā yóu mài, 116
xián mài, 112
*xián*痛, 9
Xiăo Ér Wèi Shēng Zŏng Wēi Fāng Lùn, 小儿卫生总微方论, 16
xiāo kĕ, 71, 91, 93, 96, 286
xié (pathogenic factors) and *zhèng* (healthy qi), 128
xū lĭ, 122
xū mài, 111

Y

yăn dāo mài, 116
yang, 128
yang brightness, 275
yang cheng-liu, 153
yang collapse, 80, 125
yang decline and cold exuberance, 27
yang deficiency, 13, 51, 82, 94, 96, 98, 109, 132, 135, 140, 162
yang deficiency and cold-dampness, 57
yang deficiency and water retention, 48
yang deficiency and yin dried up, 323
yang deficiency failing to transform and transport, 187
yang deficiency of the heart and kidneys, 90
yang deficiency pattern, 80, 138, 157
yang depletion, 140
yang failure causing cold to accumulate in the qi and blood, 36
yang hyperactivity, 30, 112, 162
yang jaundice, 13, 35
yang maculae, 36
yang oedema, 21, 180
yang patterns, 126
yang qi, 276
yang qi being obstructed, 54
yang unable to come out of yin, 90
yang within yin, 286
yang *zang* person, 16
yang-deficient constitution, 133
yangming, 275
yangming bowel pattern, 78
yangming channel headache, 83
yangming channel pattern of cold damage, 78
yangming channels, 19
yangming fu excess pattern, 218
yangming tidal fever, 78
yangming warm disease, 295
yang-qi deficiency, 133
yawning, 69
ye tian-shi, 288
yellow, 13
yellow and dry coating, 58, 135
yellow and fall out, 28
yellow and fetid stools, 333
yellow and foul leucorrhoea, 249, 251
yellow and greasy coating, 57, 58, 203, 295
yellow and red urine, 71
yellow and slippery coating, 57
yellow and sticky sputum, 203
yellow and sticky sputum or a rattling sound in the throat, 203
yellow and sticky tongue coating, 262
yellow and white mixed tongue coating, 325
yellow coating, 56, 60, 204, 211, 232, 233, 243, 246, 291, 317, 322
yellow colour of the skin and sclera, 230
yellow dry coating, 219, 220, 234, 236
Yellow Emperoris Inner Classic, 4, 15, 205, 238, 275, 288, 294
yellow greasy coating, 91, 215, 218, 249, 251, 253, 324, 333
yellow leucorrhoea, 99
yellow nasal discharge, 208
yellow rough coating, 57
yellow sclera, 228
yellow skin, 35
yellow skin and eyes, 249, 331
yellow skin colour and pale bulging veins on the abdominal wall, 87
yellow sputum, 269
yellow sticky coating, 230
yellow sticky sputum, 215
yellow sweat, 80
yellow thick sputum, 210, 214, 215, 244
yellow tongue coating, 160, 295
yellow urine, 199, 203, 231, 233, 236, 245, 246, 329
yellow-greasy coating, 58, 214, 252
yellowing eyes, 300
yellowing of the eyes, 300
yellowish, 71
yellowish coating, 149
yellowish complexion, 14
yellowish greasy tongue coating, 87
yellowish thick phlegm, 70
yellow-sticky coating, 230
yet complementary opposites, 138

yì, 305
Yī Xué Zhèng Zhuàn, 医学正传, 66
yǐn, 38
yin and yang, 138
yin and yang harmonised person, 16
yin cold stagnation, 167
yin collapse, 80, 125
yin damage, 51
yin deficiency, 14, 15, 30, 51, 88, 135, 140, 162, 323, 325, 328, 329
yin deficiency and dried fluid, 51
yin deficiency generating wind, 33
yin deficiency of the heart and kidney, 325
yin deficiency of the liver and kidney, 86
yin deficiency of the lung, 31
yin deficiency of the lung and kidney, 30, 63, 67
yin deficiency pattern, 78
yin deficiency resulting in vigourous fire, 23, 50, 90
yin deficiency resulting in vigourous fire and damage of body fluids, 50
yin deficiency with exuberant fire, 23
yin deficiency with internal heat, 81
yin excess, 132
yin fails to restrain yang, 241
yin fire, 323
yin fluid deficiency generating wind, 52
yin fluid exhaustion, 144
yin jaundice, 13, 35
yin maculae, 36
yin oedema, 21, 180
yin or yang collapse patterns, 64
yin patterns, 126
yin *zang* person, 16
yin-blood deficiency, 220
yin-cold congealing, 142
yin-deficiency tidal fever, 78
ying, 275
ying and blood depletion, 55
ying system, 289
ying-blood depletion, 97
yin-yang, 128
yú xiáng mài, 116
yuan (original) qi dissipation, 109
yuan qi, 163
yuan qi deficiency, 164

Z

zang organs, 129
zang qi exhaustion, 109
zang-fu organs, 129, 189
zang-fu's exuberance or decline of qi and blood, 315
zhāng mén, 127
Zhang Zhong-jing, 275
zheng qi, 135, 283
zheng qi dispelling the pathogenic qi, 55
zheng qi is overcoming the pathogenic qi, 53
zhōng fǔ, 127
zhōng jí, 127
Zhū Bìng Yuán Hòu Lùn, 诸病源候论, 4
zhuàn dòu mài, 116
zōng (gathering) qi, 29, 205
zong (gathering) qi (宗气) deficiency, 17
zong (gathering) qi fails, 331
zong qi, 65, 216
zú sān lǐ, 127

Notes

Notes

图书在版编目（CIP）数据

中医诊断学＝Diagnostics in Chinese Medicine：英文/陈家旭主编.—北京：人民卫生出版社，2011.12
国际标准化英文版中医教材
ISBN 978-7-117-14650-0

Ⅰ.①中…　Ⅱ.①陈…　Ⅲ.①中医诊断学-教材-英文　Ⅳ.①R241

中国版本图书馆 CIP 数据核字（2011）第 145578 号

门户网：www.pmph.com	出版物查询、网上书店
卫人网：www.ipmph.com	护士、医师、药师、中医师、卫生资格考试培训

中医诊断学——国际标准化英文版中医教材

主　　编：陈家旭
出版发行：人民卫生出版社（中继线 +8610-5978-7399）
地　　址：中国北京市朝阳区潘家园南里 19 号
　　　　　世界医药图书大厦 B 座
邮　　编：100021
网　　址：http://www.pmph.com
E - mail：pmph @ pmph.com
发　　行：pmphsales @ gmail.com
购书热线：+8610-5978 7399 / 5978 7338（电话及传真）
开　　本：787×1092　1/16
版　　次：2011 年 12 月第 1 版　2011 年 12 月第 1 版第 1 次印刷
标准书号：ISBN 978-7-117-14650-0/R・14651

版权所有，侵权必究，打击盗版举报电话：+8610-5978-7482
（凡属印装质量问题请与本社销售中心联系退换）